An Essential Guide to Systemic Lupus Erythematosus

An Essential Guide to Systemic Lupus Erythematosus

Edited by **Mitch Sellin**

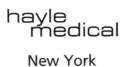

hayle
medical

New York

Published by Hayle Medical,
30 West, 37th Street, Suite 612,
New York, NY 10018, USA
www.haylemedical.com

An Essential Guide to Systemic Lupus Erythematosus
Edited by Mitch Sellin

International Standard Book Number: 978-1-63241-041-2 (Hardback)

Printed in the United States of America.

Contents

Preface

In my initial years as a student, I used to run to the library at every possible instance to grab a book and learn something new. Books were my primary source of knowledge and I would not have come such a long way without all that I learnt from them. Thus, when I was approached to edit this book; I became understandably nostalgic. It was an absolute honor to be considered worthy of guiding the current generation as well as those to come. I put all my knowledge and hard work into making this book most beneficial for its readers.

This book deals with the fundamentals and sciences of Systemic Lupus Erythematosus. It is an apt resource for scientists seeking extensive coverage of their spheres of interest. The book delves into the progress of molecular biology and how it has enhanced our comprehension of this disease. It is an important medical resource for practicing doctors coming from diverse spheres of rheumatology. It discusses cytokines, genetics, fas-pathway, toll like receptors and atherogenesis in SLE. Animal models have also been looked into. This book will be resourceful for students, researchers and physicians.

I wish to thank my publisher for supporting me at every step. I would also like to thank all the authors who have contributed their researches in this book. I hope this book will be a valuable contribution to the progress of the field.

Editor

The Scientific Basis of SLE

Cytokines and Systemic Lupus Erythematosus

Jose Miguel Urra[1] and Miguel De La Torre[2]

[1]*Immunology Service, General Hospital Ciudad Real, Ciudad Real*
[2]*Nephrology Service, Cabueñes Hospital, Asturias*
Spain

1. Introduction

Systemic lupus erythematosus (SLE) is a multisystem autoimmune disease characterized by the production of numerous autoantibodies that typically involves multiple organ systems. As opposed to lupus in animal models, SLE in humans is heterogeneous and affects different individuals with a wide range of disease courses and manifestations. The pathogenesis is still unclear, a myriad of innate and adaptative immune system aberrations in SLE have been identified as major contributors of the disease.

Cytokines are a diverse group of soluble proteins and peptides, produced and released by immune system cells , that act as humoral regulators and modulate the functional activities of individual cells and tissues, playing a pivotal role in the differentiation, maturation, and activation of various immune and no immune cells. Cytokine dysregulation is likely to play a role in the loss of immune tolerance that leads to SLE, and in the damage resulting from the disease. Many of the genes that are associated with risk for lupus are cytokines, regulators of cytokines, or downstream members of cytokine pathways.

Multiple cytokines have been implicated in the disease activity or organ involvement in SLE. Among these, IL-6, Interferon (IFN), B-lymphocyte stimulator (BlyS), IL-10, IL-17 is thought to play an important role in the creation of the characteristic milieu in SLE, which promotes B-cell survival and autoantibody production. On the other hand, also cytokines like IL-10, IL1, TNF-α , IFN, are important in development of the autoimmune injury in renal and central nervous system, the most frequently observed causes of death in patients with SLE. Moreover, recent studies strongly suggest that the cytokines, at least in part, would be implicated in the pathogenesis of accelerated atherosclerosis associated with SLE.

The knowledge of cytokines not only provides new insight into pathogenesis of SLE, but also it has allowed the development of clinical applications such as monitoring of disease and as potential therapeutic targets with the use of several biologic agents, targeting different cytokines or their receptors. Consequently, many trials of anticytokine therapies for SLE are underway.

The focus of the present chapter is to summarize the cytokines which have significant implications in the pathogenesis of SLE, the potential clinical and therapeutic use will be reviewed.

2. SLE gender susceptibility and cytokines

One feature of lupus, which also occurs with other autoimmune diseases, is the influence of gender on disease susceptibility. In fact 90% of people affected by lupus are women (Masi &

Kaslow 1978). Immunological, epidemiological and clinical evidence suggest that female sex hormones play an important role in the etiology and pathophysiology of chronic immune diseases. Abundant studies have suggested that gender differences in susceptibility to SLE are mediated by sex hormones (Rider & Abdou 2001, Cohen-Solal et al 2006, Zandman et al 2007) .The high female prevalence is most marked after puberty: while the pre-puberty female to male ratio is 3 : 1, this increases to 10 : 1 during the childbearing years and decreases again to 8 : 1 after menopause (Lahita et al 1999a). Pregnancy is frequently associated with activity and flares of the disease in SLE patients (Lahita 1999a). Also there is an increased risk of developing SLE in postmenopausal women who received estrogen hormone replacement therapy (Buyon et al 2007) and increased the risk of flares in postmenopausal patients (Straub 2007). Together these considerations indicate that estrogen may be proposed as candidates to explain the sexual dimorphism of SLE. Cytokines are intimately involved with sex hormones, as they regulate the level of sex hormones both systemically and locally, especially in the reproductive organs. The interactions between cytokines and estrogens affect important cellular activities as proliferation and apoptosis (Lahita 1999b).

Estrogens exert their effects by activation of intracellular receptors, the estrogen receptor alpha (ERα) and beta (ERβ) (Green et al 1986). In addition to its intracellular receptors have also been reported membrane receptors that correspond to full-length isoforms of both ERα and ERβ with extracellular functionality (Pedram et al 2006). Both receptors have been identified in the membrane of thymocytes and have a great importance in the proper development of the thymus (Stimson & Hunter 1980). Thus it seems that estrogen receptors influence the adequate development of T lymphocytes. It is well known that low doses of estrogen promote enhanced Th1 responses and increased cell-mediated immunity, while high doses of estrogen lead instead to increased Th2 responses and antibodies production (Maret et al 2003, Bao et al 2002). This effect of estrogens seems to be achieved through direct alteration in the Th cytokine profile from a proinflammatory (IL-2, IFN-γ) to an humoral direction (IL-4, IL-5, IL-9, IL-13). Besides the effect of estrogen on the profile of cytokines released by T cells, estrogen also increases the release of IL-1, IL-6 and TNF by monocytes/macrophages (Kramer et al 2004). SLE patients show immune-related disorders mediated through estrogens. In vitro peripheral blood mononuclear cells in SLE patients show an increase in anti-dsDNA and IL-10 in response to estrogen, and in vivo there are clear differences in hormonal and cytokine levels in SLE *vs* control pregnancies (Doria et al 2004). Although there is much indirect evidence for estrogen involvement in the lupus disease process, the direct role of estrogen/estrogen-receptor mediated pathways in regulating cytokine production in SLE patients has not as yet been clearly defined. The first evidence for a molecular marker of estrogen action in SLE was the estrogen dependent changes in lupus T-cells calcineurin that could alter cytokine regulation (Rider et al 1998). Calcineurin is the target of a class of drugs called calcineurin inhibitors, which includes cyclosporine, pimecrolimus and tacrolimus. Calcineurin induces different transcription factors as NFATs that are important in the transcription of cytokine genes. A recent study demonstrate that blocking estrogens receptor in vivo in SLE pre- menopausal women they reduced the expression of calcineurin in peripheral T cells (Abdou et al 2008). Another possible mechanism of the role of estrogen in gender susceptibility in lupus is the altered expression of its receptors. Peripheral cells of SLE patients showed increased expression of ERα mRNA and decreased expression of ERβ (Iinui et al 2007). ERs are overexpressed in CD4+ and CD8+ cells while is decreased in B cells. The decline in ERβ expression inversely correlated with SLEDAI score. In conclusion, estrogen and its ability to influence on the profiles of cytokines release and immune system regulation is a very powerful factor in the gender susceptibility described in lupus.

3. Cytokines involved in SLE

3.1 Th1/Th2 balance in SLE

The Th1/Th2 balance hypothesis emerge from observations in mice of two subtypes of CD4 T-helper cells differing in cytokine secretion patterns and other functions (Mosmann et al 1986). The concept subsequently was applied to human immunity (Mosmann et al 1989). Th1 cells release significantly INFγ and IL2, and through these mediators Th1- polarized responses are highly protective against infections especially the intracellular pathogens, because of the ability of Th1-type cytokines to activate phagocytes and enhance the cellular response. In contrast Th2 cells release mainly IL4, IL5 IL9 and IL13 and induce the *in situ* survival of eosinophils (through IL-5), promote the production by B lymphocytes of high amounts of antibodies, including IgE (through IL-4 and IL-13), as well as the growth and degranulation of mast cells and basophiles (through IL-4 and IL- 9). (figure 1)

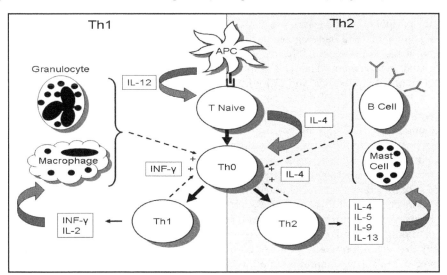

Fig. 1. Diagrammatic representation of the differentiation into Th1 or Th2 cells from naive cells.

Antigen-presenting cells interact with undifferentiated cells secreting specific cytokines that induce differentiation toward Th1 or Th2 cells. INFγ released by Th1 cells and IL4 produced by Th2 cells act as their own growth factors and cross-regulate the other differentiation.

Two features define the Th1/Th2 balance, first each cell subset produced cytokines that served as their own growth factor (autocrine effect) and second the two subsets released cytokines to cross regulate each other's development. Polarization to a subtype or another depends largely on the APC and experience on the antigen. This process is directed by the microenvironment of cytokines resulting in the antigen presentation of APC to T naive cells. A Th1/Th2 imbalance with excess of Th1 predominance appears in organ specific inflammatory diseases as arthritis, multiple sclerosis and type 1 diabetes, and instead a predominance of Th2 response has been described in allergy and systemic autoimmune diseases (Abbas et al 1996).

The roles of Th1 and Th2 cytokines in the pathogenesis of SLE are controversial. In patients with SLE, Th2 cytokines are increased (Ogawa et al 1992), whereas Th1 cytokines are decreased (Klinman & Steinberg 1995). Thus, SLE was initially considered to be a Th2 predominant disease. However different results contradict this hypothesis like that IFNγ levels in the sera of patients with SLE are significantly elevated and that there is a correlation between the severity of SLE and the amount of IFNγ secreted (Al-Janadi et al 1993). All these findings suggest that the Th1 and Th2 responses are both important in the pathogenesis of lupus associated tissue injury. SLE is a disease involving a wide spectrum of cytokines. SLE patients with arthritis have higher IFNγ levels than the other patients, and conversely, patients with serositis or CNS involvement have higher IL-4 levels (Chang et al 2002). Furthermore SLE patients with nephritis have higher Th1 cytokines in serum and urine than non-nephritis patients (Chang et al 2006). Still more a significant difference in the Th1/Th2 balance in peripheral blood exists between WHO class IV and V lupus nephritis. Th1 cells are predominant in class IV but not in class V (Akahoshi et al 1999). In class V, the number of infiltrating cells was reduced, with a large percentage of CD4 T cells producing IL4 in the peripheral blood (Masutani et al 2001).

SLE is known to be a heterogeneous disease in which a wide range of cytokines are involved, it seems the most likely that Th1 or Th2 dominance depends on the stage of the disease and involvement. The Th2 response would be related to the development and production of autoantibodies, and Th1 with immune-mediated inflammatory activity.

3.2 B-lymphocytic Stimulator (BLyS)

BlyS a member of theTNF family, is also known as the B cell–activating factor(BAFF) and appears to play an important role in the differentiation and survival of B cells (Mackay et al 2002). BlyS can be released in a soluble form or can be expressed as a transmembrane protein on a wide variety of cell types, including monocytes, activated neutrophils, T cells, and DCs and its release is upregulated by IFN-γ, IL-10, G-CSF and CD40L (Nardelli et al 2001, Moore et al 1999, Litinskiy et al 2002, Harigay et al 2008).

BLyS binds to 3 receptors, BAFF-R (BAFF receptor), TACI (transmembrane activator and calcium modulator and cyclophylin ligand anteractor), and BCMA (B-cell maturation antigen), that are differentially expressed during B cell ontogeny (Bossen & Schneider 2006, Bossen et al 2008). The stimulation of all three receptors promotes B-cell differentiation and proliferation. BLyS is the sole ligand for BAFF-R, whereas TACI and BCMA each can bind either BLyS or another TNF family ligand known as a proliferation-inducing ligand (APRIL) (Bossen et al 2008).

After maturation in the bone marrow, newly formed B cells migrate to the secondary lymphoid organs (spleen and lymph nodes). These B cells do not possess all the characteristics of fully mature B cells, and they are referred to as transitional B cells. This transitional stage is an elastic checkpoint where thresholds for negative selection are homeostatically adjusted by free BLyS concentration. At this point an upregulation of BLyS expression can result in the rescue of self-reactive B cells from elimination. This effect explains, at least in part, the greatly increased levels of autoantibody production and associated autoimmune manifestations observed in transgenic mice that overexpress BlyS (Cancro et al 2009, MacKay et al 2007, Zheng et al 2005, Miller et al 2006, Thien et al 2004)

Elevated BLyS serum levels are often observed in SLE patients and correlate with disease activity (Petri et al 2008). Experiments in mice, have been demonstrated causality between BLyS over expression and development of SLE , on the other hand, also had been documented the amelioration of clinical disease in SLE mice following treatment with BlyS antagonist (Mackay et al 1999, Petri et al 2008, Jacob et al 2006)

The primary source of BlyS secretion in SLE remains speculative, a secretion by DCs (dendritic cells), a profoundly dysregulated IFNs in SLE or an increased levels of BLyS resulting from the presentation of self antigens (derived of an defective clearance of apoptotic bodies) to innate immune cells (which express BLyS upon antigenic stimulation) are potentially mechanisms implicated (Cancro et al 2009).

Because BLyS may figure prominently in the development of SLE and it could be a valid target for SLE, therapy with BLyS antagonists have been developed. Belimumab, a fully human monoclonal Ab (IgG1) that binds soluble BLyS and inhibits its binding to TACI, BCMA, and BR3, and Atacicept (TACI-Ig) a soluble, recombinant fusion protein of the human IgG1 Fc and the extracellular domain of the TACI receptor that binds BLyS and APRIL, have been tested in clinical trials. Results from phase III trials have demonstrated the safety profile and efficacy of belimumab in controlling SLE in a broad range of patients (Navarra et al 2011).

3.3 Interferon-α

Interferon alpha (INF-α) is produced mainly by plasmocytoid dendritic cells (PDC) in response to viral infection. INF-α is not one protein, but rather a family of highly related proteins encoded on the short arm of chromosome 9, and called type I INFs. Studies in which cellular mRNAs are screened against thousands of gene sequences have demonstrated that in SLE patients the INF-α induced genes are the most overexpresed of all those assayed (Baechler et al 2003). Evidence of the effect of INF-α in SLE comes from observations on the therapeutic administration of IFN-α in various types of malignancies and hepatitis C infection. Case reports emerged describing the development of lupus associated autoantibodies and even clinical lupus (Niewold & Swedler 2005). Discontinuation of IFN-a typically resulted in remission of SLE symptoms, supporting a causal relationship with IFN-a. Only a minority of patients treated with IFN-a develop SLE (<1% of patients) , these data support the idea that IFN-a can be sufficient to induce SLE in some genetically designed individuals. In addition, SLE patients commonly harbor anti INF-α autoantibodies. Anti INF-α antibodies-positive patients have lower levels of serum type I IFN bioactivity and evidence for reduced downstream IFN-pathway and disease activity.

A very strong correlation is consistently observed between the presence of SLE-associated autoantibodies that recognize nucleic acid structures or RNA-containing protein, such as anti-Ro, anti-La, anti-Sm, anti-RNP, and anti-dsDNA and high production of INF-α (Kirou et al 2005). Also lupus patients with high serum IFNa had a significantly higher prevalence of cutaneous and renal disease in most studies (Dall'era et al 2005). It is interesting that both of these clinical manifestations share an association with a particular serology (rash with anti-Ro and nephritis with anti-dsDNA).

The principal mechanism through which INF-α is produced in SLE is through Toll-like receptors (TLR). TLR receptors is a family of receptors present in a variety of cells and that recognize characteristics ligand present in pathogens. Some TLR recognize RNA and DNA sequences of single or double chain. A quality of many cases of lupus is the production of autoantibodies against RNA or DNA containing protein complexes such as Sm, RNP, Ro, and La. Autoantibodies specific for these lupus-associated riboproteins can bind with antigens derived from apoptotic cells. The RNA/DNA found in these complexes are capable of promoting the production of IFN-a through the stimulation of TLR. Because some TLR is located in the endosomes, RNA or DNA containing complexes must access the interior of the cell before they are able to act as activators. The Fc portions of the immune complexes are recognized and internalized by cells with Fc receptors in their surface, providing a route of entry for RNA or DNA to reach TLR, resulting in interferon alpha production (Figure 2). This process is especially well established in PDCs on TLR7 and TLR9 (Båve et al 2003).

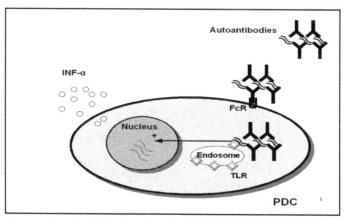

Fig. 2. Induction of INF-α in lupus. RNA/DNA containing immunecomplexes access the interior of the cell through recognition of Fc portion by Fc receptors in PDC membrane. Inside cell the RNA/DNA specific ligand are recognized by Toll-like receptors (TLR). TLR depending signals reach to the cell nucleus and induces transcription of IFN genes.

INF-α generate an effective antigen-presenting cells state by mediating maturation of dendritic cells. Thus INF-α prime the immune system for augmented sensitivity to subsequent stimuli. The activate antigen presenting cell state may also be characterized by an augmented capacity to generate a peripheral T-cell repertoire enriched in autoreactive cells. Dendritic cells are primary activators of T-cells and affect both tolerance and activation, depending of the state of dendritic cells. Dendritic cells from lupus patients are able to present self-antigens to T-cells in a stimulatory rather than regulatory manner, a process which is INF-α dependent (Blanco et al 2001). Moreover PDCs significantly enhance autoreactive B cell proliferation, autoantibody production, and survival in response to TLR activation (Ding et al 2009). Recently it has been reported that activation of the IFN signaling pathway may be linked to the risk of atherosclerosis by affecting plaque formation in patients with SLE (Li et al 2011).

In conclusion, in SLE patients, some autoantibodies are able to induce the production of INF-α. INF-α enhances the autoimmunity and immune response.

3.4 Tumor necrosis factor-α (TNF-α)

TNF-α is a pleiotropic cytokine produced by a variety of cell types including monocytes, lymphocytes and non immunological cell types in response to inflammation, infection and other environmental challenges. There are controversial results about the role of TNF in mice lupus strains. In NZB/W stain diminished production of TNF-α has been reported demonstrating the protective effect of TNF-α (Jacob & McDevitt 1988). In other strains of murine lupus an increased production of TNF-α has been described. In addition, TNF-α concentration correlates with the severity of the illness and anti-TNF therapy is profitable (Boswell et al 1988). Overall, these results show a duality in the role of TNF in lupus, one beneficial and one detrimental.

TNF-α contributes to avoiding the development of autoimmunity and autoantibody production. When introducing inhibitory TNF-α therapies in patients with diseases such as arthritis, spondyloarthropathies or Crohn disease shows the appearance of antinuclear antibodies and anti-ds DNA antibodies (De Ricke et al 2003, Garcia-Planella et al 2003). Normally these antibodies are not pathological, but in a few patients autoantibodies are associated with a SLE-like activity. TNF-α blocker induced lupus is usually benign and the symptoms resolve after TNF blockade stopped (Ramos-Casal et al 2007). It should be noted that these patients do not have the genetic background that makes them susceptible to SLE developing. When using anti-TNF therapy in SLE patients it has been found an elevation of antinuclear and anticardiolipin antibodies in most patients (Aringer et al 2007). This elevation was transient and did not produce complement consumption or lupus flare.

On the other hand numerous studies have shown that TNF blockade in SLE patients suffering from arthritis, nephritis and skin lesions were clinically effective in open clinic trials (Aringer et al 2004, Hayat el al 2007). It has found expression of TNF-α in inflamed tissue biopsies in patients with lupus, which does not occur in healthy individuals (Herrera-Esparza et al 1998), and TNF-α expression is associated with high histological disease activity (Zha et al 2009).

TNF-α performs two major functions: one as an immunoregulatory cytokine and the other as a potent mediator of inflammation. Among the immunoregulatory functions TNF-α induces the release of antiapoptotic molecules, TNF blockade may lead to increased apoptosis (Aringer et al 2007). The resulting increase in apoptotic material could explain why the emerging antibodies appear to exclusively target nuclear antigens and phospholipids, both of which are expressed on apoptotic bodies (Utz et al 1997). In addition, TNF blockade hampers the elimination of autoimmune B lymphocytes by cytotoxic T cells (Via et al 2001). All together could explain the pathways to increased lupus autoantibodies under TNF-α blockade.

The immunecomplexes generated by autoantibodies are deposited in tissues and organs. The deposit of immunecomplexes mediated inflammatory process triggered largely by TNF-α. The expression of TNF-α activates the local inflammation and tissue damage. TNF-*a* is the most important proinflammatory cytokine and a harbinger of tissue destruction, and it is at the top of a pro-inflammatory "cascade" leading to tissue damage. In contrast to the complex role of TNF-*a* in apoptosis and in immune regulation, its powerful proinflammatory effects are unequivocal. At the tissue level, TNF blockade induces remission of inflammation and hence tissue recovery. Anyway in the use of anti-TNF therapy is important to note the dual activity of this cytokine.

3.5 IL-6

IL6 is a pleiotropic cytokine, structurally, it shares homology with other cytokines: oncostatin M, IL11, leukaemia inhibitory factor, ciliary neurotrophic factor and cardiotrophin (Hirano, 1998). It was known initially as B-cell stimulatory factor 2 because it stimulates B cell growth and maturation to antibody-producing plasma cells. It is produced by a wide range of cell types including, monocytes, T cells, fibroblasts, synoviocytes and endothelial cells. IL-6 beyond his capacity of B cell activation and promotion of Ig production, play an important role in governing inflammation process (Ishihara et al., 2002).

IL-6 responses are transmitted through gp130, which serves as the universal signal-transducing receptor subunit for all IL-6-related cytokines. Although this classically occurs through IL-6 binding to its membrane-bound receptor (IL-6R), it is clear that a soluble form of the cognate IL-6 receptor (sIL-6R) affords IL-6 with an alternative mechanism of gp130 activation. This additional mode of cell activation is termed IL-6 trans-signaling and results from formation of a sIL-6R_IL-6 complex, which can directly bind cellular gp130. Because gp130 is ubiquitously expressed within tissue, trans-signaling provides IL-6 with the capacity to activate cells that would not intrinsically respond to IL-6 itself (Hibi et al., 1990; Hirano et al., 1994; McLoughlin et al., 2005). Therefore, IL-6 and gp130 signaling plays a critical role in the inflammatory process and tissue injury (Nechemia-Arbely et al., 2008).

An association between IL-6 and progression of lupus has been published for several murine models of SLE. The direct role of IL-6 in controlling autoantibody production has been demonstrated in the pristane induced model of lupus (Richards et al., 1998). On the other hand the administration of recombinant IL-6 to female NZB/W mice exacerbates the progression of glomerulonephritis (Ryffel et al., 1994). Anti IL-6 monoclonal antibody given in MRL lpr lupus prone mice, has been shown to cause a decrease in renal damage and a temporary reduction in levels of anti-dsDNA antibody production (Kiberd 1993).

Elevated levels of IL-6 have been found in the serum and in the urine of active SLE patients (Chun et al., 2007; Grondal et al., 2000; Horii et al., 1993). Raised expression of gp130, has been found in patients with active SLE, while an important reduction in the gp130 expression on B lymphocytes was observed when the activity of the disease had disappeared after readjusting its immunosuppressive treatment (De La Torre et al., 2009). Therefore, monitoring the frequency of gp130, could provide a useful tool in the diagnosis and monitoring of disease activity in patients with lupus.

Beyond the ability of IL-6 to stimulate B-lymphocyte differentiation into immunoglobulin secreting cells, IL-6 in concert with TGF-B is a critical cofactor for Th17 development, whereas the absence of IL-6 induces Foxp3, thereby specifying Treg development (Weaver et al., 2006). The two T-cell subsets play prominent roles in immune functions: Th17 cell is a key player in the pathogenesis of autoimmune diseases and protection against bacterial infections, while Treg functions to restrain excessive effector T-cell responses (Kimura et al., 2010).

Factors leading to the constitutive expression of IL-6 in SLE have not been elucidated yet, they may involve other regulator cytokines, like IL-10, or may be due, at least in part, to genetic differences (Linker et al., 1999; Tackey et al., 2004).

Recently, tocilizumab, a humanized monoclonal antibody against the α-chain of the IL-6 receptor, which prevents the binding of IL-6 to membrane bound and soluble IL-6 receptor, has been tested in SLE patients, with promising results (Illei et al., 2010).

3.6 IL-2

The cytokine IL-2 is a multifactorial cytokine. It was initially identified as a potent T cell growth factor, however, more recent data strongly indicate that IL-2 is essential for immune tolerance (Humrich et al., 2010). IL-2 constitutes a key element in the maintenance of the homeostasis between a proliferative immune response and the induction of tolerance, which supports the involvement of this cytokine in diverse autoimmunity disorders, such as SLE (Sharma et al., 2011). Predominantly produced by activated CD4+ and CD8+ T cells, IL-2 exerts its functions trough the interaction with its receptor (IL-2R) (Kammer, 2005).

It has been reported that production of IL-2 is decreased in patients with SLE (Sharma et al., 2011). Transcriptional regulators responsible for the transcription or suppression of IL-2 production are imbalanced in SLE T cells and this explains the reduced IL-2 levels found in SLE patients (Solomou et al., 2001). The decreased production of IL-2 in SLE patients most likely contributes to various immune defects such as decreased Treg production, decreased activation-induced cell death (AICD), and potentially decreased cytotoxic T lymphocytes (Lieberman & Tsokos 2010).

IL-2 signals are critical for the outcome of a CD8+ T cell response. Recently it was discovered that a strong IL-2 signal promotes the progressive acquisition of effector T cell functions (such as perforin and granzyme B expression, the hallmarks of CD8+ T cell cytotoxicity) but decreases the capacity to generate cells with memory features. By contrast, in conditions of weak IL-2 signaling, T cells fail to acquire the full program of effectors differentiation.(Pipkin et al., 2010)

IL-2 module activation-induced cell death (AICD). The activation of AICD is a mechanism of self tolerance in which apoptosis of autoreactive lymphocytes is induced after repeated stimulation. The deficiency in activation induced cell death might be related to the persistence of autoreactive T cell clones that eventually may lead to the activation of B cell subsets, with the subsequent production of autoantibodies and the development of autoimmune disorders (Gómez-Martín et al., 2009).

IL-2 is also required for the expansion and conversion of CD4+foxp3-T cells into CD4+ foxp3+ cells or regulatory T cells (Treg) (Setoguchi et al., 2005; Zheng et al., 2007;). Tregs cells, are necessary for maintaining tolerance to self antigens and they are able to do is by suppressing self-reactive T cells (Buckner , 2010). It has been well recognized that a decline in Tregs as a critical event in the development of systemic autoimmunity both mice and SLE patients (Valencia et al., 2007; Suzuki et al., 1995). On the other hand, recently IL-2 signaling has been shown to play a role in inhibiting the development of Th17 cells (Tato et al., 2007; Ma et al., 2010). Thus, the effects of IL-2 on Treg and Th17 cells may serve to promote auto-reactivity while at the same time inhibiting a counter regulatory response (discussed later).

3.7 IL-17

Interleukin 17 (IL-17) is a proinflammatory cytokine that is involved in defending the host against extracellular, some intracellular pathogens and fungi (Bettelli et al., 2008; Khader et al., 2010). IL-17 promote inflammation on several levels, as their receptors are expressed on both hematopoietic cells and non hematopoietic cells. Il-17 exerts its effects through the recruitment of monocytes and neutrophils by increasing the local production of chemokines. IL-17 can also stimulate B-cell antibody production (Hsu et al., 2008; Mitsdoerffer et al., 2010).

Recent studies have reported that production of IL-17 is abnormally high in patients with SLE. Its levels are increased in SLE sera and correlate with SLE disease activity. Moreover, the frequency of IL-17-producing T cells is increased in the peripheral blood of patients with SLE (Crispín & Toscos, 2010; Shah et al., 2010). Recent evidence indicates that a significant fraction of the IL-17 produced in SLE derives from Th17 cells and CD3+CD4-CD8- (double negative or DN) T cells (Nalbandian et al., 2009).

The identification of Th17-lineage-specific transcription factors, established Th17 cells as an independent T-cell subset. Differentiation of naïve T cells into Th17 cells depends on TGF-β and IL-6, being IL-23 essential for expansion and maintenance of pathogenic Th17 cells (Jäger & Kuchroo, 2010). Interestingly, the participation of TGF-β in the differentiation of Th17 cells places the Th17 lineage in close relationship with $CD4^+CD25^+Foxp3^+$ regulatory T cells (Tregs), as TGF-β also induces differentiation of naive T cells into $Foxp3^+$ Tregs in the peripheral immune compartment (Korn et al., 2009).

In light of this knowledge, now is the general notion that there is a reciprocal relationship between pro-inflammatory IL-17-producing Th17 cells and protective $Foxp3^+$ Tregs. The presence of pro-inflammatory cytokines like IL-6, which is induced during infection, inflammation or injury, inhibited the induction of $Foxp3^+$ Tregs and simultaneously promoted Th17-cell differentiation (Bettelli et al., 2006). On the other hand, tolerance induction was associated with decreased IL-6 production and increased TGF-β production that paralleled a reduction in the fraction of IL-17-producing T cells and a reciprocal increase in regulatory T cells (Kang et al., 2007). Therefore, some authors support the notion that therapeutic intervention in SLE should focus on therapeutic agents that can regulate the immune balance between Th17 and Treg cells rather than on those that exclusively regulate Th17 cells or a specific cytokine (Yang et al., 2011).

3.8 IL-10

Interleukin (IL)-10 is one of the most important cytokine with anti-inflammatory properties. Today it its known that the ability to synthesize IL-10 is not limited to certain T cells subsets, but is characteristic of almost all leukocytes. Very important sources in vivo appear to be mainly monocytes and macrophages as well as Th cells (Sabat et al., 2010).

IL-10 is a potent inhibitor of antigen presentation. The other profound effect of IL-10 is to inhibit the production of proinflammatory cytokines and mediators from macrophages and DCs. The major inflammatory cytokines, IL-1, IL-6, IL-12, and tumor necrosis factor (TNF), are all dramatically repressed following exposure to IL-10. On the other hand, IL-10 can costimulate B-cell activation, prolong B-cell survival, and contribute to class switching in B cells (Mosser & Zhang, 2008).

Multiple studies have reported high levels of IL-10 in SLE patients and in murine models of lupus, and this increase correlated with disease activity (Capper et al., 2004; Hagiwara et al., 1996; Houssiau et al., 1995; Park et al., 1998). However, the specificity of these findings is unclear. A recent study that investigated the role of IL-10 in a novel congenic model of lupus, B6.Sle1.Sle2.Sle3 (B6.TC) showed, that although B6.TC mice produced higher IL-10 levels that nonautoimmune control mice, an overexpression of IL-10 decreased T-cell activation, auto-antibody production and autoimmune pathogenesis (Blenman et al., 2006). Interestingly, other study has recently been shown that the presence of immune complexes and IFNα a cytokine implicated in the pathogenesis of SLE, decreases the capacity of IL-10 to suppress inflammation, limiting therefore the anti-inflammatory effect of this cytokine (Yuan et al., 2011). These results reinforce the notion that IL-10 exerts multiple functions and we must be cautious in equating high levels of IL-10 and increased pathogenesis in systemic autoimmunity (Blenman et al., 2006).

4. Cytokines in organ damage

4.1 Cutaneous lupus and cytokines

Cutaneous lupus erythematosus represents an autoimmune disease characterized by photosensitivity, apoptosis of keratinocytes and an inflammatory infiltrate in superficial and/or deep compartments of the skin. Skin disease is the second most common manifestation in SLE patients. Although clearly there is a link between the skin and systemic manifestations of SLE, often the skin may flare independently or patients may have SLE without skin disease. Treatments also may improve the skin, systemic disease, or both, suggesting that there are differences pathogenetically between skin and systemic findings in cutaneous lupus.

UV-irradiation is a well-known trigger of apoptosis in keratinocytes and there is accumulating evidence that abnormalities in the generation and clearance of apoptotic material is an important source of antigens in autoimmune diseases (Caricchio et al 2003). Phototesting studies suggest that both UVB and UVA are potentially pathogenic wavelengths, although it is clear that UVA induction requires higher doses of light relative to UVB. UV light can induce the binding of autoantibodies to selected nuclear antigens located on blebs or apoptotic bodies of skin. It has been suggested that these bleb-associated antigens may then be phagocyted, packaged, and presented to lymphocytes, thereby stimulating autoimmune responses (Casciola-Rosen & Rosen 1997). The high presence of anti-Ro antibodies in cutaneous involvement in lupus might be explained because anti-Ro antibodies might interfere with protection from UV damage as genetic knock-out of 60kD Ro resulted in an SLE-like illness in multiple strains of mice that were susceptible to UV damage (Xue et al 2003).

Exposure of keratinocytes to UVB results in the synthesis of many pro-inflammatory cytokines, including tumor necrosis factor-a (TNF-α) interleukin-1α (IL-1α), IL-6, IL-8, and IL-10 (Brink et al 2000). TNF-α is not only involved in the mediation of local inflammatory reactions within the epidermis, but may also enter the circulation and cause systemic effects. There is an association of subacute cutaneous LE with the extended HLA haplotype DRB1*03-B*08. Contained within this haplotype is the TNF2 allele, a TNFα promoter polymorphism, associated with increased TNFα production (Werth et al 2000).

UV induced injury trigger the initial chemokine production and release results in a first wave of skin-homing memory T cells and plasmacytoid dendritic cells (PDCs) via chemokine driven pathways. DNA, RNA, and immune complexes, present in skin containing apoptotic material, can serve as IFN-alpha inducers in PDCs . There is a higher frequency of PDCs in skin compared to the blood of patients with SLE, suggesting that PDCs migrate from the circulation into the skin. Under normal conditions PDCs are not able to respond to self nucleic acids, but in lupus PDCs became activated to produce INF-α by self nucleic acids in complex with autoantibodies to DNA or nucleoproteins. These immuno-complexes trigger innate activation of PDC through TLR7 and 9 and lead to sustained production of INF-α (show Figure 2) that may induce an unabated maturation of dendritic cells and the activation of autoreactive T cells. Enhanced type I IFN signaling promotes Th1-biased inflammation in cutaneous lupus. IFN-α can amplify cutaneous inflammation via the induction of chemokines that recruit potentially auto-reactive T cells into the skin. For example, IFN-α induces the production of chemokines, CXCL9, CXCL10, and CXCL11, which recruit chemokine receptor CXCR3 expressing lymphocytes, including Th1 cells and CD8+ T cells, from peripheral blood into inflamed skin (Wenzel et al 2005). Large numbers of CXCR3+ lymphocytes are detected in cutaneous lupus skin lesions. The majority of these infiltrating cells are memory T CD4+ lymphocytes. Among memory T cell subsets, CXCR3 is predominantly expressed on the surface of IFN-γ-producing Th1 cells, generating a proinflammatory effector response (Meller et al 2005). Hence, UV-irradiation may induce chemokine production and release, subsequently recruiting a first wave of skin-homing memory T cells and PDCs to sites of UV-injury which produce cytokine-mediated inflammation and tissue damage.

4.2 Neuropsychiatric SLE

Neuropsychiatric systemic lupus erythematosus (NPSLE) involves neurological manifestations seen in the central, peripheral, and autonomic nervous systems as well as psychiatric disorders in patients with SLE in which other causes have been excluded. NPSLE may occur at any time during the course of the disease, and symptoms are extremely diverse, ranging from depression, psychosis, and seizures to stroke (Committee on Neuropsychiatric Lupus Nomenclature 1999). Though the pathophysiology of NPSLE has not yet been elucidated, two mechanisms of damage, specifically those produced by autoantibodies, and inflammatory mediators, are implicated in NPSLE. The most common neuropathologic features are multifocal microinfarcts many of them due to the effect of anti-cardiolipin antibodies (Hanlyet al 1992).

Cytokines and chemokines have been implicated in the pathophysiology of NPSLE. Of the different cytokines studied, interleukin-6 (IL-6) has been shown to have the strongest positive association with NPSLE (Fragoso-Loyo et al 2007). IL-6 is a cytokine with high proinflammatory activity. IL-6 level in the CSF of NPSLE was reported to be elevated without damage of the blood-brain barrier, demonstrating an intrathecal synthesis of IL-6. In addition, the expression of IL-6 mRNA was elevated in the hippocampus and cerebral cortex, suggesting that IL-6 expression was increased within the entire CNS of NPSLE (Hirohata & Hayakawa 1999). Furthermore, when IL-6 activity was followed throughout symptom remission, they noted a decrease in CSF IL-6 activity measured indirectly, but not in serum IL-6 activity (Hirohata & Miyamoto 1990). A recent study has shown that the sensitivity and specificity of CSF IL-6 for diagnosis of lupus psychosis was 87.5% and 92.3%, respectively, indicating that CSF IL-6 might be an effective marker for the diagnosis of lupus psychosis (Hirohata et al 2009). Although some cytokines are important biomarkers of NPSLE, the mechanism for the elevated levels of cytokines is thus far unknown. Immune complexes in SLE can stimulate IFN-a and there is strong evidence in humans and in mice that IFN-a can cause neuropsychiatric manifestations. It has recently described using a bioassay containing plasmacytoid dendritic cells, that NPSLE CSF induced significantly higher IFN-a compared with CSF from patients with multiple sclerosis or other autoimmune disease controls. NPSLE CSF was 800-fold more potent at inducing IFN-a compared with paired serum, due to inhibitors present in serum (Santer et al 2009). Further immunological studies are expected to show how autoantibodies in SLE patients work to promote the cytokine storm associated with the pathophysiology of NPSLE.

4.3 Cytokines role in lupus nephropathy

Renal involvement in SLE is present in over 50% of patient with active SLE and remains a major cause of end-stage renal disease and it is associated with a greater than four-fold increase in mortality in recent series (Bernatsky et al., 2006; Boumpas et al., 1995). The pathologic manifestations of lupus nephritis (LN) are extremely diverse and may affect any or all renal compartments. The complexity of renal manifestations can be most easily approached using the World Health Organization Classification revised and updated in 2004 (Weening et al., 2004).

The picture of cytokines present in LN is already complex and no single-cell population or cytokine has been decisively identified as a key mediator. Elevated circulating levels and/or tissue mRNA transcripts for several cytokines are reported in lupus patients and mice. On the other hand, the data regarding the relative importance of Th1-type versus Th2-type cytokines are inconsistent (Foster, 2005; Theofilopoulos et al., 2001).

The development of laser-manipulated micro dissection (LMD) from clinical biopsy specimens, together with messenger RNA (mRNA) expression analysis in the targeted glomeruli or specific regions of interest, using real-time quantitative PCR, has allowed to explore the single-cell cytokine profile of the samples from the LN patients. Interestingly a recent study, using LMD and PCR analysis of renal biopsy samples from LN patients has showed a negative correlation between the level of IL-2 and renal damage while a positive correlation between IL-17 and renal damage was evidenced. Indicating that IL-2 and IL-17 play opposite roles in SLE development, suggesting that IL-2 may play a role in protecting against SLE development, while IL-17 might have a reverse effect (Wang et al., 2010). On the other hand, recent studies have highlighted the potential importance of the Th17 immune response in renal inflammatory disease. These include the identification and characterization of IL-17-producing T cells in nephritic kidneys of mice and humans, as well as evidence for the contribution of IL-17 and the IL-23/Th17 axis to renal tissue injury in LN (Turner et al., 2010; Zhang et al., 2009).

5. Conclusions

This chapter has focused in the new insights about the role of cytokine in the pathogenesis of Systemic Lupus Erythematosus. The imbalance in the levels of cytokines and their receptors found in SLE is clearly crucial to the development of the pathology of the disease. The cytokines are actively involved in both favoring the production of auto-antibodies as generating inflammation in affected tissues. Interactions between the cytokine milieus are complex and the attenuation of one cytokine would need to be approached with caution, considering effects on the cytokine network as a whole. There are still many facets of immunopathology of SLE elicited by cytokines to be elucidated. A more in-depth understanding of these cytokines may be of clinical significance in the context of devising biomarkers or therapeutic agents. Cytokine therapy, is highly probable that, in the future will take a relevant place in the therapeutic armamentarium of autoimmune disorders.

6. Acknowledgements

We thank Dr. Luis Caminal, Autoimmune Diseases Unit, Hospital Universitario Central de Asturias, sincerely for suggestions.

7. References

Abbas AK, Murphy KM, & Sher A. (1996). Functional diversity of helper T lymphocytes. *Nature* Vol 383 No 6603 (Oct 1996) pp 787-793. ISSN 0028-0836.
Abdou NI. Rider V. Greenwell C. Li X., & Kimler BF.(2008) Fulvestrant (Faslodex), an estrogen selective receptor downregulator, in therapy of women with systemic lupus erythematosus. Clinical, serologic, bone density, and T cell activation marker studies: a double-blind placebo-controlled trial. *The Journal of Rheumatology* Vol 35 No 5 (May 2008) pp 797-803.ISSN 0315-162X.
Akahoshi M, Nakashima H, Tanaka Y, Kohsaka T, Nagano S, Ohgami E, Arinobu Y, Yamaoka K, Niiro H, Shinozaki M, Hirakata H, Horiuchi T, Otsuka T, & Niho Y. (1999)   Th1/Th2 balance of peripheral T helper cells in systemic lupus

erythematosus. *Arthritis and Rheumatism* Vol 42 No 8 (Aug 1999) pp 1644–8. ISSN 0004-3591.

Al-Janadi M, Al-Balla S, Al-Dalaan A, & Raziudin S. (1993). Cytokine profile in systemic lupus erythematosus, rheumatoid arthritis and other rheumatic disease. *Journal of Clinical Immunology* Vol 13 No1 (Jan 1993) pp 58–67. ISSN 0271-9142.

Aringer M, Graninger WB, Steiner G, & Smolen JS. (2004). Safety and efficacy of tumor necrosis factor alpha blockade in systemic lupus erythematosus: an open-label study. *Arthritis and Rheumatism* Vol 50 No 10 (Oct 2004) pp 3161-3169. ISSN 0004-3591.

Aringer M, Steiner G, Graninger WB, Höfler E, Steiner CW, & Smolen JS. (2007). Effects of short-term infliximab therapy on autoantibodies in systemic lupus erythematosus. *Arthritis and Rheumatism* Vol 56 No 1 (Jan 2007) pp 274-279. ISSN 0004-3591.

Baechler EC, Batliwalla FM, Karypis G, Gaffney PM, Ortmann WA, Espe KJ, Shark KB, Grande WJ, Hughes KM, Kapur V, Gregersen PK, & Behrens TW. (2003). Interferon inducible gene expresion signature in peripheral blood cells of patients with severe Lupus. *Proceedings of the National Academy of Sciences of the United States of America* Vol 100 No 5 (Mar 2003) pp 2610-2615. ISSN 0027-8424.

Bao M. Yang Y. Jun HS, &. Yoon JW. (2002) Molecular mechanisms for gender differences in susceptibility to T cellmediated autoimmune diabetes in nonobese diabetic mice. *Journal of Immunology* Vol 168 No10 (May 15 2002) pp 5369-5375 ISSN 0022-1767.

Båve U, Magnusson M, Eloranta ML, Perers A, Alm GV, & Rönnblom L. (2003) FcγRIIa is expressed on natural IFN-α- producing cells (plasmacytoid dendritic c ells) and is required for the IFN-α production induced by apoptotic cells combined with Lupus IgG. *Journal of Immunology* Vol 171 No 6 (Sept 2003) pp 3296–3302. ISSN 0022-1767.

Bernatsky,S.;Boivin, JF; Joseph, L.; Manzi, S.; Ginzle,r E.; Gladman, DD.; Urowitz, M.; Fortín, PR.; Petri, M.; Barr, S.; Gordon, C.; Bae, SC.; Isenberg, D.; Zoma, A.; Aranow, C.; Dooley, MA.; Nived .; Sturfelt, G.; Steinsson, K.; Alarcón, G.; Senécal, JL.; Zummer, M.; Hanly, J.; Ensworth. S.; Pope, J.; Edworthy, S.; Rahman, A.; Sibley, J.; El-Gabalawy, H.; McCarthy, T.; St Pierre, Y.; Clarke, A. & Ramsey-Goldman, R. (2006) . Mortality in systemic lupus erythematosus. *Arthritis and Rheumatism* Vol. 54, No. 8, (Aug 2006), pp. 2550–2557 ISSN 0004-3591.

Bettelli, E; Oukka, M.; Kuchroo, VK. & Korn, T. (2009). IL-17 and Th17 Cells. *Annual reviews of Immunology.* Vol. 27 (2009), pp. 485-517. ISSN 0732-0582.

Bettelli, E.; Korn, T.; Oukka, M. & Kuchroo, VK. (2008) Induction and effector functions of T(H)17 cells. *Nature* Vol. 453, (Jun 2008), pp. 1051-7. ISSN 0028-0836.

Bettelli, E.; Carrier, Y.; Gao, W.; Korn, T.; Strom, TB.; Oukka, M.; Weiner, HL. & Kuchroo, VK. (2006). Reciprocal developmental pathways for the generation of pathogenic effector TH17 and regulatory T cells. *Nature* Vol. 441, (May 2006), pp. 235-8. ISSN 0028-0836.

Blanco P, Palucka AK, Gill M, Pascual V, & Banchereau J.(2001). Induction of dendritic cell diferentiation by INF-α in systemic lupus erythemotosus. *Science* Vol 294 No 5546 (Nov 2001) pp 1540-1543. ISSN 0193-4511.

Blenman, KR.; Duan, B.: Xu, Z.; Wan, S.; Atkinson, MA.; Flotte, TR.; Croker, BP. & Morel,L. (2006). IL-10 regulation of lupus in the NZM2410 murine model. *Laboratory Investigations.* Vol 86, No 11, (Nov 2006), pp. 1136-48 ISSN 0023-6837

Bossen C.; Cachero TG.; Tardivel A.; Ingold K.; Willen L.; Dobles M.; Scott ML.; Maquelin A.; Belnoue E.; Siegrist CA.; Chevrier S.; Acha-Orbea H.; Leung H.; Mackay F.; Tschopp J & Schneider P. (2008). TACI, unlike BAFF-R, is solely activated by oligomeric BAFF and APRIL to support survival of activated B cells and plasmablasts, *Blood* Vol 111 No 3 (Feb 2008), pp. 1004–1012 ISSN 0006-4971.

Bossen C, & Schneider P.(2006). BAFF.; APRIL and their receptors: structure, function and signaling. *Seminars in Immunology.* Vol 18 No 5 (Oct 2006) pp:263–75, ISSN 1044-5323.

Boswell JM; Yui MA, Burt DW, & Kelley VE. (1988). Increased tumor necrosis factor and IL-1 beta gene expression in the kidneys of mice with lupus nephritis. *Journal of Immunology* Vol 14 No9 (Nov 1988) pp 3050-3054. ISSN 0022-1767.

Boumpas, DT.; Auston, HA.; Fessler, BJ.; Balow, JE.; Klippel, JH. & Lockshin, MD. (1995). Systemic lupus erythematosus: Emerging concepts. Part I. Renal neuropsychiatric, cardiovascular pulmonary and hematologic disease. *Annals of Internal Medicine* Vol. 122, No.12, (Jun 1995), pp. 940-950. ISSN 0003-4819.

Brink N, Szamel M, Young AR, Wittern KP, & Bergemann J. (2000). Comparative quantification of IL-1beta, IL-10, IL-10r, TNFalpha and IL-7 mRNA levels in UV-irradiated human skin in vivo. *Inflammation Research* Vol 49 No 6 (Jun 2000) pp 290-296. ISSN 1023-3830.

Buckner, JH. (2010). Mechanisms of impaired regulation by CD4(+)CD25(+)FOXP3(+) regulatory T cells in human autoimmune diseases. *Nature Reviews of Immunology.* Vol. 10, No.12,(Dec 2010), pp. 849-59. ISSN 1474-1733.

Buyon JP, Petri MA, Kim MY, Kalunian KC, Grossman J, Hahn BH, Merrill JT, Sammaritano L, Lockshin M, Alarcón GS, Manzi S, Belmont HM, Askanase AD, Sigler L, Dooley MA, Von Feldt J, McCune WJ, Friedman A, Wachs J, Cronin M, Hearth-Holmes M, Tan M, & Licciardi F. (2007)The effect of combined estrogen and progesterone hormone replacement therapy on disease activity in systemic lupus erythematosus: a randomized trial. *Annals of Internal Medicine* Vol 142 No 21 (Jun 2005) pp 953–62. ISSN 0003-4819.

Cancro MP.; D'Cruz DP & Khamashta MA. (2009). The role of B lymphocyte stimulator(BLyS) in systemic lupus erythematosus. *Journal of Clinical Investigations.* Vol 119. No 5 (May 2009), pp. 1066-73 ISSN 0021-9738.

Capper, ER.; Maskill, JK.; Gordon, C. & Blakemore, AI. (2004). Interleukin (IL)-10, IL-1ra and IL-12 profiles in active and quiescent systemic lupus erythematosus: could longitudinal studies reveal patient subgroups of differing pathology?.*Clinical and Experimental Immunology.* Vol 138, No 2 (Nov 2004), pp. 348-56, ISSN 0009-9104.

Caricchio R, McPhie L, & Cohen PL. (2003). Ultraviolet B radiation-induced cell death: critical role of ultraviolet dose in inflammation and lupus autoantigen redistribution. *Journal of Immunology* Vol 171 No 11 (Dec 2003) pp 5778–86.ISSN 0022-1767.

Casciola-Rosen L, & Rosen A. (1997). Ultraviolet light-induced keratinocyte apoptosis: A potential mechanism for the induction of skin lesions and autoantibody production in LE. *Lupus.* Vol 6 No 2 pp 175-80. ISSN 0961-2033.

Chan R.W.-Y., Lai F.M.-M., Li E.K.-M., Tam L.-S., Chow K.-M., Li P.K.-T., & Szeto C.. (2006). Imbalance of Th1/Th2 transcription factors in patients with lupus nephritis.

Rheumatology (Oxford, England) Vol 45 No 8 (Aug 2006) pp 951-957. ISSN 1462-0324.

Chang DM, Su WL, & Chu SJ. (2002)The expression and significance of intracellular T helper cytokines in systemic lupus erythematosus. *Immunological Investigations* Vol 31 No 1 (Febr 2002) pp 1-12. ISSN 0882-0139.

Chun, H.Y.; Chung, J.W.; Kim, H.A.; Yun, J.M.; Jeon, J.Y.; Ye, Y.M.; Kim, S.H., Park, H.S. & Suh, C.H.J. (2007). Cytokine IL-6 and IL-10 as biomarkers in systemic lupus erythematosus. *Clinical. Immunology.* Vol. 27, No. 5, (Sep 2007), pp. 461-466. ISSN 0271-9142.

Cohen-Solal JF, Jeganathan V, Grimaldi CM, Peeva E, & Diamond B (2006) Sex hormones and SLE: influencing the fate of auto reactive B cells. *Current topics in microbiology and immunology* Vol 305 No 1 pp 67-88. ISSN 0070-217X

Committee on Neuropsychiatric Lupus Nomenclature.(1999). The American College of Rheumatology nomenclature and case definitions for neuropsychiatric lupus syndromes. *Arthritis and Rheumatism.* Vol 42 No 4 (Apr 1999) pp 599-608.ISSN 0004-3591.

Crispín, JC. & Tsokos, GC. (2010). IL-17 in systemic lupus erythematosus. *Journal of Biomedicine and Biotechnology.* (Apr 2010): 943254. ISSN 1110-7243.

Dall'era MC, Cardarelli PM, Preston BT, Witte A, & Davis JC Jr. (2005). Type I interferon correlates with serological and clinical manifestations of SLE *Annals of the rheumatic diseases* Vol. 64, no. 12 (Dec 2005) pp. 1692-1697.ISSN 0003-4967.

De La Torre, M.; Urra, J.M. & Blanco, J. (2009). Raised expression of cytokine receptor gp130 subunit on peripheral lymphocytes of patients with active lupus. A useful tool for monitoring the disease activity?. *Lupus* Vol. 18, No 3, (Mar 2009), pp. 216- 222. ISSN 0961-2033.

De Rycke L, Kruithof E, Van Damme N, Hoffman IE, Van den Bossche N, Van den Bosch F, Veys EM, & De Keyser F. (2003) Antinuclear antibodies following infliximab treatment in patients with rheumatoid arthritis or spondylarthropathy. *Arthritis and Rheumatism* Vol 48: No 4 (Apr 2003) pp 1015-1023.ISSN 0004-3591.

Ding C, Cai Y, Marroquin J, Ildstad ST, & Yan J.(2009). Plasmacytoid Dendritic Cells Regulate Autoreactive B Cell Activation via Soluble Factors and in a Cell-to-Cell Contact Manner. *Journal of Immunology* Vol 183 No 11 (Dec 1 2009) pp 7140-7149. ISSN 0022-1767.

Doria A, Ghirardello A, Iaccarino L, Zampieri S, Punzi L, Tarricone E, Ruffatti A, Sulli A, Sarzi-Puttini PC, Gambari PF, & Cutolo M.(2004)Pregnancy, cytokines and disease activity in systemic lupus erythematosus. *Arthritis and Rheumatism* Vol 51 No 6 (Dec 15 2004) pp 989-95. ISSN 0004-3591.

Foster, MH. (1999). Relevance of systemic lupus erythematosus nephritis animal models to human disease. *Seminars in Nephrology.* Vol 19, No 1 (Jan 1999), pp.12-24. ISSN 0270-9295.

Fragoso-Loyo H, Richaud-Patin Y, Orozco-Narváez A, Dávila-Maldonado L, Atisha-Fregoso Y, Llorente L, & Sánchez-Guerrero J. (2007). Interleukin-6 and chemokines in the neuropsychiatric manifestations of systemic lupus erythematosus. *Arthritis and Rheumatism.* Vol 56 No 4 (Apr 2007) pp 1242-50. ISSN 0004-3591.

Garcia-Planella E, Domènech E, Esteve-Comas M, Bernal I, Cabré E, Boix J, & Gassull MA. (2003). Development of antinuclear antibodies and its clinical impact in patients with Crohn's disease treated with chimeric monoclonal anti-TNFalpha antibodies (infliximab). *European journal of gastroenterology & hepatology* Vol 15 No 4 (Apr 2003 pp 351-354. ISSN 0954-691X .

Gómez-Martín, D.; Díaz-Zamudio, M.; Crispín, JC. & Alcocer-Varela, J. (2009) Interleukin 2 and systemic lupus erythematosus: beyond the transcriptional regulatory net abnormalities. *Autoimmunity reviews*. Vol.9, No. 1 (Sep 2009), pp. 34-9. ISSN 1568-9972.

Green GL. Gilna P. Waterfield M. Baker A. Hort Y. & Shine J. (1986). Sequence and expression of human estrogen receptor complementary DNA. *Science* Vol 231 No 4742 (Mar 1986) pp 1150-1154. ISSN 0193-4511.

Grondal, G.; Gunnarsson, I.; Ronnelid, J.; Rogberg, S.; Klareskog, L. & Lundberg, I. (2000). Cytokine production,serum levels and disease activity in systemic lupus erythematosus *Clinical and Experimental Rheumatology* Vol. 18, No. 5, (Sep-Oct 2000, pp. 565-570. ISSN 0392-856X.

Hagiwara, E.; Gourley, MF.; Lee, S. & Klinman, DK. (1996). Disease severity in patients with systemic lupus erythematosus correlates with an increased ratio of interleukin-10:Interferon- gamma-secreting cells in the peripheral blood. *Arthritis and Rheumatism* Vol. 39, No 3 (Mar 1996), pp.379-385, ISSN 0004-3591   .

Hanly JG, Walsh NM,   &bSangalang V. (1992).   Brain pathology in systemic lupus erythematosus. *Journal of Rheumatolology* Vol 19 No (May 1992) pp 732–41.ISSN 0315-162X .

Harigai M.; Kawamoto M.; Hara M.; Kubota T.; Kamatani N & Miyasaka N.(2008) Excessive production of IFN-γ in patients with systemic lupus erythematosus   and its contribution to induction of B lymphocyte stimulator/B cell-activating factor/TNF ligand superfamily-13B. *Journal of Immunology*. Vol 181:. No. 3   (Aug 2008), pp. 2211–2219, ISSN 0022-1767 .

Hayat SJ, Uppal SS, Narayanan Nampoory MR, Johny KV, Gupta R, & Al-Oun M. (2007). Safety and efficacy of infliximab in a patient with active WHO class IV lupus nephritis. *Clinical Rheumatology* Vol 26 No 6 (Jun 2007) pp 973-975. ISSN 0770-3198.

Herrera-Esparza R, Barbosa-Cisneros O, Villalobos-Hurtado R, & Avalos-Díaz E. (1998). Renal expression of IL-6 and TNFα genes in lupus nephritis *Lupus* Vol 7 No 3 (Mar 1998) pp 154–158. ISSN 0961-2033.

Hibi,M.;Murakami,M.; Saito, M.; Hirano, T.; Taga, T. & Kishimoto, T. (1990). Molecular cloning and expression of an IL-6 signal transducer, gp130. *Cell* Vol. 63. No. 6, (Dec 1990), pp. 1149-1157. ISSN 0092-8674.

Hirano, T. (1998). Interleukin 6 and its receptor: ten years later. *International reviews of Immunology* Vol. 16, (1998), pp. 249–284 ISSN 0883-0185.

Hirano, T.; Matsuda, T. & Nakajima, K. (1994). Signal transduction through gp-130 is shared among the receptor for the interleukin-6 related cytokine subfamily. *Stem Cells* Vol. 12, No. 3 (May 1994), pp. 262–277. ISSN 1066-5099.

Hirohata S, Kanai Y, Mitsuo A, Tokano Y, & Hashimoto H; NPSLE Research Subcommittee. (2009). Accuracy of cerebrospinal fluid IL-6 testing for diagnosis of lupus psychosis. A multicenter retrospective study. *Clinical Rheumatology* Vol 28 No 11 (Nov 2009) pp 1319-23. ISSN 0770-3198.

Hirohata S, & Hayakawa K. (1999). Enhanced interleukin-6 messenger RNA expression by neuronal cells in a patient with neuropsychiatric systemic lupus erythematosus. *Arthritis and Rheumatism* Vol 42 No 12 (Dec 1999) pp 2729–30. ISSN 0004-3591.

Hirohata S,& Miyamoto T. (1990). Elevated levels of interleukin-6 in cerebrospinal fluid from patients with systemic lupus erythematosus and central nervous system involvement. *Arthritis and Rheumatism.* Vol 33 No 5 (May 1990) pp 644–9. ISSN 0004-3591.

Horii, Y.; Iwano, M.; Hirata, E.; Shiiki, H.; Fujii, Y.; Dohi, K. & Ishikawa, H. (1993). Role of interleukin-6 in the progression of mesiangial proliferative glomerulonephritis. *Kidney International Suppl* Vol. 39, (Jan1993), pp. S71-5 ISSN 0098-6577.

Houssiau, FA.; Lefebvre, C.; Vanden Berghe, M.; Lambert, M.; Devogelaer,JP. & Renauld, JC. (1995). Serum interleukin 10 titers in systemic lupus erythematosus reflect disease activity. *Lupus*, Vol.4, No 5, (Oct 1995), pp. 393-5, ISSN 0961-2033

Hsu, HC.; Yang, P.; Wang, J.; Wu, Q.; Myers, R.; Chen, J.; Yi, J.; Guentert, T.; Tousson, A.; Stanus, AL.; Le, TV.; Lorenz, RG.; Xu, H.; Kolls, JK.; Carter, RH.; Chaplin, DD.; Williams, RW. & Mountz, JD. (2008). Interleukin 17-producing T helper cells and interleukin 17 orchestrate autoreactive germinal center development in autoimmune BXD2 mice. *Nature Immunology.* 2008 Vol. 9, No 2, pp. 166-75. ISSN 1529- 2908.

Humrich, JY.; Morbach, H.; Undeutsch, R.; Enghard, P.; Rosenberger, S.; Weigert. O.; Kloke, L.; Heimann, J.; Gaber, T.; Brandenburg, S.; Scheffold, A.; Huehn, J.; Radbruch, A.; Burmester, GR. & Riemekasten, G. (2010) Homeostatic imbalance of regulatory and effector T cells due to IL-2 deprivation amplifies murine lupus. *Proc Natl Acad Sci U S A.* Vol. 107, No. 1 (Jan 2010), pp. 204-9. ISSN 0027-8424.

Iinui A, Ogasawara H, Naito T, Sekigawa I, Takasaki Y, Hayashida Y, Takamori K, & Ogawa H. (2007) Estrogen receptor expression by peripheral blood mononuclear cells of patients with systemic lupus erythematosus. *Clinical Rheumatology* Vol 26 No 10 (Oct 2007) pp 1675-1678. ISSN 0770-3198.

Ishihara, K. & Hirano, T. (2002). IL-6 in autoimmune disease and chronic inflammatory proliferative disease. *Cytokine & Growth Factor Reviews.* 2002 Vol. 13, (Aug-Oct 2002), pp. 357-68. ISSN 1359-6101.

Jacob CO, & McDevitt HO. (1988). Tumour necrosis factor-alpha in murine autoimmune lupus' nephritis. *Nature* Vol 331:No 6154 (Jan 28, 1988) pp 356-358. ISSN 0028-0836.

Jacob CO.; Pricop L.; Putterman C.; Koss MN.; Liu Y.; Kollaros M.; Bixler SA.;Ambrose CM.; Scott ML & Stohl W. (2006). Paucity of clinical disease despite serological autoimmunity and kidney pathology in lupus-prone New Zealand Mixed 2328 mice defi cient in BAFF. *Journal of Immunology* Vol 177 No 4 (Aug 2006), pp. 2671-2680, ISNN 0022-1767.

Jäger, A. & Kuchroo, VK. (2010). Effector and regulatory T-cell subsets in autoimmunity and tissue inflammation. *Scandinavian Journal of Immunology.* Vol. 72, No 3, (Sep 2010), pp. 173-84. ISSN 0300-9475.

Kammer, GM. (2005) Altered regulation of IL-2 production in systemic lupus erythematosus: an evolving paradigm. *Journal of Clinical Investigations.* 2005 Vol 115, No. 4, pp. 836-40. ISSN 0021-9738.

Kang, HK.; Liu, M. & Datta SK. (2007). Low-dose peptide tolerance therapy of lupus generates plasmacytoid dendritic cells that cause expansion of autoantigen-specific regulatory T cells and contraction of inflammatory Th17 cells. *Journal of Immunology* Vol. 178, No. 2 (Jun2007), pp. 7849-58. ISSN 0022-1767.

Khader, SA. & Gopal, R. (2010). IL-17 in protective immunity to intracellular pathogens. *Virulence*. Vol. 1 No.5 (Sep-Oct 2010), pp. 423-7. ISSN 2150-5594.

Kiberd, BA. (1993). Interleukin-6 receptor blockage ameliorates murine lupus nephritis. *Journal of American Society of Nephrology* Vol. 4, No. 1, (Jul 1993), pp. 58–61 ISSN 1046-6673.

Kirou KA, Lee C, George S, Louca K, Peterson MG, & Crow MK. (2005). Activation of the interferon-α pathway identifies a subgroup of systemic lupus erythematosus patients with distinct serologic features and active disease. *Arthritis and Rheumatism* Vol 52 No 5 (May 2005) pp 1491–1503. ISSN 0004-3591.

Klinman DM, & Steinberg AD. (1995). Inquiry into murine and human lupus. *Immunological reviews* Vol 144 No (Apr 1995) pp 157–93. ISSN 0277-9366.

Kramer PR. Kramer SF., & Guan G. (2004)17 β-estradiol regulates cytokine release through modulation of CD16 expression in monocytes and monocyte-derived macrophages. *Arthritis and rheumatism* Vol 50 No 6 (Jun 2004) pp 328-337. ISSN 0004-3591.

Lahita RG. (1999) The role of sex hormones in systemic lupus erythematosus. *Current opinion in rheumatology*. Vol 11 No 5 (Sept 1999) pp 352–356. ISSN 1040-8711.

Lahita RG.(1999) Emerging concepts for sexual predilection in the disease systemic lupus erythematosus. *Annals of the New York Academy of Sciences* Vol 876: No (Jun 1999) pp 64–70. ISSN 0077-8923.

Laurence, A.; Tato, CM.; Davidson, TS.; Kanno, Y.; Chen, Z.; Yao, Z.; Blank, RB.; Meylan, F.; Siegel, R.; Hennighausen, L.; Shevach, EM. & O'shea, JJ. (2007) Interleukin-2 signaling via STAT5 constrains T helper 17 cell generation. *Immunity* Vol. 26, No. 3, (Mar 2007), pp. 371-381 ISSN 1074-7613.

Li J, Fu Q, Cui H, Qu B, Pan W, Shen N, & Bao C. (2011). Interferon-α priming promotes lipid uptake and macrophage-derived foam cell formation: A novel link between interferon-α and atherosclerosis in lupus. *Arthritis and Rheumatism*. Vol 63 No 2 (Feb 2011) pp 492-502. ISSN 0004-3591.

Lieberman, LA. & Tsokos, GC. (2010). The IL-2 defect in systemic lupus erythematosus disease has an expansive effect on host immunity. *Journal of Biomedicine and Biotechnology*. (Jun 2010) ISSN 1110-7243.

Litinskiy MB.; Nardelli B.; Hilbert DM.; He B.; Schaffer A.; Casali P. & Cerutti A. (2002). DCs induce CD40-independent immunoglobulin class switchingthrough BLyS and APRIL. *Nature Immunology*. Vol 3, No 9 (Sep 2002), pp. 822-829, ISSN 1529-2908.

Ma, J.; Yu, J.; Tao, X.; Cai, L.; Wang, J. & Zheng, SG. (2010). The imbalance between regulatory and IL-17-secreting CD4+ T cells in lupus patients. *Clinical Rheumatology*. Vol. 29, No. 11, (Nov 2010), pp. 1251-8. ISSN 0770-3198.

Mackay F.; Silveira PA & Brink R. (2007). B cells and the BAFF/APRIL axis: fast-forward on autoimmunity and signaling. *Current Opinion in Immunology*.Vol 19 No 3 (Jun 2007), pp. 327-36. ISSN 0952-7915.

Mackay F, & Browning.JL. (2002). BAFF: a fundamental survival factor for B cells. *Nature. Reviews. Immunology*. vol 2: No.7 (Jul 2002), pp.465–475, ISSN 1474-1733.

Mackay F.; Woodcock SA.; Lawton P.; Ambrose C.; Baetscher M.; Schneider P.; Tschopp J & Browning JL (1999). Mice transgenic for BAFF develop lymphocytic disorders along with autoimmune manifestations. *The Journal of Experimental Medicine* Vol 190 No 11 (Dec 1999), pp. 1697-1710, ISSN 0022-1007.

Maret A, Coudert JD, Garidou L, Foucras G, Gourdy P, Krust A, Dupont S, Chambon P, Druet P, Bayard F, & Guéry JC. (2003) Estradiol enhances primary antigen-specific CD4 T cell responses and Th1 development in vivo. Essential role of estrogen receptor-α expression in hematopoietic cells. *European journal of immunology* Vol 33 No 2 (Feb 2003) pp 512- 521. ISSN 0014-2980.

Masi AT, & Kaslow RA. (1978). Sex effects in systemic Lupus Erithematosus: A clue to pathogenesis. *Arthritis and Rheumathism* . Vol 21 No 4 (May 1978) pp 480-484. ISSN 0004-3591.

Masutani K, Akahoshi M, Tsuruya K, Tokumoto M, Ninomiya T, Kohsaka T, Fukuda K, Kanai H, Nakashima H, Otsuka T, & Hirakata H. (2001) Predominance of Th1 immune response in diffuse proliferative lupus nephritis. *Arthritis and rheumatism* Vol 44 No 9 (Sept 2001) pp 2097–106. ISSN 0004-3591.

McLoughlin, RM.; Jenkins, BJ.; Grail, D.; Williams, AS.; Fielding, CA.; Parker ,CR.; Ernst, M.; Topley, N. & Jones, SA. (2005). IL-6 trans-signaling via STAT3 directs T cell infiltration in acute inflammation *Proc Natl Acad Sci U S A.* Vol. 102, No 27, (Jul 2005), pp. 9589-94. ISSN 0027-8424.

Meller S, Winterberg F, Gilliet M, Müller A, Lauceviciute I, Rieker J, Neumann NJ, Kubitza R, Gombert M, Bünemann E, Wiesner U, Franken-Kunkel P, Kanzler H, Dieu-Nosjean MC, Amara A, Ruzicka T, Lehmann P, Zlotnik A, & Homey B. (2005). Ultraviolet radiation-induced injury, chemokines, and leukocyte recruitment: an amplification cycle triggering cutaneous lupus erythematosus. *Arthritis and Rheumatism* Vol 52 No 5 (May 2005) pp 1504-16. ISSN 0004-3591.

Miller JP.; Stadanlick JE & Cancro MP. (2006).Space, selection, and surveillance: setting boundaries with BLyS. *Journal of Immunology* Vol 176 No 11 (Jun 2006,) pp. 6405-10, ISNN 0022-1767.

Mitsdoerffer, M.; Lee, Y.; Jäger, A.; Kim, HJ.; Korn, T.; Kolls, JK.; Cantor, H.; Bettelli, E. & Kuchroo, VK. (2010). Proinflammatory T helper type 17 cells are effective B-cell helpers. *Proc Natl Acad Sci U S A.* Vol. 107, No. 32, (Aug 2010), pp.14292-7 ISSN 0027-8424.

Moore PA.; Belvedere O.; Orr A.; Pieri K.; LaFleur DW.; Feng P.; Soppet D.; Charters M.;Gentz R.; Parmelee D.; Li Y.; Galperina O.; Giri J.; Roschke V.; Nardelli B.; Carrell J.; Sosnovtseva S.; Greenfield W.; Ruben SM.; Olsen HS.;Fikes J, & Hilbert M. (1999.) BlyS: member of the tumor necrosis factor family and B lymphocyte stimulator, *Science,* Vol 285(5425). No 9 (Jul1999), pp. 260-263, ISSN 0193-4511.

Mosmann TR, & Coffman RL. (1989). TH1 and TH2 cells: different patterns of lymphokine secretion lead to different functional properties. *Annual reviews of immunology* Vol 7 pp 145-173. ISSN 0732-0582.

Mosmann TR, Cherwinski H, Bond MW, Giedlin MA, & Coffman RL. (1986). Two types of murine helper T cell clone. I. Definition according to profiles of lymphokine activities and secreted proteins. *Journal of Immunology* Vol 136 No 7 (Apr 1 1986) pp 2348-2357.ISSN 0022-1767.

Mosser, DM. & Zhang, X. (2008). Interleukin-10: new perspectives on an old cytokine. *Immunology reviews.* Vol. 226 (Dec 2008), pp. 205-18 ISSN:0105-2896.

Nalbandian, A.; Crispín, JC. & Tsokos, GC. (2009). Interleukin-17 and systemic lupus erythematosus: current concepts. *Clinical and Experimental Immunology*. Vol. 157, No 2, (Aug 2009), pp. 209-15. ISSN 0009-9104.

Nardelli B.; Belvedere O.; Roschke V.; Moore PA.; Olsen HS.; Migone TS.; Sosnovtseva S.; Carrell JA.; Feng P.; Giri JG & Hilbert DM.(2001). Synthesis and release of B-lymphocyte stimulator from myeloid cells. *Blood*. Vol 97. No 1(Jan 2001), pp. 98-204,ISSN 0006-4971.

Navarra SV.; Guzmán RM.; Gallacher AE.; Hall S.; Levy RA.; Jimenez RE.; Li EK.; Thomas M.; Kim HY.; León MG.; Tanasescu C.; Nasonov E.; Lan JL.; Pineda L.; Zhong ZJ.; Freimuth W & Petri MA; BLISS-52 Study Group. (2011). Efficacy and safety of belimumab in patients with active systemic lupus erythematosus: a randomised, placebo-controlled, phase 3 trial. *Lancet* Vol 26 No 377(Feb 2011), pp. 721-31, ISSN 0140-6736.

Nechemia-Arbely, Y.; Barkan, D.; Pizov, G.; Shriki, A.; Rose-John, S.; Galun, E. &, Axelrod, JH. (2008). IL-6/IL-6R axis plays a critical role in acute kidney injury. *Journal of American Society of Nephrology*. Vol.19, No. 6, (Jun 2008), pp.1106-15 ISSN 1046-6673.

Niewold TB, & Swedler WI.(2005) Systemic lupus erythematosus arising during interferon-alpha therapy for cryoglobulinemic vasculitis associated with hepatitis C. *Clinical Rheumatology*. Vol 24 No 2 (Ap 2005) pp 178–181. ISSN 0770-3198.

Ogawa N, Itoh M, & Goto Y. (1992). Abnormal production of B cell growth factor in patients with systemic lupus erythematosus. *Clinical and experimental immunology* Vol 89 No 1 (Jul 1992) pp 26–31. ISSN 0009-9104.

Park, YB.; Lee. SK; Kim, DS.; Lee, J.; Lee, CH. & Song, CH. (1998). Elevated interleukin-10 levels correlated with disease activity in systemic lupus erythematosus. *Clinical and experimental Rheumatology*, Vol. 16, No 3, (May-Jun 1998), pp. 283-8, ISSN 0392-856X.

Pedram A. Razandi M. & Levin R. (2006) Nature of functional estrogens receptors at the plasma membrane. *Molecular Endocrinology (Baltimore, Md.)*. Vol 20 No 9 (Sept 2006): pp 1996-2009. ISSN 0888-8809.

Petri M.; Stohl W.; Chatham W.; McCune WJ.; Chevrier M.; Ryel J.; Recta V.; Zhong J. & Freimuth W (2008). Association of plasma B lymphocyte stimulator levels and disease activity in systemic lupus erythematosus. *Arthritis and Rheumatism* Vol 58 No 8 (Aug 2008), pp 2453-2459, ISSN 0004-3591.

Pipkin, ME.; Sacks, JA.; Cruz-Guilloty, F.; Lichtenheld, MG.; Bevan, MJ. & Rao, A. (2010) Interleukin-2 and inflammation induce distinct transcriptional programs that promote the differentiation of effector cytolytic T cells. *Immunity*. Vol. 32, No 1 (Jan 2010), pp. 79-90. ISSN 1074-7613.

Ramanujam M.; Wang X.; Huang W.; Liu Z.; Schiffer L.; Tao H.; Frank D.; Rice J.; Diamond B.; Yu KO.; Porcelli S & Davidson. (2006). A.Similarities and differences between selective and nonselective BAFF blockade in murine SLE. *Journal of Clinical Investigations*, Vol 116 No 3 (Mar2006), pp. 724-734, ISSN 0021-9738.

Ramos-Casals M, Brito-Zerón P, Muñoz S, Soria N, Galiana D, Bertolaccini L, Cuadrado MJ,& Khamashta MA . (2007). Autoimmune diseases induced by TNF-tageted therapies: analysis of 233 cases. *Medicine (Baltimore)* Vol 86 No 4 (Jul 2007) pp 242-251. ISSN 0025-7974.

Richards, HB.; Satoh, M.; Shaw, M.; Libert, C.; Poli, V. & Reeves, WH. (1998). Interleukin 6 dependence of anti-DNA antibody production: evidence for two pathways of autoantibody formation in pristane-induced lupus. *The Journal of Experimental Medicine* Vol. 188, No. 5, (Sep 1998), pp. 985–990 ISSN 0022-1007.

Rider V, & Abdou NI. (2001). Gender differences in autoimmunity: molecular basis for estrogen effects in systemic lupus erythematosus. *International immunopharmacology.* Vol 1 No 6 (Jun 2001) pp 1009–1024. ISSN 1567-5769.

Rider V. Foster RT. Evans M. Suenaga R. & Abdou NI.(1998) Gender differences in autoimmune diseases: estrogen increases calcineurin expression in systemic lupus erythematosus. *Clinical immunology and immunopathology* Vol 82 No 2 (Nov 1998) pp 258-262.ISSN 0090-1229.

Ryffel, B.; Car, BD.; Gunn, H.; Roman, D.; Hiestand, P. & Mihatsch ,MJ. (1994). Interleukin-6 exacerbates glomerulonephritis in (NZB × NZW)F1 mice. *American Journal of Pathology* Vol. 144, No. 5, (May 1994), pp. 927-937 ISSN 0002-9440.

Sabat, R.; Grütz, G.; Warszawska, K.; Kirsch, S; Witte, E.; Wolf, K. & Geginat, J. (2010).Biology of interleukin-10. Cytokine& *Growth Factor reviews.* Vol. 21, No 5 (Oct 2010), pp.331-44, ISSN 1359-6101.

Santer DM, Yoshio T, Minota S, Möller T, & Elkon KB.(2009) Potent induction of IFN-alpha and chemokines by autoantibodies in the cerebrospinal fluid of patients with neuropsychiatric lupus. *Journal of Immunology.* Vol 182 No 2 (Jan 12, 2009) pp 1192–1201.ISSN 0022-1767.

Setoguchi, R.; Hori, S.; Takahashi, T. & Sakaguchi, S. (2005). Homeostatic maintenance of natural Foxp3+ CD25+CD4+ regulatory T cells by interleukin 2 and induction of autoimmune disease by IL-2 neutralization. *Journal of Experimental Medicine* Vol. 201, No. 5, (Mar 2005), pp.723–735 ISSN 0022-1007.

Shah, K.; Lee, WW.; Lee, SH.; Kim, SH.; Kang, SW.; Craft, J. & Kang, I. (2010). Dysregulated balance of Th17 and Th1 cells in systemic lupus erythematosus. *Arthritis Research and Therapy.* Vol. 12, No. 2, (2010); R53, ISSN 1478-6354.

Sharma, R.; Fu, SM. & Ju, ST. (2011) IL-2: a two-faced master regulator of autoimmunity. *Journal of Autoimmunity.* Vol. 36, N0 2, (Mar 2011), pp 91-7. ISSN 0896-8411.

Solomou, EE.; Juang, YT.; Gourley, MF.;Kammer, GM. & and Tsokos, GC. (2001).Molecular basis of deficient IL-2 production in T cells from patients with systemic lupus erythematosus. *Journal of Immunology,* Vol. 166, No. 6, (Mar 2001), pp. 4216–4222. ISSN0022-1767.

Stimson WH. & Hunter IC.(1980) Oesrtrogen induced immunoregulation mediated through the thymus. *Journal of clinical & laboratory immunology* Vol 4 No 1 (Jul 1980) pp 27-33. ISSN 0141-2760.

Straub RH. (2007) The complex role of estrogens in inflammation. *Endocrine Reviews* Vol 28 No 5 (Aug 2007) pp 521-574. ISSN 0163-769X.

Suzuki, H.; Kündig, TM.; Furlonge,r C.; Wakeham, A.; Timms, E.; Matsuyama, T.: Schmits, R.; Simard, JJ.; Ohashi, PS. & Griesser, H. (1995) Deregulated T cell activation and autoimmunity in mice lacking interleukin-2 receptor beta. *Science* Vol. 268, (Jun 1995), pp. 1472–1476. ISSN 0036-8075.

Theofilopoulos, AN.; Koundouris, S.; Kono, DH. & Lawson, BR.. (2001) The role of IFN-gamma in systemic lupus erythematosus: a challenge to the Th1/Th2 paradigm in autoimmunity. *Arthritis Research* Vol. 3, No 3, (Feb 2001), pp. 136-41 ISSN 1465-9905.

Thien M.; Phan TG.; Gardam S.; Amesbury M.; Basten A.; Mackay F, & Brink R. (2004). Excess BAFF rescues self-reactive B cells from peripheral deletion and allows them to enter forbidden follicular and marginal zone niches. *Immunity* Vol 20 No 6 (Jun 2004), pp. 785-798, ISSN 1074-7613.

Turner, JE.; Paust, HJ; Steinmetz, OM. & Panzer, U. (2010). The Th17 immune response in renal inflammation. *Kidney International*. Vol. 77, No 12, (Jun 2010), pp. 1070-5. ISSN 0085-2538.

Utz PJ, Hottelet M, Schur PH, & Anderson P. (1997). Proteins phosphorylated during stress-induced apoptosis are common targets for autoantibody production in patients with systemic lupus erythematosus. *Journal of Experimental Medicine* Vol 185 No 3 (Mar 1997) pp 843-854. ISSN 0022-1007.

Valencia, X.; Yarboro C.; Illei, G. & P. E. Lipsky, PE. (2007) Deficient CD4+CD25high T regulatory cell function in patients with active systemic lupus erythematosus., *Journal of Immunology* Vol. 178, No. 4, (2007), pp. 2579-2588 ISSN 0022-1767.

Via CS, Shustov A, Rus V, Lang T, Nguyen P, & Finkelman FD. (2001) In vivo neutralization of TNF-alpha promotes humoral autoimmunity by preventing the induction of CTL. *Journal of Immunology* Vol 167 No 12 (Dec 15 2001) pp 6821-6826. ISSN 0022-1767.

Wang, Y.; Ito, S.; Chino, Y.; Goto, D.; Matsumoto, I.; Murata, H.; Tsutsumi, A.; Hayashi, T.; Uchida, K.; Usui, J.; Yamagata, K. & Sumida, T. (2010) Laser microdissection-based analysis of cytokine balance in the kidneys of patients with lupus nephritis. *Clinical and Experimental Immunology*. Vol. 159, No 1, (Jan 2010), pp.1-10 ISSN 0009-9104.

Weening JJ.; D'Agati, VD.; Schwartz, MM.; Seshan, SV.; Alpers, CE.; Appel, GB., Balow,JE.; Bruijn ,JA.; Cook, T.; Ferrario, F.; Fogo, AB.; Ginzler, EM.; Hebert, L.; Hill, G.; Hill, P.; Jennette, JC.; Kong, NC.; Lesavre, P.; Lockshin, M.; Looi, LM.; Makino, H.; Moura, LA. & Nagata, M. (2004).The classification of glomerulonephritis in systemic lupus erythematosus revisited. *Journal of American Society of Nephrology*. Vol. 15, No 2, (Feb 2004), pp. 241-50. ISSN 1046-6673.

Wenzel J, Uerlich M, Wörrenkämper E, Freutel S, Bieber T, & Tüting T. (2005). Scarring skin lesions of discoid lupus erythematosus are characterized by high numbers of skin-homing cytotoxic lymphocytes associated with strong expression of the type I interferon-induced protein MxA. The *British journal of dermatology*. Vol 153 No 5 (Nov 2005) pp 1011-5. ISSN 0007-0963.

Werth VP, Zhang W, Dortzbach K, & Sullivan K. (2000). Association of a promoter polymorphism of TNFalpha with subacute cutaneous lupus erythematosus and distinct photoregulation f transcription. *The Journal of investigative dermatology* Vol 115 No 4 (Oct 2000) pp 726-30.ISSN 0022-202X.

Xue D, Shi H, Smith JD, Chen X, Noe DA, Cedervall T, Yang DD, Eynon E, Brash DE, Kashgarian M, Flavell RA, & Wolin SL. (2003). A lupus-like syndrome develops in mice lacking the Ro 60-kDa protein, a major lupus autoantigen. *Proceedings of the National Academy of Sciences of the United States of America*. Vol 100 No 13 (Jun 24, 2003) pp 7503-8. ISSN 0027-8424.

Yang, J.; Yang, X.; Zou, H.; Chu, Y. & Li, M. (2011). Recovery of the immune balance between Th17 and regulatory T cells as a treatment for systemic lupus erythematosus. *Rheumatology (Oxford)* (Apr 2011) ISSN 1462-0324.

Yuan, W.; DiMartino, SJ.; Redecha, PB.; Ivashkiv, LB. & Salmon, JE. (2011). Systemic lupus erythematosus monocytes are less responsive to interleukin-10 in the presence of immune complexes. *Arthritis and Rheumatism.* (Jan 2011), Vol.63, No 1, pp. 212-8. ISSN 0004-3591.

Zandman-Goddard G, Peeva E, & Shoenfeld Y (2007) Gender and autoimmunity. *Autoimmunity reviews* Vol 6 No 6 (Jun 2006) pp 366–372. ISSN 1568-9972.

Zhang, Z.; Kyttaris, VC. & Tsokos, GC. (2009). The role of IL-23/IL-17 axis in lupus nephritis. *Journal of Immunology.* Vol 183, No. 5, (Sep 2009), pp. 3160-9. ISSN 0022-1767.

Zheng Y.; Gallucci S.; Gaughan JP.; Gross JA & Monestier M.(2005) A role for B cell-activating factor of the TNF family in chemically induced autoimmunity. *Journal of Immunology* Vol 175 No 5 (Nov 2005), pp. 6163-8, ISNN 0022-1767.

Zheng, SG.; Wang, J.; Wang, P.; Gray, JD. & Horwitz, DA. (2007). IL-2 is essential for TGF-β to convert naïve CD4+CD25− cells to CD25+Foxp3+ regulatory T cells and for expansion of these cells. *Journal of Immunology* Vol. 178, No. 4 (Feb 2007), pp. 2018–2027 ISSN 0022-1767.

Zhu L, Yang X, Ji Y, Chen W, Guan W, Zhou SF, & Yu X. (2009). Up-regulated renal expression of TNF-α signalling adapter proteins in lupus glomerulonephritis. *Lupus*, Vol 18 No 2 (Feb 2009) pp 116–127. ISSN 0961-2033.

2

Genetics and Epigenetic in Systemic Lupus Erythematosus

Suad M. AlFadhli
Kuwait University
Kuwait

1. Introduction

Systemic lupus erythematosus (SLE) (OMIM #152700) is the prototype of a multiorgan autoimmune disease and still considered as a disease with an ambiguous etiology. The disease predominantly affects women during the reproductive years at a ratio of eight women per one man (Lopez, 2003). Its pathogenesis is multifactorial lying on genetic and environmental factors in which it occurs in genetically-predisposed individuals who have experienced certain environmental triggers resulting in an irreversible loss of immunologic self-tolerance. The nature of these environmental triggers is largely unknown. It is most likely that it requires a number of environmental triggers occurring together or sequentially over a limited period of time. The concept has therefore emerged of 'threshold liability' in which disease develops when a threshold of genetic and environmental susceptibility effects is reached (Jönsen,2007). Epigenetics, the control of gene packaging and expression independent of alterations in the DNA sequence, is providing new directions linking genetics and environmental factors. It has become clear that besides genetics, epigenetics plays a major role in complex diseases with complex immunological pathogenesis like lupus. Convincing evidence indicates that epigenetic mechanisms, and in particular impaired T cell DNA methylation, provide an additional factor. Interpreting the precise contribution of epigenetic factors to autoimmunity, and in particular to SLE, has become an active research area.

Herein, we will discuss our current understanding of SLE as an autoimmune disease and as a complex genetic disorder. Through the review of the current list of best validated SLE disease susceptibility candidate genes, in particular considering how the known and potential function of these genes may allow us to articulate the genetic of SLE pathogenesis. In addition we will review the effect of epigenetics on SLE pathology.

1.1 SLE, the disease

This complex autoimmune disease results on defects of multiple immunologic components of both the innate immune system and the adaptive immune system including altered immune tolerance mechanism, hyperactivation of T and B cells, decreased ability to clear immune complexes and apoptotic cells, and failure of multiple regulatory networks (Firestein, 2008). Moreover it is likely that immunological dysfunction precedes the onset of clinical disease by many years, making it a particularly challenging disease to study (Arbuckle, 2003).

SLE is a heterogeneous disease that has a diverse range of clinical symptoms, resulting from a widespread immune-mediated damage and it is presented differently from patient to patient (Arnett, 1988). The most common clinical manifestations of this disease include an are erythematous rash, oral ulcers, polyarthralgia, polyserositis, nonerosive arthritis, renal, hematologic, neurologic, pulmonary and cardiac abnormalities. Eleven criteria were identified for SLE clinical presentation, at least four of the 11 coded criteria need to be present for a clinical diagnosis of SLE (Arnett, 1988; Hochberg, 1997; Tan, 1982). Ethnic and genetic heterogeneity contributes to the complexity in SLE clinical presentation. Differently from Multiple sclerosis and although the disease is progressive in nature, no severity criteria have been developed to subgroup SLE patients (with the exception of kidney disease) (Tsao, 1998). A more detailed classification of SLE this heterogeneous disease would significantly help in its genetic analysis. Analyses conditioned on specific disease traits suggest that genetic effects arising from particular linkage regions may contribute to specific clinical or immunological features of SLE (i.e. the presence of haemolytic anaemia or the production of dsDNA antibodies) (Ramos, 2006; Hunnangkul, 2008). A similar picture has arisen from the study of mouse models. However, now it is widely accepted that SLE occurs in phases during a period of time that can be also of years. Therefore, the following steps in the development process of SLE have been suggested: i) genetic predisposition, ii) gender as an additional predisposing factor, iii) environmental stimuli which start immune responses, iv) appearance of autoantibodies, v) regulation of the autoantibodies, T and B cell fails with the development of the clinical disease, vi) chronic inflammation and oxidative damage as causes of tissue damage influencing morbidity (Gualtierotti, 2010).

1.2 Genetic contribution in the pathology of lupus

A genetic contribution to human lupus is well established. The strong genetic contribution to the development of SLE is supported by the high heritability of the disease (>66%), a higher concordance rate for SLE in monozygotic twins than in dizygotic twins or siblings (24–56% versus 2–5%, respectively) which was observed over 30 years ago, and the high sibling recurrence risk ratio of patients with SLE (between eightfold and 29-fold higher than in the general population) and up to 10% of SLE patients have a relative with lupus (Deapen, 1992). Clustering of SLE is fairly rare occurring only in 1/1000-2000 cases. Except in the rare cases of complement deficiency, the inheritance pattern of SLE does not follow simple Mendelian rules as we would expect for a single major gene effect, instead a polygenic model of susceptibility provides the best explanation for the familial clustering. Suggesting that genetic risk in most lupus patients arises from the combination of a number of relatively common variations in several different genes, each of these variations have a modest effect size, contribute to disease genesis. Despite this knowledge, however, it is a challenge to fully understand the genetic pathogenesis of the disease. This is essentially because SLE features a polygenic genetic model, which according to today's evidence may involve as many as 100 genes, and every gene only has a moderate effect size. Genetic studies can enhance our understanding of disease pathogenesis better. During the past few years, progress in biomedical science, bioinformatics, and experimental technology has given us new tools rapidly advanced our understanding of the genetic basis of systemic lupus erythematosus (SLE) and allowed a deeper investigation of SLE genetics and genomics. High throughput genotyping/sequencing platforms, high-throughput expression-level study technologies, etc., have brought forth many new insights. In particular, the genome-wide association study (GWAS) approach, with its ability to screen hundreds of thousands of SNPs across the genome without previous knowledge of candidate regions or genes, has not only supported some findings from previous candidate gene studies, but also discovered convincing evidence for novel genetic loci that may be implicated in SLE (Hardy, 2009; Hirschhorn, 2009). Although the number of genes involved in susceptibility to SLE is increasing in number with the advances in research and technology, however, the complete list of genes that fully account for disease susceptibility is not completed yet. Table1 represents the top SLE candidate genes categorized by chromosomal location.

Most of the genes proven to be associated with susceptibility to SLE are involved in three types of biological process: 1) immune complex processing, 2) toll-like receptor function and type I interferon production, and 3) immune signal transduction in lymphocytes. Several genes without an obvious immunologic function in SLE have been discovered from recent GWA studies such as: KIAA1542, PXK, XKR6, ATG5, etc. (Harley, 2008). These novel gene (loci) discoveries, which are assumed the most powerful and interesting results from GWA studies, can lead us to new pathways or mechanisms that we previously didn't know. The genetic heterogeneity between ethnic populations has been suggested to be important in SLE risk (Yang, 2009), showing the need for further GWAS in the various populations. Genetic loci for SLE in an ethnic group are not always replicated in the other ethnic groups, especially between Whites and Asians (Kim, 2009). However, some loci have been shown consistent associations across ethnicities such as; HLA-DRB1, FCGRs (FCGR2A and FCGR3A), STAT4, and IRF5, BLK, TNFAIP3, BANK1, and MECP2, providing common mechanisms in the development of SLE across ethnic groups. For example: In a large collection of different ethnic groups including European American, Korean, African American, and Hispanic American, relatively high-density genotyping across STAT1 and STAT4 genes has confirmed the association of multiple STAT4 SNPs and common risk haplotypes with SLE in multiple racial groups (Namjou, 2009).

The ethnical diversity in gene association with SLE can be explained due to various reasons: *First*, different genetic backgrounds in the various populations from different ancestries result in the different genetic risk factors for the same disease (Namjou, 2009; Kochi 2009; Tian , 2008). *Second*, SLE as most of the complex traits in human are developed by combined genetic factors and environmental factors for a long period of time. *Third*, the other explanation of inconsistency in genetic association among populations is that disease-associated SNP is unlikely to be the causal variant and rather is more likely to be in strong LD with the biologically relevant variant (Hardy, 2009; Graham, 2009). To date, since it is not feasible to test all variants of human genome even in a GWA study, the aforementioned reasons as reasonable explanation of non-reproducible genetic studies between populations.

1.3 SLE and Copy Number Variation (CNV) and Mendelian forms of SLE
1.3.1 Copy Number Variation (CNV)

CNV is exhibited in up to 12% of the human genome (Ku, 2010). Therefore, it is increasingly believed that large-scale deletion or duplication of DNA segments is a major source of human genetic variation (Ku, 2010). CNVs appear to play an important role in several common diseases (International Schizophrenia Consortium, 2008; Sebat, 2007). The relative contribution of CNVs, to the genetic component of SLE is unclear. Comprehensive studies of CNVs in SLE are expected in the coming years. Although evidences of the involvement of CNVs in SLE susceptibility are accumulating, for example; CNV was found in various genes involved in the pathology of SLE such as: the Fc receptor region (Fanciulli, 2007), Complement Factor 4 in the HLA class III region (Yang,2007), the histamine H4 receptor (HRH4) (Yu, 2010), however, a definitive role for the CNV has not been convincingly disentangled from nearby, linked risk variants (Fanciulli, 2007; Yang,2007).

1.3.2 Mendelian manner of SLE

A number of rare variants that cause SLE in a Mendelian manner have been identified throughout the years, including disruption of several complement pathway components (Harley, 1998). The Mendelian forms of SLE shed light onto pathways critical in pathogenesis, but account for only a small portion of the overall disease incidence (Harley, 1998).

2. Genes involved in the susceptibility to SLE

Herein we will describe the involvement of the key genes involved in the susceptibility to SLE. The genes will be introduced according to their location on the chromosomes.

2.1 Chromosome 1

There is considerable evidence supporting that multiple genes on this chromosome contribute to the development and expression of SLE (Tsao, 2000).

2.1.1 Fcγ receptors: FCGR2A, FCGR3A, FCGR2B and FCGR3B, (1q23-24)

The Fragment crystallizable receptors (FcRs) Fcγ receptor family (FCGRs: FCGR2A (CD32a); FCGR2B (CD32b); FCGR3A (CD16a) and FCGR3B (CD16b)) are a heterogeneous group of hematopoeitic cell surface glycoproteins that bind to the Fc region of immunoglobulins and facilitate the efficiency of antibody-antigen interactions with effector cells of the immune system. These receptors regulate a variety of cellular and humoral immune responses including phagocytosis, immune complex clearance, degranulation, antibody-dependent cellular cytotoxicity, transcriptional regulation of cytokine and chemokine expression, and B cell activation. The cellular distribution and Ig isotype (IgA, IgD, IgE, IgG and IgM) specificity influence the regulatory roles of Fc receptors. In broad terms, FcγRs can be classified into high or low affinity receptors based on their affinity for IgG or into activating (FcγRI, FcγRIIA/C, FcγRIII) or inhibitory (FcγRIIB) receptors based on their signaling activity and associated functions as they stimulate or inhibit immune functions such as phagocytosis, cytotoxicity, degranulation, antigen presentation and cytokine production via immune tyrosine activating or inhibitory motifs (ITAM or ITIM). In humans, three major classes of IgG-receptor have been described; FcγRI (CD64), FccRII (CD 32), and FcγRIII (CD16). These classes can be further sub-divided into discrete isoforms such as FcγRIIA, FcγRIIB, FcγRIIC, FcγRIIIA and FcγRIIIB that exhibit significant differences in their affinity for individual IgG sub-classes and tissue distribution. One of the difficulties of studying the Fcγ-receptor region on chromosome (1q23-24) is the high level of sequence similarity between each of the Fcγ-receptor genes suggests that the whole Fcγ-receptor gene cluster arose from the duplication of a single ancestral gene. Another complicating factor at this locus is the presence of copy number variation (CNV).

In human patients as well as in experimental animal models, FcγRs have been implicated in immune dysfunction and the development of autoimmunity. The best correlation between impaired FcγRs function and autoimmune pathogenesis is seen in systemic lupus. Various functional variants in FCγR2A, FCγR2B, and FCγR3A have been identified as risk factors for SLE (Nimmerjahn, 2008). These variants might lead to the defective clearance of immune complexes from the circulation therefore will contribute to the deposition in tissues such as the kidney and blood vessels (Lehrnbecher, 1999a; Tsokos, 2001).

FcγRIIA receptor contains ITAM on cell membranes of neutrophils, monocytes, macrophages, dendritic cells and platelets. It is the major receptor for the IgG2 subclass, which is a poor activator of classical complement pathway. It is the only FcR for clearing IgG2-bound immune complexes. The association of FCGR2A alleles with SLE has been studied intensively in several populations (Brown, 2007). Mutations in FCGRs have been shown to alter the function of monocytic cells and B-lymphocytes. For example; the nonsynonymous SNP which result in the substitution of Arginine at amino acid position 131 (R131) of FCGR2A (R131; rs1801274) to Histidine within the ligand binding domain of FcγRIIa diminishes binding to IgG2 results in impaired IgG2-mediated phagocytosis (Parren, 1992a,b; Warmerdam, 1991a,b; Clark, 1991; Salmon, 1996). FcγRIIA R131, might contribute to the risk of proliferative lupus nephritis by activating phagocytes, releasing proinflammatory cytokines and reduced clearance of immune complexes (ICs) (Bredius, 1993; Karassa, 2002). Karassa *et al.* conducted a meta-analysis regarding this polymorphism which included 17 studies, involving a total of 3114 SLE patients and 2580 non-SLE controls of European, African, and Asian descent, demonstrating that the R131 allele was associated with SLE (Karassa, 2002). In other studies conducted in Asians, it has been shown that the FCGRIIA-R131 allele was correlated with certain disease phenotypes. Kobayashi *et al.* studied Japanese SLE patients with or without periodontitis, and found that the R allele was significantly correlated (Kobayashi, 2007). Siriboonrit *et al.* also found in a Japanese cohort that the R allele was significantly increased in patients with lupus nephritis (Siriboonrit, 2003). In various ethnic groups (Europeans, African Americans and Koreans), R131 (rs1801274) showed inconsistent association with susceptibility to SLE, lupus nephritis, or both (Duits, 1995; Yap, 1999; Chen, 2004; Salmon, 1996; Song, 1998). Ethnic differences, disease heterogeneity, genotyping error due to extensive sequence homology among FCGR genes and random fluctuations in small samples might explain these inconsistent associations.

FcγR3IIIA receptor contains ITAM on cell surfaces of natural killer (NK) cells, monocytes, and macrophages. FcγR3A alleles with differential affinity for IgG1 and IgG3 have also been shown to be associated with SLE patients from ethnically diverse groups (Yap, 1999). The nonsynonymous SNP, where valine (V158) of FcγRIIIA changes to phenylalanine (F158) (rs396991) was shown to reduce the IgG1-, IgG3-, and IgG4-binding capacity of the receptor compared to V/V homozygotes. This polymorphism, normally termed FcγRIIIA-176 F/V or FcγRIIIA-158 F/V when excluding the leader sequence, was first reported to be of significant correlation with SLE in the Asian population (Japanese) by Kyogoku et al (Tsuchiya, 2005). Studies in human cohorts have shown that SLE is significantly associated with both alleles, R131 and F158, that encode lower affinity isoforms of FcγRIIA and FcγRIIIA respectively (Lehrnbecher, 1999b). F158 homozygotes bind IgG1- and IgG3-containing ICs less efficiently than V 158 homozygotes, and confers less efficient clearance of ICs than other alleles was associated with SLE susceptibility(Koene, 1998). However, the association between FcγR3A-V/F158 polymorphism and susceptibility to SLE and/or lupus nephritis has been variable in several studies (Tsao, 2004). A meta-analysis of more than 1,000 subjects in each of the three categories (SLE without or without renal involvement, and non-SLE controls) has concluded that the F158 allele confers a 1.2-fold risk for developing lupus nephritis in patients of European, African, and Asian descent but not for SLE susceptibility without renal involvement (Karassa, 2003).

The FcγRIIA-R131 and FcγRIIIA-F158 are often inherited together on the same chromosome as a single-risk haplotype for SLE (Magnusson, 2004). The presence of multiple risk alleles might interact to enhance the risk for SLE (Sullivan, 2003). The relative importance of FcγR2A-H/R131 and FcγR3A-V/F158 to disease progression might depend on the IgG subclass of pathogenic auto antibodies in an individual patient.

A novel polymorphism in FCGR3A, the rs403016 located in the Exon 3 which causes a non-synonymous substitution, the FCGR3A-72R/S, has been found to be associated with SLE in a Chinese SLE cohort, where the R allele contributes to disease susceptibility (Ye, 2006; Pan, 2008).

In a meta-analysis carried out by Lehrnbecher et. al., the development of SLE was significantly associated with the alleles encoding the low affinity isoforms of both FcγRIIA (FcγRIIA-R/R131) and FcγRIIIA (FcγRIIIA-F/F158) (Lehrnbecher, 1999b). More recently, a similar meta-analysis study carried out by Karassa and colleagues found that an FcγRIIA-R/H131 polymorphism represents a significant risk factor for the development of SLE but had no clear effect on susceptibility for lupus nephritis in a large patient cohort (Karassa, 2002).

Lower level evidence exists for a non-synonymous mutation in FcγRIIIA proposed to alter IgG binding affinity, a promoter SNP in FCGR2B that alters transcription factor binding and receptor expression and, in Asian populations, a non-synonymous SNP in exon 6 of FCGR2B suggested to influence B-cell activation (Brown, 2007).

FcγRIIB: FCGR2B receptor is expressed on B cells, dendritic cells, monocytes/macrophages, and mast cells. It contains an ITIM that regulates B-cell survival and proliferation by down-modulating B-cell receptor signaling, and by decreasing antibody-mediated phagocytosis in macrophages (Daeron, 1997).

A nonsynonymous SNP in the transmembrane domain of FcγRIIB (Ile187Thr) that alters the inhibitory function of FcγRIIB on B cells is associated with SLE in Asian populations,(Kyogoku, 2002; Siriboonrit, 2003; Chu, 2004) but not in other populations partly owing to their low allele frequencies (Li, 2003; Kyogoku, 2004; Magnusson, 2004). The FcγR2B encoded by the Thr187 allele results in impaired inhibition of B-cell activation and promotes autoimmunity (Floto, 2005). A functional promoter haplotype (-386G/-120T) of FcγRIIB that confers increased transcription of FcγRIIB has been associated with 1.6-fold risk for SLE in Caucasian Americans (Su, 2004). This haplotype is not in LD with FcγRIIA and FcγRIIIA polymorphisms and is likely to have an independent association with SLE (Kyogoku, 2002).

FcγRIIIB: FCGR3B is expressed solely on neutrophils. It lacks an ITAM domain, so the transmission of intracellular signals is likely to involve cooperation with other transmembrane proteins. Of particular interest are data suggesting that this is achieved through an interaction with complement receptor 3/integrin α_M (Krauss, 1994; Poo, 1995; Stockl, 1995). It is considered low affinity receptor for the Fc region of immunoglobulins gamma. It binds to complexed or aggregated IgG and also monomeric IgG. Contrary to FCγR3A, is not capable to mediate antibody-dependent cytotoxicity and phagocytosis. It may serve as a trap for immune complexes in the peripheral circulation which does not activate neutrophils.

Six SNPS exist in FCGR3B, underlying three different allotypic variants of FCGR3B (NA1, NA2 and SH). The association reported by Hatta *et a.l.*(Hatta, 1999) between the NA2 allotype and SLE in a Japanese population has not been replicated, suggesting that the association between SLE and this genomic region might be influenced by other genetic variations. Both duplication and deficiency of FCGR3B were reported in normal individuals (Clark, 1990; Koene, 1998). The inheritance pattern of FCGR3B in some families affected by SLE has suggested that the copy number variation might be the underlying condition.

The number of copies of FCGR3B in a cell can vary from none to four, with a gene-dose effect that reduced FcγRIIIB copy number being a risk factor for glomerulonephritis in SLE patients. In addition, FCGR3B copy number varies significantly with non-Mendelian inheritance, suggesting that the association of FCGR3B copy number with lupus nephritis is an independent risk factor (Aitman, 2006). Since human FCGR3B is expressed mainly in neutrophils, and it is postulated that SLE patients with low FCGR3B copy number have reduced neutrophil expression, which leads to reduced glomerular clearance of immune complexes, and brings forth susceptibility to SLE and other autoimmune disorders. This observation supports that copy number polymorphism at orthologous regions of diverse genomes is associated with immunologically related disease. It also suggests that genome plasticity, manifested by gene duplication/deletion and copy number polymorphism, is a common cause of genetically complex phenotypes. Fc receptor-like genes (FCRLs): FCLs clustered at 1q21–22 encode proteins that are structurally homologous classical FCGRs. To enhance our understanding of the functional roles of *Fcγ* receptors in SLE, an integrated approach to simultaneously assess CNVs, allotypic variants, SNPs and the functional diversity of these receptors in large-scale case–control studies including multiple ethnic populations is needed to dissect the relative contribution of various variants in this complex FCGR locus to SLE.

2.2 Protein tyrosine phosphatase non-receptor 22 (PTPN22) (1p13)

PTPN22 is a negative regulator for T-cell signal transduction in cellular immunity. It is considered to be the strongest common genetic risk factor for human autoimmunity besides the major histocompatibility complex (MHC) and as an important candidate gene in SLE. A number of candidate gene studies found (SNP rs2476601) R620W polymorphism in the proximal protein-rich SH3-binding domain (+1858T/C), to be associated with the increased risk of SLE (Orozco, 2005). This has been confirmed in a meta-analysis (Lea, 2011) and SLE GWA analysis. This polymorphism was found to be associated with several autoimmune diseases in Caucasians, including T1D, autoimmune thyroid disease, RA and SLE, but not with multiple sclerosis (MS). SNP rs2476601 is not polymorphic in Koreans and Japanese and almost absent in African populations (Gregersen, 2006) while it is more common in northern Europeans (8–15%) compared with southern Europeans (2–10%) (Gregersen, 2009). Suggesting the presence of genetic heterogeneity across various ethnicities.

The lymphoid tyrosine phosphatase protein (LYP), which is encoded by *PTPN22*, is known to regulate immunological synapse formation. LYP is involved in the down-regulation of T-cell activation through its interaction with a negative regulator of TCR signaling C-terminal Src tyrosine kinase (Csk); this interaction is prevented by the arginine to tryptophan amino acid substitution consequent upon the associated mutation rs2476601 R620W (C1858T) (Begovich, 2004; Bottini, 2004).

One would expect this R620W substitution to result in increased T-cell signaling and activation; however, experimental evidence suggests the opposite with TCR signaling actually reduced in cells carrying the tryptophan variant protein (Vang, 2005). A number of explanations have been proposed including an effect of the mutation on the tyrosine phosphatase activity of LYP, or an effect on the binding of other ligands or the conformation of LYP in response to these ligands (Vang, 2008). At a cellular level the mechanism by which reduced T-cell activation may actually increase the potential for autoimmunity remains a matter for speculation, although the suppression of regulatory T-cells is a possibility (Vang, 2008). A connection between PtPn22 and the type I IFN pathway has been suggested on the basis of elevated serum IFN-α activity and decreased tumor necrosis factor (TNF) levels in patients with SLE carrying the rs2476601 risk allele (Kariuki, 2008). By contrast, another *PTPN22* polymorphism, the loss-of-function mutation Arg263Gln in the catalytic domain (R263Q), leads to reduced phosphatase activity of PtPn22, and, therefore, increases the threshold for TCR signaling has been associated with protection against SLE in European-derived populations (Orru, 2009).

2.3 Interleukin 10 (IL 10) 1q32.1

IL-10 is an important immunoregulatory cytokine in man with both immunosuppressive and immunostimulatory properties (Mosmann, 1994). It is characterized with anti-inflammatory and stimulatory activities, and plays a critical role in the regulation of cellular and humoral immune responses. IL-10 is also involved in the pathology of human autoimmune disease (Llorente, 1994; Cash, 1995; Perez, 1995), particularly in the dysregulation of B-cell function in systemic lupus erythematosus leading to autoantibody production (Itoh, 1995; Llorente, 1995). In addition, its ability to induce T-cell anergy (Luscher, 1994) and inhibit major histocompatibility complex class-I expression (Matsuda, 1994) may be important in its apparent contribution to tumor-related immunosuppression (Kim, 1995; Suzuki, 1995; Fortis, 1996).

It has been known that IL10 production is under strong genetic influence (Westendorp, 1997). Two CA-repeat microsatellites, IL10R (-4 kb) (GeneBank accession number AF295024) and IL10G (-1.1 kb) (GeneBank accession number X78437), and single nucleotide polymorphisms (SNPs) were reported in IL10 promoter that has potential association with IL10 production. These SNPs are located at positions -A3575T, -A2849G, -A2763C, -A1082G, -C819T, and -A592C from the transcription start site. It has been known that -A1082G, -C819T, and -A592C combined to form three haplotypes; GCC, ACC, and ATA linked with different IL10 expression level (Crawley, 1999).

IL-10 has been associated in the pathogenesis of SLE; Increased *IL10* production by peripheral blood B cells and monocytes from patients with SLE is known to correlate with disease activity (Hagiwara, 1996), increased IL-10 productions promotes B-cell hyperactivity and autoantibody production (Llorente, 1995). The association between IL10 promoter haplotypes (defined by three SNPs in the *IL10* promoter region -627C→A, -854C→T and -1117G→A. These single base-pair substitutions produce three different haplotypes, GCC, ACC and ATA,) (Turner, 1997; Eskdale, 1997a) and SLE has been have been reported in European, Hispanic American and Asian populations (Eskdale, 1997b; Mehrian, 1998; Chong, 2004). A large-scale replication study in populations from the USA and Sweden has confirmed *IL10* as a SLE susceptibility locus (Gateva, 2009). However, they were found to have significant association with lupus nephritis.

Levels of IL-10 secretion have been correlated to specific IL10 promoter polymorphisms; a study has shown that the SNP haplotypes in the distal promoter of IL-10 correlate with different IL-10 production phenotype in normal individuals, and high IL-10 haplotype is associated with SLE in African-Americans, which may be a part of their genetic susceptibility to SLE. A meta-analysis of 15 IL-10 studies has shown that the G11 allele is associated with SLE in whole studied populations, and among the promoter SNPs, −A1082G polymorphism, which is found in Asian population only, was also associated with SLE (Nath, 2005). Based on these analyses, IL-10 polymorphisms confer SLE risk in an ethnicity-specific manner (Gateva, 2009; Eskdale, 1997; Mehrian, 1998; Chong, 2004).

2.4 Complement receptor 1 (CR1, CD35), (1q32)

Genome scans have shown linkage (lod score >1.0) at chromosome 1q32, which contains complement components, like complement receptor 1 (**CR1**), complement receptor 2 (CR2), and C4b-binding protein (C4BP) genes and IL10 family members; IL10, IL19, IL20, and IL24, which play a significant role in the pathogenesis of SLE (Johanneson, 2002; Tsao, 1999). The C3b/C4b complement receptor (Gene ID: 1378) (CR1, CD35) is a polymorphic transmembrane single chain glycoprotein expressed on red cell surface binds to C3b and C4b and clears circulating C3- and C4-bearing immune complexes containing (Dykman, 1984).

Functional and structural polymorphisms of CR1 have been reported. The functional polymorphism determines the quantitative expression of CR1 on erythrocytes, i.e. HH, HL, and LL (H = allele correlated with high expression, L = low) (Wilson, 1986). The structural polymorphism exists in its molecular size (Dykman, 1983). The extracellular portion of the CR1 molecule consists of three to five groups of seven short consensus repeats termed long homologous repeats (LHR). The most frequent type of CR1 (F or A) is comprised of four extracellular LHRs and expresses one binding site for C4b and two binding sites for C3b (Wong, 1983). The S (or B) variant of CR1 is characterized by additional C3b binding site on a fifth LHR (Wong, 1989). A meta-analysis for the CR1 functional polymorphisms in SLE shows no significant association of CR1 L allele, L/L genotype, and L/L+L/H genotypes with SLE. However, the same meta-analysis of CR1 structural polymorphisms suggested an association of CR1 S (structural variant of CR1) to be associated with SLE in Caucasians (Nath, 2005).

2.5 Tumor necrosis factor (ligand) SuperFamily, member 4(TNFSF4), 1q25

TNFSF4 (also known as OX40L; 1q25) encodes a cytokine that is expressed on CD40-stimulated B cells, activated antigen-presenting cells (APCs) and vascular endothelial cells. Also its unique receptor, TNFRSF4 (also known as OX40; 1p36), is primarily expressed on activated CD4+ T cells. Their interaction induces the production of CD28-independent co-stimulatory signals to activate CD4+ T cells (Baum, 1994). OX40L-mediated signaling inhibits the generation and function of IL-10-producing CD4+ type 1 regulatory T cells, but induces B-cell activation and differentiation, as well as IL-17 production in vitro (Ito, 2006a; Li, 2008).

These two tumor necrosis factor (TNF) superfamily members (OX40L and OX40) located within proximal intervals showing genetic linkage with SLE (Cunninghame, 2008; Chang, 2009; delGado-Vega, 2009).TNFSF4 has been identified as a susceptibility gene for SLE in multiple studies. Protective and risk haplotypes at TNFSF4 were identified in a study of two cohorts from Minnesota and UK, a haplotype in the upstream region of TNFSF4, marked by SNPs rs844644 and rs2205960, has been shown to correlate with increased cell surface TNFSF4 expression and TNFSF4 transcript and to be associated with SLE (Graham, 2008).

Associations between some *TNFSF4*-tagging SNPs and an increased risk for SLE have been confirmed in GWAS in Chinese populations and in a European replication study; these results were also replicated in four independent SLE datasets from Germany, Italy, Spain and argentine. It has not been fully established how TNFRSF4/ TNFSF4 interactions influence T-cell subset profiles. Most evidence suggests a bias towards a Th2 pattern of cytokine release, although there is also evidence for a down-regulation of regulatory T-cell subsets (Ito, 2006b; Lane, 2000). There is also good evidence that signaling through TNFSF4 can induce B-cell activation and differentiation (Stuber, 1995&1996). TNFRSF4/ TNFSF4 signaling is therefore bi-directional, and the precise immunological consequences of this complex pathway are yet to be clarified. Further studies are needed to localize causal variants and to understand how these polymorphisms affect the pathogenesis of SLE.

2.6 C-reactive protein (CRP), 1q23.2
CRP is a sensitive marker of inflammation. The genes for CRP (CRP) map to 1q23.2 within an interval linked with SLE in multiple populations. It is hypothesized that polymorphism of CRP gene contributes to susceptibility to systemic lupus erythematosus (SLE).
Basal levels of CRP were influenced independently by two polymorphisms at the CRP locus, CRP 2 and CRP 4. Furthermore, the latter polymorphism was linked/associated with SLE and antinuclear autoantibody production. Thus, the polymorphism associated with reduced basal CRP was also associated with the development of SLE.
CRP is normally involved in phagocytosis of apoptotic debris and immune complexes in innate immune response. Defective clearance of products of apoptosis may be the source of autoantigens in SLE, and such phenomenon may also be enhanced by FcγR2A polymorphisms, with FcγR2 receptor being the main receptor for CRP (Bharadwaj, 1999).
During the active phase of SLE, despite the presence of marked tissue inflammation, CRP levels are abnormally low due to reduced synthesis (Russell, 2004). Family-based studies of association and linkage have identified the minor allele of rs1205 in the 3'UTR SNP of CRP to be associated with SLE and antinuclear antibody production (Russell, 2004), and the number of CA repeats correlated with disease risk in a Spanish cohort (Russell, 2004). Also, a single dose of CRP has recently shown to reverse lupus nephritis and nephrotoxic nephritis in mice, suggesting the acute-phase response of CRP may hinder tissue inflammation and damage (Rodriguez, 2005). These results are promising, and future investigation of this gene will not only allow better understanding of the genetic influence of CRP but also its pathophysiology and possible therapeutic options.
Two of several polymorphisms in the CRP gene, designated CRP2 (G/C) and CRP4 (G/A) have been demonstrated to have an impact on baseline serum concentration of CRP, with the C- and A-alleles being associated with lower concentrations (Russell, 2004). Furthermore, the CRP4 A-allele was shown to confer increased susceptibility to SLE in 586 families (P=0.006) (Russell, 2004). The A allele at *CRP* 4 had a relatively high frequency in European and Asian-Indian populations (~0.3) and was present in Afro-Caribbean families too, but at a lower frequency (0.14).

2.7 Poly(ADP-ribose) polymerase (PARP), (1q41–42)
PARP is an enzyme (PARP-1 EC 2.4.2.30) is induced by DNA strand breaks caused by several agents and utilizes NAD to form polyADPR, bound to acceptor proteins. It is responsible for DNA repair, proliferation, stress response, apoptosis, and genomic stability (Oliver, 1999). The involvement of PARP-1 in autoimmune diseases has been suggested

especially in systemic lupus erythematosus (SLE) due to the decreased levels of activity and mRNA in SLE patients (Haug 1994). Autoantibodies to PARP are frequently found in patients affected with autoimmune diseases, some of which may prevent caspase-3-mediated PARP cleavage during apoptosis, resulting in the accumulation of autoimmune cells (Decker, 2000). On chromosome 1q41–q42 a 15-cM region has been linked with susceptibility to SLE (Tsao, 1997), this linkage has been confirmed in several independent studies. In a family-based TDT analysis, PARP alleles had skewed transmission to affected offspring, but this finding is not consistent in other multi-ethnic studies (Tsao, 1999). A polymorphic CA tandem repeat within the PARP promoter region suggested to affect transcription activity has been associated with SLE in some but not other similar studies (Oei, 2001). A study investigated the association of PARP promoter CA tandem repeats polymorphisms with SLE susceptibility in Taiwan. Nine alleles ranging from 12 to 20 repeats were disclosed. No statistically significant association with SLE susceptibility was found in this population however; PARP microsatellite polymorphisms demonstrate associations with clinical subphenotypes such as discoid rash and arthritis, anti-cardiolipin IgG and anti-ds-DNA antibody production. These indicate that PARP CA repeats may play a key role in lupus pathogenesis involving DNA repair of cell damage and consequent autoantibody production. Tsao *et al* demonstrated a skewed transmission of PARP alleles in a family study with the PARP CA8 allele as susceptible and the PARP CA14 allele as a protector of lupus transmission (Tsao, 1999).

In a Korean study, PARP polymorphisms could not prove any statistically significant association with the risk of SLE was observed, however, they found that two single-nucleotide polymorphisms (SNPs -1963A/G and +28077G/A) were significantly associated with an increased risk of nephritis, and one non-synonymous variant [+40329T/C (V762A)] was also significantly associated with an increased risk of arthritis, while the -1963A/G polymorphism showed a protective effect on arthritis in Korean SLE patients (Hur, 2006).

2.8 Toll-like receptor 5 (TLR5), 1q41–q42

At least 10 different *TLR* have been cloned from the human genome to date. Toll-like receptors (TLR) are type I transmembrane proteins contain an extracellular leucine-rich region involved in pathogen recognition and a conserved intracellular Toll/IL-1 receptor domain that activates a signaling pathway. Stimulation of the TLR pathway ends in NF-κB activation and transcription of immune response genes, such as cytokines and chemokines. TLRs play an important role in the activation and regulation of both adaptive and innate immunity. They are considered as excellent candidate genes for genetic susceptibility studies for autoimmune diseases. TLR5 is a critical regulator of inflammatory pathways and maps to chromosome 1q41. Activation of TLR5 triggers production of proinflammatory cytokines, such as IL-6, which, in turn, can stimulate B cells to proliferate, differentiate, and secrete antibodies. Dysregulation of this process may lead to excessive production of cytokines as well as autoantibodies (Dean, 2000).

It was hypothesized that the stop codon variant C1174T (rs5744168) (Arginine to a stop codon at position 392 (R392X) in TLR5, is associated with susceptibility to SLE. This hypothesis was tested by using a TDT in a Caucasian SLE cohort and found that the TLR5 stop codon polymorphism, but not other TLR5 alleles, is associated with protection from developing SLE as subjects with 1174T produced less proinflammatory cytokines (IL-6, TNF-α, and IL-1β) (Hawn, 2003; Hawn, 2005). In addition the same group found that this association was most pronounced in individuals who are seronegative for anti-dsDNA autoantibodies (Tsao, 1999; Hawn, 2005). TLR5^{R392X} may provide protection from SLE by decreasing production of proinflammatory cytokines during infection with flagellated bacteria, which may influence formation of the adaptive immune response. These results suggest a role for the innate immune response in the development of SLE that involves flagellated bacterial infections.

3. Chromosome 2

Locus 2q32- q37 encodes the Programmed cell death 1 gene (PDCD1), Cytotoxic T-lymphocyte associated protein 4 (CTLA4) and STAT4 transcription factor. All were proven to be associated to susceptibility to SLE.

3.1 Programmed cell death 1 gene (PDCD1/ CD279) (2q37)

PDCD1 codes for an immunoreceptor, PD-1, member of the CD28/CTLA4/ICOS co-stimulatory receptor family that bears an inhibitory immunoreceptor tyrosine-based motif (ITIM). It is expressed on activated T- and B-cell surfaces to regulate their peripheral tolerance (Agata 1996; Finger, 1997). PDCD1 is upregulated in T cells following activation, and inhibits TCR signaling and T/B cell survival. It is considered a strong candidate for SLE association.

The human *PDCD1* has an intron enhancer which contains binding sites for other transcription factors that are involved in lymphocyte development and T cell differentiation. PDCD single nucleotide polymorphism (SNP) (PD1.3A, the minor A allele of 7146 G/A) in this intron enhancer alters a binding site for the runt-related transcription factor (RUNX1). The PDCD1 enhancer has a very high GC content (from 50 to 75%). The A allele of the PDCD1 enhancer SNP changes a potential methylation site from CpG to CpA that is surrounded by many other potential methylation sites. Methylation is a known mechanism of regulation of gene activity (Avni, 2000). Whether methylation is involved in the regulation of PDCD1 is under investigation. Changes in methylation can condition the developmental stage of PDCD1 expression.

SNP 7146 G/A was shown to be association with SLE susceptibility and its contribution to SLE development was confirmed in Europeans and Mexicans by inducing lymphocytic hyperactivity in these patients (Prokunina, 2002). PDCD-1 polymorphisms may be a shared genetic factor for multiple autoimmune diseases in humans, and the cellular function leading to disease onset awaits further investigation. PDCD1 7209 CT or 7209 TT genotype exhibited 3.28-fold increased risk of SLE in the Polish and Taiwanese populations (Mostowska, 2008).

The most logical explanation of the mechanism of disease susceptibility for PDCD1 was suggested by Alarcón-Riquelme M *et al* (Alarcón-Riquelme, 2003); The stated: "So what effects could the aberrant function or expression of PDCD1 have in early lymphocyte differentiation that may lead to autoimmune disease, in particular SLE? It mainly depends on at what stage of differentiation does the RUNX1–PDCD1 interaction take place whether it occurs before clonal receptor rearrangements or after. As PDCD1 seems to act during positive selection in the thymus, at least in the mouse, this leads us to suggest that the human mutation may be promoting positive selection of early autoreactive progenitors, leading to an increased "susceptibility" to expand autoreactive T or B cells after antigenic stimuli, however the amount of information to date on PDCD1 in lymphocyte development and its regulation is still an open question".

3.2 Cytotoxic T-lymphocyteassociated protein 4 (CTLA4), (2q33)

CTLA4 is a structural homologue of CD28. It is a negative costimulatory molecule that inhibits T cell activation, and may help to limit T cell responses under conditions of inflammation and prevents autoimmune diseases by promoting anergy. It competes with the binding of CD28 on antigen presenting cells (APCs), and transduces inhibitory signals by activation of serine/threonine phosphatases. Genetic variability in CTLA4 has been implicated in the development of several autoimmune diseases including SLE (Matsushita, 1999). SLE patients have increased levels of soluble CTLA-4. A single nuclear polymorphism (SNP) CT60A/G within the 3'UTR of CTLA4 decreased the production of a spliced variant with inhibitory activity, which indicates the importance of CTLA-4 in providing protection against autoimmunity (Ueda, 2003).

SLE in Caucasians, CTLA-4 polymorphisms of its promoter and exon-1 regions was found to be associated to SLE. Later, in a Chinese cohort, the CTLA-4 promoter (-1722 T/C) polymorphism showed positive evidence (Liu, 2001 & Xu, 2004). However, several genetic studies investigating CTLA-4 polymorphisms and SLE have been negative. Among the positive studies, different mutations were identified within the CTLA4 promoter (−1722T/C, −1661A/G, −319C/T) and exon 1 (+49G/A) in various ethnic groups (Lee, 2005). More work is needed to delineate the genetic relationship between CTLA-4 and SLE.

3.3 Signal transducer and activator of transcription 4 protein (STAT4), (2q32)

STAT4 play key roles in the interferon and Th1 signaling pathway through mediating responses to IL-12 in lymphocytes, and regulates T helper cell differentiation. STAT4 also is known to mediate signals induced by immunologically relevant cytokines including, like IRF5, the Type 1 IFNs (Darnell, 1994 & Watford, 2004). In response to these cytokines, STAT4 activation plays an important role in directing a Th1 T-cell response, and mediates the production of Th1-type cytokines such as IFN-α (Morinobu, 2002; Nguyen, 2002; Nishikomori, 2002). In addition, STAT4 signaling also mediates type 1 IFN signaling in antigen-presenting cells, and may be necessary for the production of IFN-α by these cells (Frucht, 2003 & Fukao, 2001).

STAT4 variation and SLE risk was initially reported in 2007 from a case–control association study (Remmers, 2007). This was subsequently confirmed in both GWA studies. Three SNPs in STAT4, rs7574865, rs11889341, and rs10168266, were then shown to be in significant association with SLE in a Japanese population, with the rs7574865 T allele, in the third intron of STAT4, showing the strongest significance. Interestingly, this rs7574865 risk variant is associated with a more severe SLE phenotype that is characterized by disease onset at a young age (<30 years), a high frequency of nephritis, the presence of antibodies towards double stranded DNA, (Taylor, 2008; Kawasaki, 2008; Sigurdsson, 2008) and an increased sensitivity to IFN-α signaling in peripheral blood mononuclear cells (Kariuki, 2009). In a meta-analysis including Europeans and Asian patients of SLE and RA, the rs7574865 T allele was found to be consistently associated with both diseases (Ji, 2010). Possible functional relevance of risk STAT4 variant has recently strongly suggested by in vivo experiment in SLE patients, in which risk variant of STAT4 (T allele; rs7574865) was simultaneously associated with both lower serum IFN-a activity and greater IFN-α induced gene expression in PBMC in SLE patients.

A risk haplotype (spanning 73 kb from the third intron to the seventeenth exon of STAT4) common to European, Americans, Koreans and Hispanic Americans was also identified

(Namjou, 2009). Functionally, either type I IFN or interleukin (IL)-12 induces phosphorylation of STAT4, which has a signal transduction role in these pathways. Individuals carrying one or more risk alleles of both IRF5 and STAT4 have an increased risk for SLE, suggesting a genetic interaction between these two genes (Sigurdsson, 2008).

The important roles of STAT4 in both innate immunity and Th1 immune response, recent enormous body of evidence of consistent association of STAT4 with SLE in multiple racial groups indicates that a risk variant or a certain risk haplotype of STAT4 has a crucial role in SLE pathogenesis that has yet to be completely determined and could provide new therapeutic targets for SLE and the other autoimmune diseases in future.

4. Chromosome 3

4.1 Phox homology (PX) domain Kinase (PXK), (3p14.3)

PXK is of unknown function. PXK domain containing serine/threonine kinase and act as modulator of Na, K-ATPase enzymatic and ion pump activities (Mao, 2005). It was identified as a novel candidate gene for systemic lupus erythematosus (SLE) from genome-wide association studies (GWAS) in Caucasians (Suarez-Gestal, 2009). The association of PXK rs6445975 with SLE observed in Caucasians was not replication study in Hong Kong Chinese and Koreans (Kim, 2011; Yu, 2011; Yang, 2009). It is possible that PXK has different genetic contribution on SLE between Caucasians and Asians and that the gene is associated with disease subphenotypes rather than with overall susceptibility.

5. Chromosome 4

5.1 BANK, BLK and LYN

All three of these genes play a critical role in controlling the activation of B cells following signaling through the B-Cell Receptor (BCR). Following ligand binding and BCR aggregation, an early intracellular event is the recruitment and activation of Src-family protein tyrosine kinases, including BLK and LYN, which mediate further intracellular signaling. The exact role of these kinases in determining cellular events has yet to be determined with certainty.

5.2 B-cell scaffold protein with ankyrin repeats (BANK1), (4q24)

BANK1 is a B-cell scaffold protein that is tyrosine phosphorylated through the B-cell receptor (BCR) upon B-cell activation, which in turn associates with the tyrosine kinase *Lyn* (Src family of tyrosine kinase) and the calcium channel *IP3R* which results in calcium ion release from the stores of the endoplasmic reticulum (Yokoyama, 2002 & Kozyrev, 2008). *BANK1* is thought to alter B cell activation to increase SLE risk. Polymorphisms in *BANK1* may cause B-cell hyper-responsiveness.

GWAS in European-derived populations have identified associations of *BANK1* and *LYN* with susceptibility to SLE (Kozyrev, 2008 & Guo, 2009). For BANK1 three functional variants with either a non-synonymous SNP (rs10516487; Arg61His), a branch point-site SNP (rs17266594; located in an intron) or a SNP in the ankyrin domain (rs3733197; Ala383Thr) might contribute to the sustained activation of B-cell receptors and the subsequent B-cell hyperactivity that is commonly observed in SLE (Kozyrev, 2008). However, the best functional evidence was found for rs17266594, which altered a branch point upstream of exon 2, resulting in the generation of a novel short isoform, but little quantitative difference in *BANK1* expression overall. With the exception of the rs10516487 SNP of *BANK1*, which showed a weak association with SLE in an Asian GWAS, the remaining SNPS of *BANK1* have not been confirmed in either Chinese or Asian GWAS, partly owing to the low frequencies of the SNPS in these populations (Chang, 2009).

6. Chromosome 5

6.1 TNIP1 (Tumor necrosis factor α-induced protein 3 (TNFAIP3) interacting protein 1), also known as ABIN (A20-binding inhibitor of NF-κB)-1, (5q32-q33.1)

TNIP1 expression is induced by NF-κB, and in turn, overexpression of TNIP1 inhibits NF-κB activation by TNF (Verstrepen, 2009). TNIP1 was shown to inhibit TNF-induced apoptosis independently of A20 (Oshima, 2009). Two recent GWAS revealed association of TNIP1 intronic SNPs rs7708392 and rs10036748, which are in strong linkage disequilibrium (LD) with SLE in the Caucasian (European-American and Swedish) and Chinese Han populations, respectively (Han, 2009 & Gateva, 2009). Association of TNIP1 with SLE was also confirmed in a Japanese population.

To date, at least 11 splice variants of *TNIP1*have been identified (Verstrepen, 2009). Presence of alternative exon 1A and 1B, as well as splice variants lacking exon 2, has been described. Because rs7708392 is located between exon 1B and exon 2, it is possible that this SNP may influence the usage of the splicing isoform. It is also possible that other causative SNPs in tight LD with rs7708392 may exist. Such a possibility would be addressed by resequencing the entire *TNIP1* gene. *TNIP1* is a shared SLE susceptibility gene in the Caucasian and Asian populations, but the genetic contribution appeared to be greater in the Asians because of the higher risk allele frequency in the population.

7. Chromosome 6

7.1 Major Histocompatibility Complex (MHC), (6p21.31)

A body of evidence has been collected to establish the pivotal role of major histocompatibility complex (MHC) in immune tolerance. The classical MHC locus (6p21.3) 3.6Mb contains at least 250 expressed genes. This locus is divided into the Class I and II regions that encode the antigen-presenting HLA proteins and Class III MHC that contains 58 genes, located between Class I and II regions, only some its genes are of potential immunological interest (e.g. TNF-α and TNF-β, C4A, C4B and C2) and others which have poorly defined function. There is particularly strong linkage disequilibrium between genetic markers in this region which is strongly association with SLE in all GWA studies. It is therefore difficult to establish whether any associated variant is functional or simply observed due to linkage disequilibrium with functional polymorphisms elsewhere. It was as early as 1971 that Grumet *et al.* reported possible relationship between the HLA genes and SLE (Grumet, 1971). MHC alleles on 6p11–21 have shown the most significant association. Although the genetic structure of the MHC makes it a particularly challenging region to study, significant progress has been made over the last year.

The Class II HLA genes are of particular importance, which encode antigen-presenting molecules that play a pivotal role in T-cell immunity. Most evidence has highlighted the DR loci, which are one of the Class II HLA gene complexes. The HLA-DRB1 gene is of particular importance in SLE. For the HLA-DRB1 gene, the serotype of DR2 holds the strongest evidence of disease association. Three class-II-containing-SLE-risk haplotypes (DRB1*1501

(DR2)/DQB1*0602, DRB1*0301) (DR3)/DQB1*0201, and DRB1*0801 (DR8)/DQB1*0402) are consistently associated with SLE in Caucasian populations by family-based TDT (van der Linden, 2001).

Within the MHC class III region, there are genes that encode TNF-α and -β, lymphotoxin-β, complement components C2 and C4, and heat shock protein 70 (Hsp70). In particular, TNFs, C2, and C4 have been implicated in SLE susceptibility. TNF-α is a multifunctional proinflammatory cytokine involved in regulating a wide spectrum of biological processes including cell proliferation, differentiation, and apoptosis, while TNF-β mediates a variety of inflammatory, immunostimulatory, and antiviral responses. Polymorphisms in these genes have been implicated in SLE susceptibility (Pan 2011 & Bettinotti, 1993).

Complement component genes within the MHC class III region include C2, C4A, C4B, and factor B. These genes are closely linked and are usually inherited as a group known as complotype. Deficiencies in complement pathway genes C2, C4, C1q and C3 appear to cause SLE in some people (Kallel-Sellami, 2008). Polymorphisms in C2, C4A and C4B are in linkage disequilibrium with HLA-B and HLA-DR alleles (Alper, 2007) and may predispose to SLE. Also the complete deficiencies of the early components are highly associated with human SLE (Yu, 2007). A homozygous deficiency in one of the early complement components, including C1q, C1r, C1s and C4 in the classical activation pathway, alone can be strong enough to cause the disease, a situation similar to a single gene defect in an autosomal recessive disease. Respectively, 93% and 78% of patients with complete C1q and C4 deficiencies eventually develop SLE or a lupus-like disease (Yu, 2007 & Botto, 2002). In addition, the concordance rates for siblings with homozygous deficiency of C1q or C4 to develop SLE are 90% and 80%, respectively, which are even higher than the rate in monozygotic twins (26–60%) with other genetic defects (Tsao, 2008). Complete deficiency of complement C4 is among the strongest genetic risk factors for human systemic lupus erythematosus (SLE). Further work will be required to determine the effect arising from C4A. C4 is the most polymorphic protein of the complement system. It is encoded by two genes, C4A and C4B, which have minor sequence differences. The resulting proteins have different functional characteristics, with C4A better able to bind immune complexes (Schifferli, 1986). The C4 genes are inherited in a discrete 'RCCX module', which contains one C4 gene (either C4A or C4B) along with three neighboring genes (RP, CYP21 and TNX) (Yang, 1999). The Class III MHC carries between one and four copies of this module; hence each diploid genome has between two and eight C4 genes, which may be either C4A or C4B (Yang, 2007). Carrying less than two copies of C4A has been identified as a risk factor for SLE (Yang, 2007).

The common European haplotype AH8.1 carries multiple variants that have been associated with SLE including DRB1*0301 (DR3), the TNF -308A allele and the C4A complement null allele. Many studies were unable to break down this haplotype below a 1Mb interval covering most of the Class II and II regions (Alper, 2007).

7.2 PR domain containing 1, with ZNF domain - APG5 autophagy 5-like (PRDM1-ATG5 region), (6q21)

PRDM1 acts as a repressor of beta-interferon gene expression. The protein binds specifically to the PRDI (positive regulatory domain I element) of the beta-IFN gene promoter. While, the ATG5 candidate gene function is still obscure and needed to be determined however, both known to play important roles in immunity. Genome-wide association studies suggested the PRDM1-ATG5 gene region as a systemic lupus erythematosus (SLE)-

associated locus both in Caucasian and Asian populations, presumably through upregulating gene expression (Zhou, 2011; Harley, 2008; Gateva, 2009; Han, 2009).

Significant positive correlations with ATG5 expression were identified, suggesting ATG5 as a candidate gene in the region (Harley, 2008). Later GWAS from a Chinese population denied the association between polymorphisms in *ATG5* and SLE, but replicated the association between the intergenic region of *PRDM1-ATG5* (rs548234 and rs6568431) and SLE ((Han, 2009). At the same time, from Caucasian replication data, both *PRDM1* (rs6568431) and *ATG5* (rs2245214) were suggested as candidate genes, because rs6568431 was more close to *PRDM1* and rs6568431 has an r^2 of less than 0.1 with rs2245214. Meta-analysis consolidated the association between rs548234 and SLE (p=1.28×10^{-16}).

7.3 Tumor necrotic factor α-induced protein 3 (TNFAIP3), 6q23

The gene product of *TNFAIP3* is a zinc-finger A20 protein, a ubiquitin-modifying enzyme, which is essential for proteasome degradation and termination of proinflammatory responses mediated by nuclear factor kappa B, thereby preventing inflammation. In humans, genetic surveys have suggested a role for *TNFAIP3* in susceptibility to complex genetic autoimmune disorders, including systemic lupus erythematosus (SLE) (Graham, 2008; Musone, 2008; Bates, 2005; Han, 2009).

Genetic association between variants in *TNFAIP3* and SLE suggest that alterations in activity and/or expression of *TNFAIP3* influence SLE pathophysiology (Graham, 2008; Musone, 2008; Bates, 2005; Han, 2009). Independent genetic associations of SLE and *TNFAIP3* in European-ancestry (EA) subjects have been localized to a region 185 kb upstream of *TNFAIP3* that was first identified with rheumatoid arthritis (Plenge, 2007; Thomson, 2007; Plenge, 2007), a region 249 kb downstream of *TNFAIP3* and a 109 kb haplotype spans the *TNFAIP3* coding region (Musone, 2008; Bates, 2005; Han, 2009) that includes a suggested causal coding variant in exon 3 (rs2230926 T>G; F127C) that reduces the ability of A20 to attenuate NF-κB signaling (Musone, 2008).

Evidence for association with SLE was observed also for a variant within *TNFAIP3* (rs5029939, GWAS *P* value = 2.55×10^{-8}) and two flanking SNPs (rs10499197, GWAS *P* value = 2.11×10^{-6}; rs7749323, GWAS *P* value = 9.63×10^{-7}) in strong LD with rs5029939 (r2>0.95). A SNP located ~185 kb upstream of *TNFAIP3* reported to be associated with risk for RA (204,206) (rs6920220) demonstrated modest association in the SLE GWAS dataset (GWAS P value = 0.01)

By fine mapping and genomic resequencing in ethnically diverse populations Adrianto I *et al*, fully characterized the *TNFAIP3* risk haplotype and isolated a novel TT>A polymorphic dinucleotide (deletion T followed by a T to A transversion) associated with SLE in subjects of European (*P* = 1.58 × 10^{-8}) and Korean (*P* = 8.33 ×10$-$10) ancestry (Adrianto, 2011). This variant, located in a region of high conservation and regulatory potential, bound a nuclear protein complex comprised of NF-κB subunits with reduced avidity. Furthermore, compared with the non-risk haplotype, the haplotype carrying this variant resulted in reduced *TNFAIP3* mRNA and A20 protein expression. These results establish this TT>A variant as the most likely functional polymorphism responsible for the association between *TNFAIP3* and SLE (Adrianto, 2011).

One hundred and twenty seven (127) SNPs in the region of *TNFAIP3* on 6q23 and 347 ancestry informative markers (AIMs) in five diverse ethnic populations were analyzed by Adrianto I *et al*, They discovered a peak associations in European and Asian populations were seen at markers rs6932056 and rs4896303 in 38 kb and 30 kb downstream of *TNFAIP3*, respectively (Adrianto, 2011).

8. Chromosome 7

8.1 Interferon regulatory factor 5 gene (IRF5), 7q32

IRF5 is one of the key genes of the interferon (IFN)-α pathway. IRF5 is a transcription factor that is responsible for the innate immune response during viral infection. IRF5 is important for trans-activation of type 1 IFN and IFN-responsive genes and for the production of pro-inflammatory cytokines interleukins such as; IL-6, IL-12, and tumor necrosis factor-α (TNF)] after toll like receptor (TLR) signaling induced by immune complexes containing self-antigens and nucleic acids (Takaoka, 2005). *IRF5* is one of the most strongly and consistently SLE-associated loci outside the MHC region in various ethnic groups and was detected using both candidate gene and GWAS approaches (Lee, 2009). Interest in type 1 (IFN-α and -β) IFN pathways was stimulated by the discovery that there is a general up-regulation IFN-inducible genes in SLE (Baechler, 2003 & Bennett, 2003). The best current genetic model proposes an SLE risk haplotype carrying multiple functional SNPs. Several SNPs in IRF5 (rs2004640, rs752637, rs729302, rs10954213etc.) were first found to be associated with SLE in Caucasians (Niewold, 2008; Kim, 2009).

In vitro functional evidence exists for at least two of these polymorphisms at SNP (rs2004640) creates a novel splice site in exon1B allowing the expression of a novel IRF5 isoform (Graham, 2006 & Sigurdsson, 2005) while the second polymorphism (rs10954213) located in the 3′ UTR creates a functional polyadenylation site and hence a shorter and more stable gene transcript (Cunninghame, 2007). To our knowledge, the most consistent evidence of association for this gene with SLE, across different populations including, was observed in the rs2004640 T allele. A meta-analysis has been conducted to study the association of the rs2004640 T allele with SLE; it included 12 studies in Europeans and Asians, it has been concluded that this polymorphism is associated with SLE susceptibility across different ethnic groups (Lee, 2009). In addition, the gene has a polymorphic 30 bp indel (insertion/deletion) in exon 6, which contributes to the diversity in the isoform pattern of IRF5, and a 5 bp indel near the 5′UTR upstream of exon 1A (Sigurdsson, 2008 & Dideberg, 2007).

To understand how IRF5 variants may predispose to SLE we need to understand the physiological role of the Type 1 IFN pathways. The majority of cells produce Type 1 IFNs as part of their early response to viral infection. Particularly large amounts are produced by plasmacytoid dendritic cells, perhaps stimulated by the recognition of viral RNA and DNA through TLR7 and TLR9. In SLE, it is possible that this is also triggered in response to inadequately cleared nucleic acid antigens released from apoptotic cells (Ronnblom, 2002). Type 1 IFNs exert a multitude of downstream effects on the immune system. Perhaps critically, they stimulate Th1 pathways and sustain activated T cells, while also lowering the threshold for B-cell activation through the B-cell receptor (BCR) and promoting B-cell survival and differentiation (Ronnblom, 2002; Braun, 2002; Le Bon, 2001; Marrack, 1999). It can therefore be seen that genetic variants that prolong or alter the actions of IRF5 could result in a prolonged proinflammatory response, and potentially break immunological tolerance. Interestingly, IRF5 signaling has also been shown to play a role in the regulation of cell cycle and apoptosis raising the possibility that susceptibility variants of IRF5 exert their effects at multiple levels (Barnes, 2003).

8.2 Ikaros zinc finger 1(IKZF), 7p12.2

IKZF1 encodes a lymphoid restricted zinc finger transcription factor named Ikaros, which is critically important for the normal development of all lymphoid cells. It regulates lymphocyte differentiation and proliferation (Georgopoulos, 1994), as well as self-tolerance through regulation of B-cell receptor signaling (Wojcik, 2007). Data derived from both GWAS and large replication studies identified *IKZF1* as a novel SLE susceptibility locus in Chinese and European-derived populations (Han, 2009). Yap et al. reported that IKZF1 was involved in the regulation of STAT4 in human T cells, which suggested that STAT4 and IKZF1 might cooperate with each other and play roles in the development of SLE (Yap, 2005). Hu W. *et al*, demonstrated that *IKZF1* mRNA expression levels in PBMCs from patients with SLE were significantly lower than those in healthy controls (Hu, 2011).

Association of SLE and disease phenotype with IKZF1 was studied in Chinese Han origin SLE patients were the allele frequency of rs4917014 (IKZF1) was significantly different in two subphenotypes: renal nephritis (p=0.02) and malar rash (p=0.00038) (He, 2010).

9. Chromosome 8

Several studies have revealed association of SLE susceptibility to different genes within a 700 kb region of locus 8p23.1 (Hom, 2008; Graham, 2008; Harley, 2008). This region contains several candidate genes, including BLK, XKR6, FAM167A/C8orf13 and C8orf12, these genes were in significant linkage disequilibrium (LD), making it difficult to determine whether the different reports are detecting the same association signal. Budarf ML *et al.* found significant association to both the BLK (rs2618476) and XKR6 (rs6985109) genes (Budarf, 2011). Although these two SNPS are separated by 620 kb, there is relatively strong correlation between them (r^2=0.39), allowing the possibility that they may represent the same signal. Here in we will review the evidence of association of both genes BLK, XKR6 with susceptibility to SLE (Budarf, 2011).

9.1 B lymphoid tyrosine kinase (BLK), 8p23.1

BLK encodes a nonreceptor tyrosine-kinase of the src family of proto-oncogenes, which mediates intracellular signaling and influences cell proliferation and differentiation. The human BLK gene was mapped to chromosome 8 at p23.1, and is expressed only in B lymphocytes (Drebin, 1995). The protein has a role in B-cell receptor signaling, B-cell development and tolerance of B cells (Reth, 1997). B cell receptor (BCR) signaling requires a tight regulation of several protein tyrosine kinases and phosphatases, and associated co-receptors. Break of the balance between positive and negative signaling molecules likely modifies the BCR signaling thresholds. Such alterations, together with other factors, may contribute to the disruption of selftolerance in SLE.

BLK has apparently become one of the most important and consistent non-MHC gene for SLE and the other autoimmune diseases across multiple ethnic groups and is one of three key genes (BLK, LYN and BANK) involved in BCR signaling found to be strongly associated with SLE proves the importance of this pathway in disease pathogenesis. B-lymphoid tyrosine kinase (BLK) was one of the top hit in more than one GWA analyses, while LYN was associated with high significance in the International Consortium for Systemic Lupus Erythematosus (SLEGEN) study only. BLK has been implicated in the pathogenesis of SLE and has been investigated in numerous ethnically diverse studies.

GWAS in European-derived populations identified a SNP (rs13277113; located in the promoter region of BLK, maps to the intergenic region between *FAM167A*/C8orf13 and

BLK), of which allele A is associated with reduced expression of *BLK* but increased expression of *FAM167A* (previously referred to as C8orf13) in patients with SLE (Ito, 2010). Another *BLK* SNP (rs2248932), located 43 kb downstream of rs13277113, is also associated with SLE where the risk C allele of rs2248932 was associated with the lower levels of BLK mRNA expression (Zhang, 2010).

Both SNPs have subsequently been confirmed as SLE-associated in Asian populations (Zhang, 2010 & Ito, 2009). Genotyping SNP rs2248932 in SLE patients of Chinese Han confirmed that SNP rs2248932 in BLK gene was significantly associated with SLE (P = 1.41 x 10-8). The association of BLK in Chinese SLE patients was consistent with a dominant model. In contrast to the Caucasian, this risk allele was the major allele in the Chinese Han; the risk allele frequency was higher in Chinese Han than in Caucasian. No association was found between this SNP and any subphenotype of SLE.   Fan *et al* performed a meta-analysis to test the association of two SNPs rs13277113 and rs2248932. A significant associations of rs13277113 and SLE were observed for dominant model (AA + AG vs. GG, OR: 1.518), and recessive model (AA vs. AG + GG, OR: 1.553); so were rs2248932 and SLE for dominant model (TT + TC vs. CC, OR: 1.34), and recessive model (TT vs. TC + CC, OR: 1.34) (Fan, 2010).

9.2 X Kell blood group precursor-related family, member 6 (XKR6), 8p23.1

XKR6, a member of a novel family of PDZCBM containing proteins sharing homology with the *C. elegans* gene *ced-8*, which has been implicated in regulating the timing of apoptosis (Giallourakis, 2006). *XKR6* contains an intronic microRNA, hsa-miR-598, which is highly expressed in human peripheral blood mononuclear cells, especially activated B-cells (Lawrie, 2008). Dissecting the relative contribution of XKR6 to SLE risk is likely to be a complicated undertaking, especially given that a polymorphic inversion under apparent selection pressure on 8p23 encompasses the *XKR6*, *C8orf12*, *C8orf13*, and *BLK* genes, all of which have been implicated in SLE risk in GWAS studies (Deng, 2008).

9.3 Yamaguchi sarcoma viral (v-yes-1) related oncogene homolog' LYN, 8q12.1

LYN is a Src-tyosine kinase involved in B cell activation by phosphorylating the ITAM domain of the BCR-associated Ig α/β signaling molecules, in turn recruiting and activating the tyrosine kinase SYK, which initiates multiple activating signals. LYN also mediates inhibitory signals by phosphorylating inhibitory receptors such as CD22 and FcγRIIb and may therefore have a critical role as a modulator of B-cell activation thresholds. In the Genome wide association studies (GWAS) of SLE, three B cell signaling molecules *BLK, LYN* and *BANK1* (Hom, 2008; Kozyrev, 2008) were found to be associated with SLE. The best characterized functionally is LYN among the other two kinases *(BANK, BLK)* shown to be associated with SLE. These data suggest that aberrant regulation of B cell signaling may be one mechanism for generating hyper-responsive B cells, which might lead to aberrant B cell development, selection and ultimately influence the production of autoantibodies. Expression of Lyn is significantly decreased in both resting and BCR stimulated peripheral blood B cells from two-thirds of SLE patients compared to controls (Liossis, 2001). Further, statistically significant alterations at the transcriptional level were confirmed by a 2.5-fold decrease in Lyn mRNA in SLE patients compared to healthy individuals. Another group analyzed the level and subcellular distribution of Lyn in SLE

B cells and found that slightly more than half of the SLE patients analyzed had reduced levels of Lyn protein, which was subsequently determined to be due to increased ubiquitination of the protein. Functional differences in LYN ubiquitination have been also associated with SLE risk (Flores-Borja, 2005).

Two SNPs, rs7829816 and rs2667978, showed significant association in some of the cohorts tested, but failed to consistently replicate in all cohorts (Harley, 2008). Lu R. *et al* has performed one of the largest studies to examine the possible genetic association of *LYN* with SLE in multiple large populations of different ancestries (European-derived, African American and Korean). Their study has replicated a previously observed association with rs7829816 (Harley, 2008), however, data from Lu R. *et al* study suggested that this association is not a dominant lupus effect. The strongest and most consistent association found in this study was at rs6983130, which is within the first intron at the 5' end near the primary transcription initiation site. This SNP showed the strongest association in the European-American female population. A strong gender influence was found with this SNP when analyzing only female subjects. Rs6983130 also showed associations with autoantibodies which is strongly associated with the development of SLE, specifically anti-dsDNA, anti-chromatin, anti-52 kDa Ro and anti-Sm.

10. Chromosome 10

10.1 Mannose-Binding Lectin (MBL), (10q11.2-21)

MBL is very similar to C1q in its structure and function. It is an important element of the innate immune system. MBL comprises a trimer of three identical polypeptides, and several trimmers further combine to form a bouquet-like structure (Holmskov, 1994). MBL recognizes carbohydrate patterns, found on the surface of a large number of pathogenic micro-organisms, including bacteria, viruses, protozoa and fungi and initiates the lectin pathway for opsonization and clearance of pathogens in an antibody-independent manner.

MBL gene comprising four exons and there is only one single functional gene. The normal structural MBL alleles is named A, while the common designation for the 3 variant structural allele B (Gly54Asp), C (Gly57Glu) and D (Arg52Cys) are O. MBL expression is influenced by polymorphic sites in the upstream part of the MBL gene nucleotides substitutions at positions -550, -221 and +4. Absent or low levels of serum MBL is a result of these polymorphisms and might be associated with the development of SLE (Takahashi, 2005 & Pradhan, 2010). Case-control genetic studies of MBL polymorphism were performed in various Ethnic groups. MBL genotyping in SLE confirmed that the MBL functional variants are associated with SLE (Ramasawmy, 2008). Serum MBL levels fluctuate during the course of SLE disease activity and MBL genotypes have been found to be useful in assessing the risk of infection during immunosuppressive treatment the majority of the SLE patients receive.

Two possible explanations for associations between MBL deficiency and occurrence of SLE were proposed (Korb, 1997): (a) MBL can bind to and initiate uptake of apoptotic cells into macrophages (Ogden, 2001 & Okada, 2002), and abnormal clearance of apoptotic cells caused by MBL deficiency may result in overexpression of autoantigens; (b) viral infection is believed to be one of the causes of SLE (Okada, 2002), and MBL deficiency may lead to more frequent infections.

11. Chromosome 11

11.1 Interferon regulatory factor 5 /PHD and RING-finger domains 1(IRF7/ PHRF1) locus, 11p15.5

IRF7 is a transcription factor that can induce transcription of IFNa and in turn IFNa-induced genes downstream of endosomal TLRs, similar to IRF5 (Barnes, 2004). A SNP near IRF7 was found to be associated with SLE susceptibility in the International Consortium for SLE Genetics (SLEGEN) genome-wide association study (Harley, 2008). The associated SNP (rs4963128) was located 23 kb telomeric to IRF7 in a gene of unknown function named PHD and RING-finger domains 1 (PHRF1; also known as KIAA1542 or CTD-binding SR-like protein rA9). This SNP was in high linkage disequilibrium ($r^2 = 0.94$) with the rs702966 SNP in IRF7 (Harley, 2008). The PHRF1 gene contains PHD-finger and RING-finger domains, and has not been functionally characterized to date. PHD and RING-finger domains both chelate zinc ions, and PHD domains are frequently found in proteins which mediate protein–protein interactions in the cell nucleus (Bienz, 2006).

There is a hypothesizes that the SLE-associated variant discovered in the IRF7/PHRF1 locus in the SLEGEN study (International Consortium for Systemic Lupus Erythematosus Genetics, 2008) could be due to a polymorphism in IRF7 that predisposes to increased IFNa production. Then, Salloum R. *et al* have proven this hypothesis by analyzing serum IFNa in SLE patients as a quantitative trait to determine associations with haplotype-tagging SNPs in the IRF7/PHRF1 locus (Salloum, 2009). In a joint analysis of European American and Hispanic American subjects, the rs702966 C allele was associated with the presence of anti–double-stranded DNA (anti-dsDNA) antibodies ($P=0.0069$). The rs702966 CC genotype was only associated with higher serum levels of IFNa in European American and Hispanic American patients with anti-dsDNA antibodies (joint analysis $P = 4.1 \times 10^{-5}$) (International Consortium for Systemic Lupus Erythematosus Genetics, 2008). However, the rs702966 C allele was not associated with anti-dsDNA in the African American subjects, and no other significant associations were seen in this group. In African American patients, the rs4963128 T allele downstream of IRF7 was associated with the presence of anti-Sm antibodies ($P = 0.0017$), where subjects with the rs4963128 CT and TT genotypes had higher IFNa levels than those with the CC genotype ($P = 0.0012$). The striking differences observed within the African American cohort separated by the presence or absence of anti-Sm antibodies suggest 2 independent patterns of association with IRF7/PHRF1 variants, which cannot be explained by European admixture at the locus. It is possible that the rs4963128 T allele marks a particular element in African-derived chromosomes that associates with anti-Sm antibodies and is not present in the other ancestral backgrounds (Salloum, 2009). Salloum R. *et al* hypothesized that the rs702966 C allele and elements in linkage with it may function similarly across all ancestral backgrounds, although the effect of the anti-Sm–rs4963128 T allele interaction on serum levels of IFNa in African Americans is independent of the effect at the rs702966 C allele (Salloum, 2009).

12. Chromosome 16

12.1 *Integrin αM* (ITGAM), 16p11.2

ITGAM is a single-pass type I membrane protein predominantly expressed primarily on neutrophils, macrophages and dendritic cells that is involved in various adhesive interactions to stimulated endothelium, and also in the phagocytosis of complement coated particles. Together with integrin chain β2, *ITGAM* forms a functionally active heterodimer, the integrin αMβ2 molecule to form the cell surface receptor, known as complement receptor 3 (CR3) or Mac-1, can bind a variety of ligands including intercellular adhesion molecule 1 (ICAM-1), the C3bi fragment of activated complement C3, fibrinogen, and factor X. ITGAM is perhaps more familiarly known as CD11b or CR3, and it thereby takes part in the uptake of complement-coated particles and the clearance of immune complexes.

The identification of ITGAM as a major susceptibility gene was perhaps the greatest surprise of the GWA analyses because it has been subject to expression studies in the past with little convincing evidence for a role in SLE (Harley, 2008 & Hom, 2008). A non-synonymous SNP in ITGAM, rs1143679, functional mutation results in an Arg77His (R77H), was first associated in European and African descendants SLE patients, where the G allele contributes to disease susceptibility (Nath, 2008 & Han, 2009). This amino acid does not lie within any known ligand binding site, but may alter the confirmation of the I/A domain to which many ligands do bind. This variant could therefore influence leucocyte trafficking mediated via ICAM-1, or equally it could influence the CR3-mediated uptake of apoptotic cells or immune complexes. Functional data is awaited with interest. However, the consistent association of rs1143679 was not replicated in Asian population (Korean and Japanese) because this SNP was monomorphic for 'G' allele (Han, 2009). This result suggests that the genetic association of ITGAM with SLE is unlikely in Asians. However, another group studied Chinese SLE patients living in Hong Kong and found that rs1143679 was associated with SLE, and another related SNP in the gene, rs1143683, was also identified (Yang, 2009). Therefore, it needs to be confirmed in larger number of SLE case–controls in Korean and Japanese populations.

12.2 Deoxyribonuclease DNase I, 16p13.3

DNase I may be the most important nuclease for the removal of DNA from nuclear antigens. Several lines of evidence suggest that defects in DNase I activity play a role in SLE pathogenesis. Studies in SLE patients and in mouse models support the involvement of DNase I among the genes involved in the clearance of apoptotic cells. The first evidence was reported by Chitrabamrung et al. (Chitrabamrung, 1981) more than two decades ago. These authors found decreased DNaseI activity in patients with SLE. It has been shown that a DNaseI knockout mouse develops a lupus-like syndrome (Napirei, 2000) and a nonsense mutation on the DNASEI gene leading to a non-functional protein has been identified in two Japanese girls with SLE. These girls had very low DNaseI activity and high titers of anti-nucleosome and anti-double-stranded DNA (dsDNA) antibodies. Subsequent analysis of several series of SLE patients from different populations showed that this mutation is extremely rare. Bodan˜o A et al., have described two Spanish SLE patients with very low serum DNase I activity harboring three new mutations in the DNASEI coding sequence that account for the reduced enzymatic activity (Bodan˜ o, 2004). The frequency of these new mutations was below 1% both in SLE patients and in the population. Bodan˜o A. et al. also found other DNASEI single-nucleotide polymorphisms (SNPs) but there was no evidence suggesting a functional role for them. These studies support the involvement of DNase I in the pathogenesis of SLE.

In a Korean SLE population, 16 SNPs from the DNaseI were studied using a case–control approach. In parallel, common autoantibodies were also examined for the same population. None of the SNPs were in significant association with SLE, however, a non-synonymous SNP in exon 8, namely rs1053874 (which was also known as +2373A/G, and which causes Gln244Arg substitution), was significantly associated with an increased risk of the production of anti-RNP and anti-dsDNA (Shin, 2004). However, the same SNP (+2373A/G) has shown association between the GG allele and SLE susceptibility in Spanish population, but no association with the majority of antinuclear antibodies (anti-dsDNA, anti-ssDNA and anti-RNP) and no effect on DNase I activity (Bodaño , 2006). This discrepancy could be related to heterogeneity between the populations.

13. Chromosome 17

13.1 Monocyte chemo-attractant protein 1 (MCP1), 17q11.2-12

MCP-1, currently also designated CCL2, encodes a β-chemokine that recruits monocyte, eosinophils, and memory T cells to inflammatory sites, to regulate adhesion molecule expression and T-cell functions in acute and possibly chronic inflammation (Charo, 2004). Evidence in human and animal studies suggests a significant role of MCP-1 in the progression of glomerular and tubulointerstitial injuries and glomerulonephriti in patients with SLE (Stahl, 1993; Rovin, 1996; Saitoh, 1998; Rovin 1998). In particular, MCP-1 has been shown to be pathogenic for kidney injury in murine lupus nephritis (Shimizu, 2004), and reported to be involved in glomerulonephritis in SLE patients, in which elevation of serum MCP-1 correlates with disease activity (Tesar, 1998). An increased urine MCP-1 (uMCP-1) level was detected in SLE patients during active renal disease (Rovin, 2005).

SNP (rs1024611) -2518A/G and G/G in MCP1 promoter region may modulate the levels of MCP-1 expression and increased susceptibility to SLE and lupus nephritis in patients from North America (Tucci, 2004). However, the Involvement of the MCP-1 –2518 A>G promoter polymorphism in SLE development and its contribution to some clinical manifestations of SLE remains controversial (Tucci, 2004; Aguilar, 2001; Hwang, 2002; Kim, 2002; Brown, 2007; Liao, 2004; Ye, 2005). In a Spanish study for example, −2518G polymorphism is noted to be associated with cutaneous vasculitis but not SLE or lupus nephritis as genotyping of −2518A/G polymorphism shows no difference in allelic or genotype frequencies in SLE patient and healthy controls (Aguilar, 2001). Further investigation is needed to delineate if ethnic heterogeneity contributes to this gene polymorphism and SLE susceptibility.

14. Chromosome 19

14.1 Tyrosine kinase 2 (TYK2), 19p13.2

TYK2 is part of the Janus kinase that binds to the interferon (IFN)-α receptor (IFNAR), on the cell surface of IFN-producing cells. Binding of IFN-α to its receptor, leads to the phosphorylation and therefore activation of TYK2 (Richter, 1998). Active TYK2 then phosphorylates IFNAR to allow binding of STAT3 and STAT5 (David, 2002) which leads to expression of IFN-α. Deficiency of TYK2 leads to defects of multiple cytokine pathways, including type I interferon, IL-6, IL-10, IL-12, and IL-23, and to impaired T-helper type 1 differentiation and accelerated T helper type 2 differentiation (Minegishi, 2006). More research needed to clarify which of these pathways is critically affected by the TYK2 risk allele.

TYK2 gene has been linked to the formation of anti-dsDNA antibodies of Caucasian SLE patients (Namjou, 2002). TYK2 rs2304256 was associated with increased risk of discoid lupus erythematosus ($P=0.012$). In a joint linkage and association study of 44 SNPs in 13 genes from type I IFN pathway in the Scandinavian population, TYK2 and interferon regulatory factor 5 (IRF5) genes displayed strong association with SLE susceptibility (Sigurdsson, 2005).

The most remarkable result from this study has probably been the association signal observed with the rs2304256 nonsynonymous SNP of TYK2 (OR = 0.79) because this has been a controversial SLE genetic factor. The rs2304256 SNP introduces a valine to phenylalanine change in the Janus homology domain 4 of *TYK2* whose functional relevance has not yet been tested. This nonsynonymous SNP showed the strongest association among the 11 TYK2 SNPs studied in Scandinavian families (Sigurdsson, 2005), but was not associated in a study of UK families (Cunninghame, 2007). This latter study, however, found association with another TYK2 SNP (rs12720270) that was not associated in the Scandinavian study. Finally, the International Consortium for Systemic Lupus Erythematosus Genetics (SLEGEN) GWA study excluded association with the rs12720270 SNP (the rs2304256 SNP was not included in the GWA panels)(International Consortium for Systemic Lupus Erythematosus Genetics, 2008).

TYK2 single nucleotide polymorphisms (SNPs), rs2304256, rs12720270 and rs280519, were genotyped in the Japanese population by Kyogoku C *et. al.* in a case-control association study. Linkage disequilibrium (LD) among TYK2 SNPs was examined and no association was revealed with SLE therefore it was concluded that TYK2 is not a genetic risk factor for SLE in a Japanese population (Kyogoku, 2009).

15. Chromosome X

15.1 Interleukin-1 receptor-associated kinase 1/Methyl-CpG-binding Protein 2 locus (IRAK1/MECP2), Xq28

IRAK1, a serine–threonine protein kinase, regulates multiple pathways in both innate and adaptive immune responses by linking several immune-receptor- complexes to TNF receptor-associated factor 6 in mouse models of lupus, *Irak1* is shown to regulate nuclear factor κB (NFκB) in TCR signaling and Toll/interleukin-1 receptor (TLR) activation, as well as the induction of IFN-α and IFN-γ, (Jacob, 2009) implicating IRAK1 in SLE. In a study of four different ethnic groups, multiple SNPs within *IRAK1* were associated with both adult-onset and childhood-onset SLE (Jacob, 2009). The identified polymorphism C203S in IRAK1 is not in any known functional domain, therefore it was suggested that the association may actually be with its neighbor, methyl-CpG-binding protein 2 (*MECP2*).

MECP2 is an X-linked gene located in a region of LD with *IRAK1*, encoding a protein that represses transcription from methylated promoters, has also been associated with lupus. Polymorphisms in *MECP2* may have relevance to the epigenetic DNA methylation changes found in lupus and discussed below. There is evidence for altered methylation in SLE, (Webb, 2009) as well as differential expression of potentially methylated genes, (Pan, 2009) although, as with *IRAK1*, a contributing causative SNP is not immediately obvious. Indeed, it is possible that both of these strong candidates contribute to the effect.

A large replication study in a European-derived population confirmed the importance of this region (*IRAK1–MECP2*) to SLE. The location of *IRAK1* and *MECP2* on the X chromosome raises the possibility that gender bias of SLE might, in part, be attributed to sex chromosome genes. Further work is required to identify the causal variants (Sestak, 2011).

15.2 Toll-like receptor (TLR7), Xp22.2

TLR7, the protein encoded by this gene is a member of the Toll-like receptor (TLR) family which is single transmembrane cell-surface receptors expressed on many types of cells including macrophages and dendritic cells, plays a fundamental role in pathogen recognition and activation of innate immunity. TLRs generally exist as homodimers. They are highly conserved from Drosophila to humans and share structural and functional similarities. TLR are activated by molecules associated with biological threat and are highly specific towards evolutionary conserved entities on microbes, such as bacterial cell-surface lipopolysaccharides, flagella and unmethylated CpG islands.

Activation of toll-like receptors initiates downstream signaling cascades, initially via the adapter molecules MyD88, Trap, Trif and Tram, leading to NF-kappa-B activation, cytokine secretion and the inflammatory response, regulate intracellular kinases and gene expression. The signaling cascade coupled to toll-like receptor activation is very similar to that of interleukin-1 receptor (IL-1R) activation. It has been suggested that some toll-like receptors may have endogenous ligands, such as Hsp60 and fibrinogen, and this has promoted speculation that endogenous toll-like receptor activators may have a pathological role in autoimmune disease. TLRs play an important role in the pathogenesis of SLE (Vollmer, 2005 & Christensen, 2006). The role of nucleic acid binding TLR7 has become quite apparent in both SLE animal models and human patients. This receptor promotes autoantibodies and cytokines responsible for chronic inflammation (Christensen, 2007 & Savarese, 2008). A recent fine mapping of the 23-kb TLR7 region using 11 SNPs in 1434 SLE cases of Eastern Asian descent versus 1591 controls showed the association of two TLR7 SNPs with SLE (rs5935436 in the promoter, $p=1.8 \times 10^{-3}$; rs3853839 in the 3'-UTR, $p=6.7 \times 10^{-4}$) (in press).

16. Epigenetics involvement in the pathology of SLE

The controversy, we came cross in the previous section, in the association of immunologically related genes with susceptibility to SLE and the incomplete concordance in monozygotic twins affected with SLE, while they carry the same SLE susceptibility genes, are clear indications that genetics is not the only factor that influences susceptibility to SLE. This means that some non-genetic factors can modify gene expression through epigenetic mechanisms, potentially contributing to SLE. The field of epigenetics is rapidly growing especially in studying autoimmune diseases. Epigenetics is the study of heritable modifications in gene function that alter the phenotype without modifying the genetic sequence, these modifications result in the activation or complete/partial gene silencing (Hirst, 2009). It is becoming clear that epigenetic modifications contribute to a variety of pathogenetic processes in which environmental and genetic factors are involved. Much of the variability in severity, organ involvement, and response to therapy among patients with systemic lupus erythematosus (SLE) is blamed on differences in gene expression. That, in turn, is due to epigenetic mechanisms, one of the "master regulators" of gene expression.

Accumulating epidemiological, clinical, and experimental evidence supports the conclusion of the critical role of epigenetic factors in immune programming. Compelling evidence has been gathered supports a role for epigenetic alterations in the pathogenesis of SLE. For example, inhibiting DNA methylation in normal CD4+ T cells induces autoreactivity, and these autoreactive cells promote autoantibody production. Furthermore, transferring hypomethylated T cells into syngeneic mice causes a lupus-like disease (Richardson, 1990 & Yung 1997). Understanding this mechanism provides the basis for clarifying how the complex interactions of the genome and epigenome shape immune responses and maintain immune tolerance to self-antigens.

In this section we will discus, in brief, some of the epigenetics mechanisms that are involved in the SLE pathogenesis. These mechanisms play an essential role in gene regulation

Gene	locus	function	P-values	ORs
PTPN22	1p13	T-cell signaling	$<1\times10^{-5}$ - 5.2×10^{-6}	1.49-1.53
FCGR2A	1q21-23	Immune complex clearance Fc Receptor	0.0016 - 6.78×10^{-7}	1.30-1.35
FCGR3B	1q23.3	Immune complex clearance Fc Receptor	2.7×10^{-8}	2.21c
FcGR3A	1q23.3	Immune complex clearance Fc Receptor		1.6
CRP	1q23.2	sensitive marker of inflammation	6.4×10^{-7}	
TNFSF4	1q25.1	T-cell signaling	over: 1.91×10^{-6}	over: 1.63 (T/U) and 1.28b
NMNAT2	1q25.3	Catalyzes the formation of NAD(+)from nicotinamide mononucleotide (NMN) and ATP.	1×10^{-10}	1.18
IL10*	1q31–q32	1q24	$4.0\times10 -8$	1.2
TLR5	1q41-q42	innate immunity		
STAT4	2q33	TLR–IFN signaling	2.8×10^{-9} - 8.96×10^{-14}	1.53-1.50
PDCD1 (CD279)	2q37	pro-B-cells differentiation		1.2
CTLA4 (CD152)	2q33.2	transmits an inhibitory signal to T cells		
PXK	3p14.3	Bind and modulates both Na, K-ATPase enzymatic and ion pump activities	7.10×10^{-9}	1.25
BANK1	4q24	B-cell signaling	3.7×10^{-7}	1.38
TNIP1	5q33	TNF–NFκB signaling		1.3
The MHC	6p21.3	T-cell signaling	2.71×10^{-21}- 1.7×10^{-52}	2.01-2.36
ATG5	6q21		1.36×10^{-7}	1.19
PRDM1	6q21	B-cell signaling	$1.74\times10 -8$	1.3
TNFAIP3	6q23	TNF–NFκB signaling	2.9×10^{-12}	1.7
IRF5	7q32	TLR–IFN signaling	1.65×10^{-11} - 3.61×10^{-19}	1.54-1.72
ICA1	7p21.3		1.90×10^{-7}	1.32
IKZF1	7p12	B-cell signaling		1.4
BLK	8p23.1	T-cell signaling	1×10^{-10} -7×10^{-10}	1.22-1.39
XKR6	8p23.1		2.51×10^{-11}	1.23
LYN	8q12.1		5.4×10^{-9}	1.30
C8orf12	8p23.1	miscRNA gene	4.00×10^{-10}	1.22
BLK–FAM167A–XKR6 locus	8p23.1	B-cell signaling	1.7×10^{-8}	1.2-1.6
MBL	10q11.2-21	element of the innate immune system		
KIAA1542 (near IRF7)	11p15.5	Interferon and TLR7/9 Signaling	3.00×10^{-10}	1.28
ITGAM	16p11.2	Neutrophil activity	3×10^{-11} - 1.61×10^{-23}	1.33-1.62

CD226	18q22.3	member of the Ig-superfamily		
TYK2	19p13.2	Janus kinases (JAKs) protein interferon signaling pathway		
UBE2L3	22q11.2	encodes a member of the E2 ubiquitin-conjugating enzyme	7.53×10^{-8}	1.22
SCUBE1	22q13.2	adhesive molecule	1.21×10^{-7}	1.28
MECP2	Xq28	Chromosomal protein that binds to methylated DNA	1.2×10^{-8}	1.39
IRAK1	Xq28	responsible for IL1-induced upregulation of the transcription factor NF-kappa B		
TLR7	Xp22.2	innate immunity		

Table 1. Top SLE candidate genes categorized by chromosomal location.

through covalent modifications of DNA and histones, and determine regional chromatin structure with consequences on gene expression. We will also discuss the involvement of MicroRNAs (miRNAs) as an epigenetic factor involved in the pathology of SLE.

16.1 Histone covalent modification

The basic chromatin subunit is the nucleosome, which consists of DNA wrapped twice around a histone core. Nucleosomes are then organized into higher order structures forming chromatin fibers (Felsenfeld 2003). Chromatin in its native form is tightly compacted and inaccessible to transcription factors and the transcription initiation machinery. However, histone "tails" protrude from the nucleosome, and are covalently modified by *acetylation, methylation, phosphorylation, ubiquitination, and SUMOylation* (SUMO (small ubiquitin-related modifier) (Felsenfeld 2003). These modifications serve as signals, referred to as the "histone code", that initiate a number of processes including the localized remodeling of chromatin from a compact, transcriptionally silent configuration to a more open structure accessible to the transcription initiation machinery.

16.2 DNA methylation and autoimmunity
DNA methylation refers to the methylation of cytosines in CpG pairs (cytosine and guanine residues separated by a phosphate, which links the two nucleosides together in DNA). Most CpG pairs in the mammalian genome are methylated, with some unmethylated pairs found in the regulatory elements of active genes. Most unmethylated CpGs are found in GC-rich sequences, termed CpG islands. CpG islands contain multiple binding sites for transcription factors, and serve as promoters for the associated gene. Methylation of these promoters can lead to gene silencing where transcriptionally active chromatin is characterized by unmethylated DNA. Convincing evidence indicates that DNA can be actively demethylated and therefore affect gene expresssion. For example, several CpG pairs in the *IL-2* promoter demethylate within 20 minutes of T-cell stimulation, prior to initiation of DNA synthesis (Bruniquel, 2003).

DNA methylation is catalyzed by the enzyme DNA methyltransferases (DNMTs) while and histone acetylation is controlled by histone acetylases (HATs) and deacetylases (HDACs). It is hypothesized that the processes of DNA methylation and histone deacetylation work together through the formation of DNMT/HDAC transcriptional repressor complexes that work in silencing gene expression through establishing a repressive chromatin environment

(Cameron, 1999). However, DNMTs and HDACs lack DNA-binding domains, and are therefore dependent on transcription factors (TFs) for their recruitment to DNA. Zhao M *et al.* set out a study to uncover mechanisms underlying the hypomethylation and hyperacetylation of genes involved in lupus autoimmunity by investigating the involvement of specific TFs. They assessed the activities of 225 TFs in CD4+ T cells from SLE patients relative to healthy controls using a newly developed screening method (Qiao, 2008), and found that the activity of regulatory factor X 1 (RFX1) is significantly downregulated in SLE CD4+ T cells (Zhao, 2010). Follow-up analyses confirmed the result of Zhao M *et al.* study and further revealed that both the expression and activity of RFX1 protein are reduced in SLE CD4+ T cells. Zhao M *et al* (Zhao, 2010) also provided evidence indicating that RFX1 recruits the co-repressors HDAC1 and DNMT1 to the promoter region of CD11a and CD70, thus regulating their expression in CD4+ T cells. Taken together, our findings indicate that reduction of RFX1 plays an important role in inducing autoreactivity and autoantibody overstimulation in SLE.

In addition, DNA hypomethylation appears to induce CD4+ T cell autoreactivity and the inhibition of DNA methylation with 5-azacytidine caused CD4+ T-cell autoreactivity. This lupus-like autoimmunity correlated with overexpression of ITGAL (CD11a) and TNFSF7 (CD70) (Lu, 2002 & 2005). CD11a and CD70 overexpression in these CD4+ T cells is associated with hypomethylation of their respective promoters (Lu, 2002 & 2005). CD11a is the alpha chain of the heterodimeric integrin lymphocyte function-associated antigen-1 (LFA-1) (CD11a/CD18) (ITGAL/Integrin beta-2). Overexpressing LFA-1 by transfection caused an identical autoreactivity (Yung, 1996).LFA-1 plays a central role in adhesive interactions between T cells and other immune system cells including macrophages, dendritic cells and B cells. This protein is also essential for the recruitment of leukocytes into sites of inflammation, antigen-specific T cell activation, helping B cell, as well as alloreactive, cytotoxic T cell and natural killer responses (Shimaoka & Springer, 2003). LFA-1 deficient lupus mice have significantly increased survival, decreased anti-DNA autoantibody formation, and reduced glomerulonephritis (Kevil, 2004). CD70 is expressed on activated T cells and increases pokeweed mitogen (PWM)-stimulated immunoglobulin (Ig) G synthesis, indicating B cell costimulatory functions (Kobata, 1995). Demethylated, autoreactive CD4+ T cells overstimulate antibody production by B cells and kill macrophages (Richardson, 2007), relaeasing apoptotic nuclear material that stimulates lupus-like autoantibodies (Denny, 2006). T-cell hypomethylation correlates with disease activity in SLE, suggesting that DNA hypomethylation may be a key player in the pathogenesis of the disease (Corvetta, 1991).

Furthermore, CD4+ lymphocytes undergo global histone H3 and H4 deacetylation and consequent skewed gene expression. Although multiple lines of evidence highlight the contribution of epigenetic alterations to the pathogenesis of lupus in genetically predisposed individuals, many questions remain to be answered. Attaining a deeper understanding of these matters will create opportunities in the promising area of epigenetic treatments.

16.3 MicroRNAs (miRNAs) and autoimmunity

MicroRNAs (miRNAs) are newly discovered, small (about 23-nucleotide), noncoding ribonucleic acids (RNAs) that function in the posttranscriptional regulation of about 30% of mRNAs by binding to their 3'-untranslated region (3'-UTR), thus targeting them for degradation or translational repression. miRNA are known to regulate cellular processes such as apoptosis, cell cycle, differentiation, and immune functions. The powerful gene regulatory role of miRNAs is now well recognized, where the recent discovery of the gene-regulatory role of miRNAs has led to a paradigm shift in the understanding of expression and function of the mammalian genome. The field of miRNA research gained widespread attention with the recognition of aberrant expression and/or function of miRNAs in a broad range of human diseases including autoimmune diseases (Pauley, 2009).

Recent research evidence has emerged showing the critical role of miRNAs not only for the development of the immune system but also for the function of both innate and adaptive arms of the immune system (Taganov, 2007; Xiao, 2009; Gantier, 2007; O'Connell, 2010; Lodish, 2008; Sonkoly, 2008; Baltimore, 2008). Using state of the art quantitative mass spectrometry two investigators measured the response of thousands of proteins after introducing microRNAs into cultured cells and after knockdown mir-223 in mouse neutrophils. Their results are consistent with each other and demonstrate that changes in the level of a single miRNA may have a significant impact on the levels of hundreds to thousands of proteins (Baek, 2008). These important studies are the first to show the impact of microRNAs on the proteome which indicated that for most interactions microRNAs act as rheostats to make fine-scale adjustments to protein output (Baek, 2008 & Selbach, 2008). Tang et al have shown that miR-146 regulates the level of at least TRAF6, IRAK1, STAT-1, and IFN regulatory factor 5 (IRF-5), all of which are important for the IFN pathway (Tang, 2009). The reported reduction of miR-146 in PBMCs from SLE patients (Tang, 2009) will likely affect the levels of these factors significantly and contribute to overexpression of type I IFN and, thus, disease activity.

It is intriguing that independent studies have demonstrated an increased level of miR-146 in RA patients, but a decreased level in SLE patients, as compared with healthy controls. Given that RA and SLE are both systemic rheumatic diseases, one may be surprised by the finding that miR-146 levels are contradictory in these diseases, and yet, it should not be surprising, since this may simply be reflecting a difference in the overall cytokine profiles between the two diseases, with type I IFN playing a dominant role in SLE, whereas TNFα, interleukin-1 (IL-1), and IL-6 are the principle cytokines in RA. In the coming years, one can expect research reports on miRNA expression in many other autoimmune diseases, as well as more-complete profiling data, with disease activity correlations or a lack thereof.

17. References

Adrianto I, Wen F, Templeton A, Wiley G, King JB, Lessard CJ, Bates JS, Hu Y, Kelly JA, Kaufman KM, Guthridge JM, Alarcón-Riquelme ME; BIOLUPUS and GENLES Networks, Anaya JM, Bae SC, Bang SY, Boackle SA, Brown EE, Petri MA, Gallant C, Ramsey-Goldman R, Reveille JD, Vila LM, Criswell LA, Edberg JC, Freedman BI, Gregersen PK, Gilkeson GS, Jacob CO, James JA, Kamen DL, Kimberly RP, Martin J, Merrill JT, Niewold TB, Park SY, Pons-Estel BA, Scofield RH, Stevens AM, Tsao BP, Vyse TJ, Langefeld CD, Harley JB, Moser KL, Webb CF, Humphrey MB, Montgomery CG, Gaffney PM. Association of a functional variant downstream of TNFAIP3 with systemic lupus erythematosus. Nat Genet. 2011;43(3):253-8.

Aguilar F., Gonz´alez-Escribano MF, ´anchez-Rom´an JS, and N´u˜nez-Rold´an A. "MCP-1 promoter polymorphism in Spanish patients with systemic lupus erythematosus," Tissue Antigens, vol. 58, no. 5, (2001) pp. 335–338.

Aitman TJ, Dong R, Vyse TJ et al. Copy number polymorphism in Fcgr3 predisposes to glomerulonephritis in rats and humans. Nature 2006;439:851–855

Alarcón-Riquelme ME, Prokunina L. Finding genes for SLE: complex interactions and complex populations. J Autoimmun. 2003;21(2):117-20.

Alper CA, Awdeh Z, Raum D, Yunis EJ. Complement genes of the major histocompatibility complex (complotypes), extended haplotypes and disease markers. Biochem Soc Symp. 1986;51:19-28.

Arbuckle MR, McClain MT, Rubertone MV et al. Development of autoantibodies before the clinical onset of systemic lupus erythematosus. N Engl J Med 2003;349:1526–33.

Arnett FC, Edworthy SM, Bloch DA et al. The American Rheumatism Association 1987 revised criteria for the classification of rheumatoid arthritis. Arthritis Rheum 1988;31:315–24.

Baechler EC, Batliwalla FM, Karypis G et al. Interferon-inducible gene expression signature in peripheral blood cells of patients with severe lupus. Proc Natl Acad Sci USA 2003;100:2610–5.

Baek D, Villen J, Shin C, Camargo FD, Gygi SP, Bartel DP. The impact of microRNAs on protein output. Nature 2008;455:64–71.

Baltimore D, Boldin MP, O'Connell RM, Rao DS, Taganov KD. microRNAs: new regulators of immune cell development and function. Nat Immunol 2008;9:839–45.

Barnes BJ, Kellum MJ, Pinder KE, Frisancho JA, Pitha PM. Interferon regulatory factor 5, a novel mediator of cell cycle arrest and cell death. Cancer Res 2003;63:6424–31.

Barnes BJ, Richards J, Mancl M, Hanash S, Beretta L, Pitha PM. Global and distinct targets of IRF-5 and IRF-7 during innate response to viral infection. J Biol Chem 2004;279:45194–207.

Bates JS, et al. Meta-analysis and imputation identifies a 109 kb risk haplotype spanning TNFAIP3 associated with lupus nephritis and hematologic manifestations. Genes Immun. 2009; 10:470–7.

Baum PR, Gayle III RB, Ramsdell F, Srinivasan S, Sorensen RA, Watson ML et al. Molecular characterization of murine and human OX40/OX40 ligand systems: identification of a human OX40 ligand as the HTLV-1-regulated protein gp34. EMBO J 1994; 13: 3992–4001.

Begovich AB, Carlton VE, Honigberg LA et al. A missense single-nucleotide polymorphism in a gene encoding a protein tyrosine phosphatase (PTPN22) is associated with rheumatoid arthritis. Am J Hum Genet 2004;75:330–7.

Bennett L, Palucka AK, Arce E et al. Interferon and granulopoiesis signatures in systemic lupus erythematosus blood. J Exp Med 2003;197:711–23.

Bettinotti MP, Hartung K, Deicher H, Messer G, Keller E, Weiss EH, Albert ED. Polymorphism of the tumor necrosis factor beta gene in systemic lupus erythematosus: TNFB-MHC haplotypes. Immunogenetics. 1993;37(6):449-54.

Bharadwaj D, Stein MP, Volzer M, Mold C, Du Clos TW. The major receptor for C-reactive protein on leukocytes is fcgamma receptor II. J Exp Med 1999;190:585–590

Bienz M. The PHD finger, a nuclear protein-interaction domain. Trends Biochem Sci 2006;31:35–40.

Bodaño A, Amarelo J, Gonza´ lez A, Go´ mez-Reino JJ, Conde C. Novel DNASEI mutations related to systemic lupus erythematosus. Arthritis Rheum 2004;50:4070–73.

Bodaño A, González A, Ferreiros-Vidal I, Balada E, Ordi J, Carreira P, Gómez-Reino JJ, Conde C. Association of a non-synonymous single-nucleotide polymorphism of DNASEI with SLE susceptibility. Rheumatology (Oxford). 2006;45(7):819-23.

Bottini N, Musumeci L, Alonso A et al. A functional variant of lymphoid tyrosine phosphatase is associated with type I diabetes. Nat Genet 2004;36:337-8.

Botto M, Walport MJ. C1q, autoimmunity and apoptosis. Immunobiology 2002;205:395-406.

Braun D, Caramalho I, Demengeot J. IFN-alpha/beta enhances BCR-dependent B cell responses. Int Immunol 2002;14:411-9.

Bredius, RG, de Vries CE, Troelstra A, van Alphen L, Weening RS, van de Winkel JG, Out TA.. Phagocytosis of Staphylococcus aureus and Hemophilus influenzae type B opsonized with polyclonal human IgG1 and IgG2 antibodies. Functional hFcγ RIIa polymorphism to IgG2. J. Immunol. 1993;151, 1463-1472.

Brown EE, Edberg JC, Kimberly RP. Fc receptor genes and the systemic lupus erythematosus diathesis. Autoimmunity 2007;40:567-81.

Brown KS, Nackos E, Morthala S, Jensen LE, Whitehead AS, and Von Feldt JM, "Monocyte chemoattractant protein-1: plasma concentrations and A(−2518)G promoter polymorphism of its gene in systemic lupus erythematosus," Journal of Rheumatology, vol. 34, no. 4, pp. (2007) 740–746.

Bruniquel D and Schwartz RH. Selective, stable demethylation of the interleukin-2 gene enhances transcription by an active process. Nat Immunol 2003;4:235–240.

Budarf ML, Goyette P, Boucher G, Lian J, Graham RR, Claudio JO, Hudson T, Gladman D, Clarke AE, Pope JE, Peschken C, Smith CD, Hanly J, Rich E, Boire G, Barr SG, Zummer M; GenES Investigators, Fortin PR, Wither J, Rioux JD. A targeted association study in systemic lupus erythematosus identifies multiple susceptibility alleles. Genes Immun. 2011;12(1):51-8.

Cameron EE, Bachman KE, Myohanen S, Herman JG and Baylin SB. Synergy of demethylation and histone deacetylase inhibition in the re-expression of genes silenced in cancer, Nat Genet 21 (1999), pp. 103–107.

Cash, J. J., Splawski, J. B., Thomas, R., McFarlin, J. F., Schulze-Koops, H., Davis, L. S., Fujita, K. and Lipsky, P. E. Elevated interleukin-10 levels in patients with rheumatoid arthritis. Arthritis Rheum. 1995;38, 96–104.

Chang YK, Yang W, Zhao M, et al. Association of BANK1 and TNFSF4 with systemic lupus erythematosus in Hong Kong Chinese. Genes Immun. 2009 Jul;10(5):414-20

Chang YK, Yang W, Zhao M, et al. Association of BANK1 and TNFSF4 with systemic lupus erythematosus in Hong Kong Chinese. Genes Immun 2009; 10: 414–420.

Charo IF and Taubman MB, "Chemokines in the pathogenesis of vascular disease," Circulation Research, vol. 95, no. 9, (2004) pp. 858–866,.

Chen JY, Wang CM, Tsao KC, Chow YH, Wu JM, Li CL, Ho HH, Wu YJ, Luo SF.. Fcγ receptor IIa, IIIa, and IIIb polymorphisms of systemic lupus erythematosus in Taiwan. 2004;Ann. Rheum. Dis. 63, 877–880.

Chitrabamrung S, Rubin L, Tan EM. Serum deoxyribonuclease I and clinical activity in systemic lupus erythematosus. Rheumatol Int 1981;1:55-60.

Chong, w. P. et al. Association of interleukin-10 promoter polymorphisms with systemic lupus erythematosus. Genes Immun. 2004;5, 484–492

Chong, w. P. et al. Association of interleukin-10 promoter polymorphisms with systemic lupus erythematosus. Genes Immun. 2004;5, 484–492.

Christensen SR and Shlomchik MJ, "Regulation of lupus-related autoantibody production and clinical disease by Toll-like receptors," Seminars in Immunology, vol. 19, no. 1, (2007) pp.11-23.

Christensen SR, Shupe J, Nickerson K, Kashgarian M, Flavell RA, and Shlomchik MJ. Toll-like receptor 7 and TLR9 dictate autoantibody specificity and have opposing inflammatory and regulatory roles in a murine model of lupus. Immunity 2006;25: 417–428.

Chu ZT, Tsuchiya N, Kyogoku C, Ohashi J, Qian YP, Xu SB, Mao CZ, Chu JY, Tokunaga K. Association of Fcγ receptor IIb polymorphism with susceptibility to systemic lupus erythematosus in Chinese: a common susceptibility gene in the Asian populations. Tissue Antigens 2004;63, 21–27.

Clark MR, Stuart SG, Kimberly RP, Ory PA, Goldstein IM. A single amino acid distinguishes the high-responder from the low-responder form of Fc receptor II on human monocytes. Eur J Immunol 1991;21:1911–6.

Clark, MR., Liu, L., Clarkson, SB., Ory, PA. & Goldstein, IM. An abnormality of the gene that encodes neutrophil Fc receptor III in a patient with systemic lupus erythematosus. J. Clin Invest. 1990;86, 341–346.

Corvetta A, Della Bita R, Luchetti MM, Pomponio G. 5-Methyl-cytosine content of DNA in blood, synovial monnuclear cells and synovial tissue from patients affected by autoimmune rheumatic diseases. J Chromatogr 1991;566:481-91.

Crawley E, Woo P, Isenberg DA. Single nucleotide polymorphic haplotypes of the interleukin-10 5' flanking region are not associated with renal disease or serology in Caucasian patients with systemic lupus erythematosus. Arthritis Rheum. 1999;42(9):2017-8

Cunninghame Graham DS, Akil M, Vyse TJ: Association of polymorphisms across the tyrosine kinase gene, TYK2 in UK SLE families. Rheumatology (Oxford) 2007;46:927-930.

Cunninghame Graham DS, Graham RR, Manku H, et al. Polymorphism at the TNF superfamily gene TNFSF4 confers susceptibility to systemic lupus erythematosus. Nat Genet 2008; 40(1):83-89.

Cunninghame Graham DS, Manku H, Wagner S et al. Association of IRF5 in UK SLE families identifies a variant involved in polyadenylation. Hum Mol Genet 2007;16:579–91.

Daeron M. Fc receptor biology. Annu Rev Immunol 1997;15:203–234

Darnell JE Jr, Kerr IM, Stark GR. Jak-STAT pathways and transcriptional activation in response to IFNs and other extracellular signaling proteins. Science 1994;264:1415–21.

David M. Signal transduction by type I interferons. Biotechniques 2002(Suppl.):58–65.

Dean, G. S., Tyrrell-Price, J., Crawley, E.&Isenberg, D. A. Ann. Rheum. Dis. 2000;59, 243–251.

Deapen D, Escalante A, Weinrib L, Horwitz D, Bachman B, Roy-Burman P, Walker A, Mack TM. A revised estimate of twin concordance in systemic lupus erythematosus. Arthritis Rheum. 1992;35(3):311-8.

Decker P, Isenberg D, Muller S. Inhibition of caspase-3-mediated poly(ADP-ribose) polymerase (PARP) apoptotic cleavage by human PARP autoantibodies and effect on cells undergoing apoptosis. J Biol Chem 2000;275:9043–9046

delGado-Vega AM, Abelson AK, Sanchez E, et al. Replication of the TNFSF4 (OX40L) promoter region association with systemic lupus erythematosus. Genes Immun 2009; 10(3):248-253.

Deng L, Zhang Y, Kang J, Liu T, Zhao H, Gao Y, Li C, Pan H, Tang X, Wang D, Niu T, Yang H, Zeng C. An unusual haplotype polymorphism on human chromosome 8p23 derived from the inversion polymorphism. Hum Mutat 2008;10:1209–16.

Denny MF, Chandaroy P, Killen PD, Caricchio R, Lewis EE, Richardson BC, et al. Accelarated macrophage apoptosis induces autoantibody formation and organ damage in systemic lupus erythematosus. J Immunol 2006;176:2095-104.

Dideberg V, Kristjansdottir G, Milani L, Libioulle C, Sigurdsson S, Louis E, Wiman AC, Vermeire S, Rutgeerts P, Belaiche J, Franchimont D, Van Gossum A, Bours V, Syvänen AC. An insertion-deletion polymorphism in the interferon regulatory Factor 5 (IRF5) gene confers risk of inflammatory bowel diseases. Hum Mol Genet. 2007;16(24):3008-16.

Drebin JA, Hartzell SW, Griffin C, Campbell MJ, Niederhuber JE. Molecular cloning and chromosomal localization of the human homologue of a B-lymphocyte specific protein tyrosine kinase (blk). Oncogene 1995;10(3):477–486

Duits A, Bootsma H, Derksen RH, Spronk PE, Kater L, Kallenberg CG, Capel PJ, Westerdaal NA, Spierenburg GT, Gmelig-Meyling FH. Skewed distribution of IgG Fc receptor IIa (CD32) polymorphism is associated with renal disease in systemic lupus erythematosus patients. Arthritis Rheum. 1995;38,1832–1836.

Dykman TR, Cole JL, Iida K, Atkinson JP. Polymorphismof human erythrocyte C3b/C4b receptor. Proc Natl Acad Sci USA 1983;80:1698–1702

Dykman TR, Hatch JA, Atkinson JP. Polymorphism of the human C3b/C4b receptor. Identification of a third allele and analysis of receptor phenotypes in families and patients with systemic lupus erythematosus. J Exp Med 1984;159:691–703

Eskdale J, Kube D, Tesch H, Gallagher G. Mapping of the human IL10 gene and further characterization of the 5' Xanking sequence. Immunogenetics 1997a;46:120–128.

Eskdale J., wordsworth, P., Bowman, S., Field, M. Gallagher, G. Association between polymorphisms at the human IL-10 locus and systemic lupus erythematosus. Tissue Antigens 1997b, 49, 635–639.

Fan Y, Tao JH, Zhang LP, Li LH, Ye DQ. Association of BLK (rs13277113, rs2248932) polymorphism with systemic lupus erythematosus: a meta-analysis. Mol Biol Rep. 2010 Dec 9. [Epub ahead of print]

Fanciulli M, Norsworthy PJ, Petretto E et al. FCGR3B copy number variation is associated with susceptibility to systemic, but not organ-specific, autoimmunity. Nat Genet 2007; 39: 721–3.

Felsenfeld G and Groudine M. Controlling the double helix. Nature 2003;421: 448–453.

Firestein GS. Kelley's textbook of rheumatology. Philadelphia (USA): W.B. Saunders Company; 2008. p1233.

Flores-Borja F, Kabouridis PS, Jury EC, Isenberg DA, Mageed RA. Decreased Lyn expression and translocation to lipid raft signaling domains in B lymphocytes from patients with systemic lupus erythematosus. Arthritis Rheum. 2005; 52(12):3955-65.

Floto RA, Clatworthy MR, Heilbronn KR, Rosner DR, MacAry PA, Rankin A, Lehner PJ, Ouwehand WH, Allen JM, Watkins NA, Smith KG. Loss of function of a lupus associated FcγRIIb polymorphism through exclusion from lipid rafts. Nat. Med. 2005;11, 1056–1058.

Fortis C, Foppoli M, Gianotti L, Galli L, Citterio G, Consogno G, Gentilini O. and Braga M. Increased interleukin-10 serum levels in patients with solid tumours. Cancer Lett. 1996;104, 1–5.

Frucht DM, Fukao T, Bogdan C, Schindler H, O'Shea JJ, Koyasu S. IFN-gamma production by antigen-presenting cells: mechanisms emerge. Trends Immunol 2001;22:556–60.

Fukao T, Frucht DM, Yap G, Gadina M, O'Shea JJ, Koyasu S. Inducible expression of Stat4 in dendritic cells and macrophages and its critical role in innate and adaptive immune responses. J Immunol 2001;166:4446–55.

Gantier MP, Sadler AJ, Williams BR. Fine-tuning of the innate immune response by microRNAs. Immunol Cell Biol 2007;85: 458–62.

Gateva V, Sandling JK, Hom G, et al. A large-scale replication study identifiesTNIP1, PRDM1, JAZF1, UHRF1BP1 and IL10 as risk loci for systemic lupus erythematosus. Nat Genet 2009;41 : 1228–33 .

Gateva V, Sandling JK, Hom G, Taylor KE, Chung SA, Sun X, Ortmann W, Kosoy R, Ferreira RC, Nordmark G, Gunnarsson I, Svenungsson E, Padyukov L, Sturfelt G, Jönsen A, Bengtsson AA, Rantapää-Dahlqvist S, Baechler EC, Brown EE, Alarcón GS, Edberg JC, Ramsey-Goldman R, McGwin G Jr, Reveille JD, Vilá LM, Kimberly RP, Manzi S, Petri MA, Lee A, Gregersen PK, et al: A large-scale replication study identifies TNIP1, PRDM1, JAZF1, UHRF1BP1 and IL10 as risk loci for systemic lupus erythematosus. Nat Genet 2009; 41:1228-1233.

Gateva, V. et al. A large-scale replication study identifies TNIP1, PRDM1, JAZF1, UHRF1BP1 and IL10 as risk loci for systemic lupus erythematosus. Nat. Genet. 2009;41, 1228–1233.

Gateva, V. et al. A large-scale replication study identifies TNIP1, PRDM1, JAZF1, UHRF1BP1 and IL10 as risk loci for systemic lupus erythematosus. Nat. Genet. 2009;41, 1228–1233.

Georgopoulos K, Bigby M, Wang JH, Molnar A, Wu P, Winandy S, Sharpe A. The Ikaros gene is required for the development of all lymphoid lineages. Cell 1994;79:143–156.

Giallourakis C, Cao Z, Green T, Wachtel H, Xie X, Lopez-Illasaca M, Daly M, Rioux J, Xavier R. A molecular-properties-based approach to understanding PDZ domain proteins and PDZ ligands. Genome Res 2006;16:1056–72.

Graham DS, Graham RR, Manku H, Wong AK, Whittaker JC, Gaffney PM et al. Polymorphism at the TNF superfamily gene TNFSF4 confers susceptibility to systemic lupus erythematosus. Nat Genet 2008; 40: 83–89.

Graham RR, Cotsapas C, Davies L, Hackett R, Lessard CJ, Leon JM et al. Genetic variants near TNFAIP3 on 6q23 are associated with systemic lupus erythematosus. Nat Genet 2008; 40: 1059–1061.

Graham RR, Hom G, Ortmann W, Behrens TW. Review of recent genome-wide association scans in lupus. J Intern Med 2009; 265:680–688.

Graham RR, Kozyrev SV, Baechler EC et al. A common haplotype of interferon regulatory factor 5 (IRF5) regulates splicing and expression and is associated with increased risk of systemic lupus erythematosus. Nat Genet 2006;38:550–5.

Gregersen PK, and Olsson LM. Recent advances in the genetics of autoimmune disease. Annu. Rev. Immunol. 2009;27, 363–391.

Gregersen, PK., Lee, HS., Batliwalla, F, Begovich, AB. PTPN22: Setting thresholds for autoimmunity. Sem. Immunol. 2006;18, 214–22.

Grumet FC, Coukell A, Bodmer JG, Bodmer WF, McDevitt HO. Histocompatibility (HL-A) antigens associated with systemic lupus erythematosus. A possible genetic predisposition to disease. N Engl J Med 1971; 285: 193–196.

Gualtierotti R, Biggioggero M, Penatti AE, Meroni PLUpdating on the pathogenesis of systemic lupus erythematosus. Autoimmun Rev. 2010;10(1):3-7.

Guo L, Deshmukh H, Lu R, et al. Replication of the BANK1 genetic association with systemic lupus erythematosus in a European-derived population. Genes Immun 2009; 10: 531–538.

Hagiwara E, Gourley M., Lee S, Klinman DK. Disease severity in patients with systemic lupus erythematosus correlates with an increased ratio of interleukin-10: interferon-γ-secreting cells in the peripheral blood. Arthritis Rheum. 39, 379–385 (1996).

Han S, Kim-Howard X, Deshmukh H, et al. Evaluation of imputation-based association in and around the integrin-alpha-M (ITGAM) gene and replication of robust association between a non-synonymous functional variant within ITGAM and systemic lupus erythematosus (SLE). Hum Mol Genet 2009;18: 1171–1180.

Han J, Zheng H, Cui Y, Sun L, Ye D, Hu Z, Xu J, Cai Z, Huang W, Zhao G, Xie H, Fang H, Lu Q, Xu J, Li X, Pan Y, Deng D, Zeng F, Ye Z, Zhang X, Wang Q, Hao F, Ma L, Zuo X, Zhou F, Du W, Cheng Y, Yang J, Shen S, Li J, Sheng Y, Zuo X, Zhu W, Gao F, Zhang P, Guo Q, Li B, Gao M, Xiao F, Quan C, Zhang C, Zhang Z, Zhu K, Li Y, Hu D, Lu W, Huang J, Liu S, Li H, Ren Y, Wang Z, Yang C, Wang P, Zhou W, Lv Y, Zhang A, Zhang S, Lin D, Li Y, Low H, Shen M, Zhai Z, Wang Y, Zhang F, Yang S, Liu J, Zhang X. Genome-wide association study in a Chinese Han population identifies nine new susceptibility loci for systemic lupus erythematosus. Nat Genet. 2009;41(11):1234-7.

Han JW, Zheng HF, Cui Y, Sun LD, Ye DQ, Hu Z, Xu JH, Cai ZM, Huang W, Zhao GP, Xie HF, Fang H, Lu QJ, Xu JH, Li XP, Pan YF, Deng DQ, Zeng FQ, Ye ZZ, Zhang XY, Wang QW, Hao F, Ma L, Zuo XB, Zhou FS, Du WH, Cheng YL, Yang JQ, Shen SK, Li J, et al: Genome-wide association study in a Chinese Han population identifies nine new susceptibility loci for systemic lupus erythematosus. Nat Genet 2009; 41:1234-1237.

Hardy J, Singleton A. Genomewide association studies and human disease. N Engl J Med 2009; 360: 1759–1768.

Harley JB, Alarcon-Riquelme ME, Criswell LA, Jacob CO, Kimberly RP, Moser KL, et al. Genomewide association scan in women with systemic lupus erythematosus identifies susceptibility variants in ITGAM, PXK, KIAA1542 and other loci. Nat Genet 2008;40(2):204–10.

Harley JB, Moser KL, Gaffney PM, Behrens TW. The genetics of human systemic lupus erythematosus. Curr Opin Immunol 1998; 10: 690–6.

Hatta Y, Tsuchiya N, Ohashi J, Matsushita M, Fujiwara K, Hagiwara K, Juji T, Tokunaga K. Association of Fcγ receptor IIIB, but not of Fcγ receptor IIA and IIIA polymorphisms with systemic lupus erythematosus in Japanese. Genes Immun. 1999;1, 53–60.

Haug BL, Lee JS, Sibley JT. Altered poly-(ADP-ribose) metabolism in family members of patients with systemic lupus erythematosus. J Rheumatol 1994;21:851–856

Hawn TR, Wu H, Grossman JM, Hahn BH, Tsao BP, Aderem A. A stop codon polymorphism of Toll-like receptor 5 is associated with resistance to systemic lupus erythematosus. Proc Natl Acad Sci U S A. 2005;102(30):10593-7.

Hawn, T. R., Verbon, A., Lettinga, K. D., Zhao, L. P., Li, S. S., Laws, R. J., Skerrett, S. J., Beutler, B., Schroeder, L., Nachman, A., et al. J. Exp. Med. 2003;198, 1563–1572.

He CF, Liu YS, Cheng YL, Gao JP, Pan TM, Han JW, Quan C, Sun LD, Zheng HF, Zuo XB, Xu SX, Sheng YJ, Yao S, Hu WL, Li Y, Yu ZY, Yin XY, Zhang XJ, Cui Y, Yang S. TNIP1, SLC15A4, ETS1, RasGRP3 and IKZF1 are associated with clinical features of systemic lupus erythematosus in a Chinese Han population. Lupus. 2010;19(10):1181-6.

Hirschhorn JN. Genomewide association studies–illuminating biologic pathways. N Engl J Med 2009;360: 1699–1701.

Hirst M, and Marra MA. 2009. Epigenetics and human disease. Int. J. Biochem Cell Biol. 41: 136–146.

Hochberg, M. C. Updating the American College of Rheumatology revised criteria for the classification of systemic lupus erythematosus. Arthritis Rheum. 1997;40, 1725.

Holmskov U, Malhotra R, Sim RB, Jensenius JC. Collectins: collagenous C-type lectins of the innate immune defense system. Immunol Today. 1994;15:67–74.

Hom G, Graham RR, Modrek B, Taylor KE, Ortmann W, Garnier S et al. Association of systemic lupus erythematosus with C8orf13-BLK and ITGAM-ITGAX. N Engl J Med. 2008 Feb 28;358(9):900-9.

Hu W, Sun L, Gao J, Li Y, Wang P, Cheng Y, Pan T, Han J, Liu Y, Lu W, Zuo X, Sheng Y, Yao S, He C, Yu Z, Yin X, Cui Y, Yang S, Zhang X. Down-regulated expression of IKZF1 mRNA in peripheral blood mononuclear cells from patients with systemic lupus erythematosus. Rheumatol Int. 2011;31(6):819-22.

Hunnangkul S, Nitsch D, Rhodes B et al. Familial clustering of non-nuclear autoantibodies and C3 and C4 complement components in systemic lupus erythematosus. Arthritis Rheum 2008;58:1116–24.

Hur JW, Sung YK, Shin HD, Park BL, Cheong HS, Bae SC. Poly(ADP-ribose) polymerase (PARP) polymorphisms associated with nephritis and arthritis in systemic lupus erythematosus. Rheumatology (Oxford). 2006;45(6):711-7.

Hwang SY, Cho ML, Park B, et al.,"Allelic frequency of the MCP-1 promoter −2518 polymorphism in the Korean population and in Korean patients with rheumatoid arthritis, systemic lupus erythematosus and adult-onset Still's disease," European Journal of Immunogenetics, vol.29, no.5,(2002) pp.413–416.

International Consortium for Systemic Lupus Erythematosus Genetics (SLEGEN), Harley JB, Alarcón-Riquelme ME, Criswell LA, Jacob CO, Kimberly RP, Moser KL, Tsao BP, Vyse TJ, Langefeld CD, Nath SK, Guthridge JM, Cobb BL, Mirel DB, Marion MC, Williams AH, Divers J, Wang W, Frank SG, Namjou B, Gabriel SB, Lee AT, Gregersen PK, Behrens TW, Taylor KE, Fernando M, Zidovetzki R, Gaffney PM, Edberg JC, Rioux JD, Ojwang JO, James JA, Merrill JT, Gilkeson GS, Seldin MF, Yin H, Baechler EC, Li QZ, Wakeland EK, Bruner GR, Kaufman KM, Kelly JA. Genome-wide association scan in women with systemic lupus erythematosus identifies susceptibility variants in ITGAM, PXK, KIAA1542 and other loci. Nat Genet. 2008;40(2):204-10

International Schizophrenia Consortium. Rare chromosomal deletions and duplications increase risk of schizophrenia. Nature 2008; 455: 237–41.

Ito I, Kawaguchi Y, Kawasaki A, Hasegawa M, Ohashi J, Kawamoto M, Fujimoto M, Takehara K, Sato S, Hara M, Tsuchiya N. Association of the FAM167A-BLK region with systemic sclerosis. Arthritis Rheum. 2010 Mar;62(3):890-5.

Ito T, Wang YH, Duramad O, Hanabuchi S, Perng OA, Gilliet M et al. OX40 ligand shuts down IL-10-producing regulatory T cells. Proc Natl Acad Sci USA 2006a; 103: 13138–13143.

Ito, I. et al. Replication of the association between the C8orf13-BLK region and systemic lupus erythematosus in a Japanese population. Arthritis Rheum. 2009;60, 553–558.

Itoh K, and Hirohata S, The role of IL-10 in human B cell activation, proliferation, and differentiation.J. Immunol. 1995;154, 4341–4350.

Jacob CO, Zhu J, Armstrong DL, Yan M, Han J, et al. Identification of IRAK1 as a risk gene with critical role in the pathogenesis of systemic lupus erythematosus. Proc. Natl Acad. Sci. USA 2009;106, 6256–6261.

Ji JD, Lee WJ, Kong KA, et al. Association of STAT4 polymorphism with rheumatoid arthritis and systemic lupus erythematosus:a meta-analysis. Mol Biol Rep 2010; 37(1): 141-7.

Johanneson B, Lima G, von Salome J, Alarcon-Segovia D, Alarcon-Riquelme ME. A major susceptibility locus for systemic lupus erythematosus maps to chromosome 1q31. Am J Hum Genet 2002;71:1060–1071

Jönsen A, Bengtsson AA, Nived O, Truedsson L, Sturfelt G. Gene-environment interactions in the aetiology of systemic lupus erythematosus. Autoimmunity. 2007;40(8):613-7.

Kallel-Sellami M, Laadhar L, Zerzeri Y, Makni S. Complement deficiency and systemic lupus erythematosus: consensus and dilemma. Expert Rev Clin Immunol. 2008;4(5):629-37.

Karassa FB, Trikalinos TA, Ioannidis JP. Role of the Fcgamma receptor IIa polymorphism in susceptibility to systemic lupus erythematosus and lupus nephritis: a meta-analysis. Arthritis Rheum. 2002;46:1563–1571

Karassa FB, Trikalinos TA, Ioannidis JP. The Fc gamma RIIIA-F158 allele is a risk factor for the development of lupus nephritis: a meta-analysis. Kidney Int 2003;63:1475–82

Kariuki, SN. et al. Cutting edge: autoimmune disease risk variant of STAT4 confers increased sensitivity to IFN-α in lupus patients in vivo. J. Immunol. 2009;182, 34–38.

Kariuki, SN, Crow MK, and Niewold TB. The PTPN22 C1858T polymorphism is associated with skewing of cytokine profiles toward high interferon-α activity and low tumor necrosis factor α levels in patients with lupus. Arthritis Rheum. 2008;58, 2818–23.

Kawasaki, A. et al. Role of STAT4 polymorphisms in systemic lupus erythematosus in a Japanese population: a case-control association study of the STAT1-STAT4 region. Arthritis Res Ther. 2008;10(5):R113.

Kelley VR and Rovin BH, "Chemokines: therapeutic targets for autoimmune and inflammatory renal disease," Springer Seminars in Immunopathology, vol. 24, no. 4, (2003) pp. 411–421.

Kevil CG, Hicks MJ, He X, Zhang J, Ballantyne CM and Raman C et al., Loss of LFA-1, but not Mac-1, protects MRL/MpJ-Fas(lpr) mice from autoimmune disease, Am J Pathol 165 (2004), pp. 609–616.

Kim EM, Bang SY, Kim I, Shin HD, Park BL, Lee HS, Bae SC. Different genetic effect of PXK on systemic lupus erythematosus in the Korean population. Rheumatol Int. 2011 Jan 18. [Epub ahead of print]

Kim HL, Lee DS, Yang SH, et al., "The polymorphism of monocyte chemoattractant protein-1 is associated with the renal disease of SLE," American Journal of Kidney Diseases, vol. 40, no. 6, (2002) pp. 1146–1152.

Kim I, Kim YJ, Kim K, et al. Genetic studies of systemic lupus erythematosus in Asia: where are we now? Genes Immun 2009; 10: 421–432.

Kim I, Kim YJ, Kim K, Kang C, Choi CB, Sung YK, Lee HS, Bae SC.. Genetic studies of systemic lupus erythematosus in Asia: where are we now? Genes Immun 2009; 10:421–432.

Kim J, Modlin RL, Moy RL, Dubinett SM, McHugh T, Nickloff BJ and Uyemura K. IL-10 production in cutaneous basal and squamous cell carcinomas. A mechanism for evading the local T cell immune response. J. Immunol. 1995;155, 2240–47.

Kobata T, Jacquot S, Kozlowski S, Agematsu K, Schlossman SF and Morimoto C, CD27–CD70 interactions regulate B-cell activation by T cells, Proc Natl Acad Sci U S A 92 (1995), pp. 11249–11253.

Kobayashi T, Ito S, Yasuda K, Kuroda T, Yamamoto K, Sugita N, Tai H, Narita I, Gejyo F, Yoshie H. The combined genotypes of stimulatory and inhibitory Fc gamma receptors associated with systemic lupus erythematosus and periodontitis in Japanese adults. J Periodontol. 2007;78(3):467-74.

Kochi Y, Suzuki A, Yamada R, Yamamoto K. Genetics of rheumatoid arthritis: underlying evidence of ethnic differences. J Autoimmun 2009; 32: 158–162.

Koene HR, Kleijer M, Roos D, de Hasse M and Von dem Borne AE, FcγRIIIB gene duplication: evidence for presence and expression of three distinct FcγRIIIB genes in NA(1+,2+)SH(+) individuals. Blood 1998;91, 673–679.

Koene, H. R. et al. The FcγRIIIA-158F allele is a risk factor for systemic lupus erythematosus. Arthritis Rheum. 1998;41,1813–1818.

Korb LC, Ahearn JM. C1q binds directly and specifically to surface blebs of apoptotic human keratinocytes: complement deficiency and systemic lupus erythematosus revisited. J Immunol 1997;158:4525–8.

Kozyrev SV, Abelson AK, Wojcik J, Zaghlool A, Reddy MV Linga, Sanchez E, et al. Functional variants in the B-cell gene BANK1 are associated with systemic lupus erythematosus. Nat Genet. 2008;40(2):211–216.

Krauss JC, PooH, Xue W, Mayo-Bond L, Todd RF III, Petty HR. Reconstitution of antibody-dependent phagocytosis in fibroblasts expressing Fc gamma receptor IIIB and the complement receptor type 3. J Immunol 1994;153:1769–77.

Ku CS, Loy EY, Salim A, Pawitan Y, Chia KS. The discovery of human genetic variations and their use as disease markers: past, present and future. J Hum Genet. 2010;55(7):403-15.

Kyogoku C, Dijstelbloem HM, Tsuchiya N, Hatta Y, Kato H, Yamaguchi A, Fukazawa T, Jansen MD, Hashimoto H, van de Winkel JG, Kallenberg CG, Tokunaga K. Fcγ receptor gene polymorphisms in Japanese patients with systemic lupus erythematosus: contribution of FCGR2B to genetic susceptibility. Arthritis Rheum. 2002;46, 1242–1254.

Kyogoku C, Morinobu A, Nishimura K, Sugiyama D, Hashimoto H, Tokano Y, Mimori T, Terao C, Matsuda F, Kuno T, Kumagai S. Lack of association between tyrosine kinase 2 (TYK2) gene polymorphisms and susceptibility to SLE in a Japanese population. Mod Rheumatol. 2009;19(4):401-6.

Kyogoku C., Tsuchiya N., wu H., Tsao BP and Tokunaga K. Association of Fcγ receptor IIA, but not IIB and IIIA, polymorphisms with systemic lupus erythematosus: a family-based association study in Caucasians. Arthritis Rheum. 2004;50, 671–673.

L.R. Finger, J. Pu, R. Wasserman, R. Vibhakar, E. Louie, R.R. Hardy et al. The human PD-1 gene: complete cDNA, genomic organization, and developmentally regulated expression in B cell progenitors. Gene 197 (1997) pp. 177–187.

Lane P. Role of OX40 signals in coordinating CD4T cell selection, migration, and cytokine differentiation in T helper (Th)1 and Th2 cells. J Exp Med 2000;191:201–6.

Lawrie CH, Saunders NJ, Soneji S, Palazzo S, Dunlop HM, Cooper CD, Brown PJ, Troussard X, Mossafa H, Enver T, Pezzella F, Boultwood J, Wainscoat JS, Hatton CS. MicroRNA expression in lymphocyte development and malignancy. Leukemia 2008;22:1440–1446.

Le Bon A, Schiavoni G, D'Agostino G, Gresser I, Belardelli F, Tough DF. Type I interferons potently enhance humoral immunity and can promote isotype switching by stimulating dendritic cells in vivo. Immunity 2001;14:461–70.

Lea WW, Lee YH. The association between the PTPN22 C1858T polymorphism and systemic lupus erythematosus: a meta-analysis update. Lupus. 2011;20(1):51-7.

Lee YH, Harley JB, Nath SK. CTLA-4 polymorphisms and systemic lupus erythematosus (SLE): a meta-analysis. Hum Genet 2005; 116: 361–367.

Lee YH, Song GG. Association between the rs2004640 functional polymorphism of interferon regulatory factor 5 and systemic lupus erythematosus: a meta-analysis. Rheumatol Int 2009; 29:1137–1142.

Lehrnbecher T, Foster CB, Zhu S, et al. (1999a) Variant genotypes of the low-affinity Fcgamma receptors in two control populations and a review of low-affinity Fcgamma receptor polymorphisms in control and disease populations. Blood 94 (12), 4220–32.

Li J, Li L, Shang X, Benson J, Merle Elloso M, Schantz A et al. Negative regulation of IL-17 production by OX40/OX40L interaction. Cell Immunol 2008; 253: 31–37.

Li X, Wu J, Carter RH, Edberg JC, Su K, Cooper GS, Kimberly RP. A novel polymorphism in the Fcγ receptor IIB (CD32B) transmembrane region alters receptor signaling. Arthritis Rheum. 2003;48, 3242–3252.

Liao CH, Yao TC, Chung HT, See LC, Kuo ML and Huang JL. "Polymorphisms in the promoterregion of RANTES and the regulatory region of monocyte chemoattractant protein-1 among Chinese children with systemic lupus erythematosus," Journal of Rheumatology, vol. 31, no. 10, (2004) pp. 2062–2067.

Liossis SN, Solomou EE, Dimopoulos MA, Panayiotidis P, Mavrikakis MM, Sfikakis PP. B-cell kinase lyn deficiency in patients with systemic lupus erythematosus. J Investig Med. 2001; 49(2):157–65.

Liu MF, Wang CR, Lin LC, Wu CR. CTLA-4 gene polymorphism in promoter and exon-1 regions in Chinese patients with systemic lupus erythematosus. Lupus 2001; 10: 647–649.

Llorente L, Zou W, Levy Y, Richaud-Patin Y, Wijdenes Y, Alcocer-Varela J, Morel-Fourrier B, Brouet J., Alarcon-Segovia D, Galanaud P. et al. Role of interleukin 10 in the B lymphocyte hyperactivity and autoantibody production of human systemic lupus erythematosus. J. Exp. Med. 1995;181, 839–844.

Llorente L., Richaud-Patin Y., Fior R., Alcocer-Varela J., Wijdnes J., Morel-Fourrier B., Galanaud P. & Emilie P. In vivo production of interleukin-10 by non-T cells in rheumatoid arthritis, Sjögren's syndrome, and systemic lupus erythematosus. A potential mechanism of B lymphocyte hyperactivity and autoimmunity.Arthritis Rheum. 1994;37, 1647–1655.

Lodish HF, Zhou B, Liu G, Chen CZ. Micromanagement of the immune system by microRNAs. Nat Rev Immunol 2008;8:120–30.

Lopez P, Mozo L, Gutierrez C, Suarez A. Epidemiology of systemic lupus erythematosus in a northern Spanish population: gender and age influence on immunological features. Lupus 2003;12:860-865.

Lu Q, Kaplan M, Ray D, Ray D, Zacharek S and Gutsch D et al., Demethylation of ITGAL (CD11a) regulatory sequences in systemic lupus erythematosus, Arthritis Rheum 46 (2002), pp. 1282–1291.

Lu Q, Wu A and Richardson BC, Demethylation of the same promoter sequence increases CD70 expression in lupus T cells and T cells treated with lupus-inducing drugs, J Immunol 174 (2005), pp. 6212–6219.

Luscher U, Filgueira L, Juretic A, Zuber M, Luscher L, Heberer M and Spagnoli GC. The pattern of cytokine gene expression in freshly excised human metastatic melanoma suggests a state of reversible anergy of tumor-infiltrating lymphocytes.Int. J. Cancer 1994;57, 612–619.

Magnusson V, Johanneson B, Lima G, Odeberg J, Alarcon- Segovia D, Alarcon-Riquelme ME, SLE Genetics Collaboration Group. Both risk alleles for FcgammaRIIA and FcgammaRIIIA are susceptibility factors for SLE: a unifying hypothesis. Genes Immun 2004;5:130–137

Magnusson V, Zunec R, Odeberg J, Sturfelt G, Truedsson L, Gunnarsson I, Alarcón-Riquelme ME.. Polymorphisms of the Fcγ receptor type IIB gene are not associated with systemic lupus erythematosus in the Swedish population. Arthritis Rheum. 2004;50(4):1348-50.

Mao, H., Ferguson, T. S., Cibulsky, S. M., Holmqvist, M., Ding, C., Fei, H., Levitan, I. B. MONaKA, a novel modulator of the plasma membrane Na,K-ATPase. J. Neurosci. 2005;25: 7934-7943.

Marrack P, Kappler J, Mitchell T. Type I interferons keep activated T cells alive. J Exp Med 1999;189:521–30.

Matsuda M, Salazar F, Petersson M, Masucci G, Hansson J, Pisa, Zhang, QC, Masucci MG and Kiessling R. Interleukin 10 pretreatment protects target cells from tumor- and allo-specific cytotoxic T cells and downregulates HLA class I expression.J. Exp. Med. 1994;180, 2371–2376.

Matsushita M, Tsuchiya N, Shiota M, et al. Lack of a strong association of CTLA-4 exon 1 polymorphism with the susceptibility to rheumatoid arthritis and systemic lupus erythematosus in Japanese: an association study using a novel variation screening method. Tissue Antigens 1999; 54: 578–584.

Mehrian, R. et al. Synergistic effect between IL-10 and bcl-2 genotypes in determining susceptibility to SLE. Arthritis Rheum. 1998;41, 596–602.

Minegishi Y, Saito M, Morio T, Watanabe K, Agematsu K, Tsuchiya S, Takada H, Hara T, Kawamura N, Ariga T, Kaneko H, Kondo N, Tsuge I, Yachie A, Sakiyama Y, Iwata T, Bessho F, Ohishi T, Joh K, Imai K, Kogawa K, Shinohara M, Fujieda M, Wakiguchi H, Pasic S, Abinun M, Ochs HD, Renner ED, Jansson A, Belohradsky BH, et al.: Human tyrosine kinase 2 deficiency reveals its requisite roles in multiple cytokine signals involved in innate and acquired immunity. Immunity 2006;25:745-755

Morinobu A, Gadina M, Strober W et al. STAT4 serine phosphorylation is critical for IL-12-induced IFN-gamma production but not for cell proliferation. Proc Natl Acad Sci USA 2002;99:12281-6.

Mosmann, T. R. Properties and functions of interleukin-10. Adv. Immunol. 1994;56, 1–26.

Mostowska M, Wudarski M, Chwalińska-Sadowska H, Jagodziński PP. The programmed cell death 1 gene 7209 C>T polymorphism is associated with the risk of systemic lupus erythematosus in the Polish population. Clin Exp Rheumatol. 2008;26(3):457-60.

Musone SL, et al. Multiple polymorphisms in the TNFAIP3 region are independently associated with systemic lupus erythematosus. Nat Genet. 2008; 40:1062–4

Namjou B, Nath SK, Kilpatrick J et al. Genome scan stratified by the presence of anti-double-stranded DNA (dsDNA) autoantibody in pedigrees multiplex for systemic lupus erythematosus (SLE) establishes linkages at 19p13.2 (SLED1) and 18q21.1 (SLED2). Genes Immun 2002;3(Suppl 1):S35–S41

Namjou B, Sestak AL, Armstrong DL, et al. High-density genotyping of STAT4 reveals multiple haplotypic associations with systemic lupus erythematosus in different racial groups. Arthritis Rheum 2009; 60: 1085–1095.

Napirei M, Karsunky H, Zevnik B, Stephan H, Mannherz HG, Mo'ro'y T. Features of systemic lupus erythematosus in Dnase 1-deficient mice. Nature Genet 2000;25:177–81.

Nath SK, Han S, Kim-Howard X, et al. A nonsynonymous functional variant in integrin-alpha(M) (encoded by ITGAM) is associated with systemic lupus erythematosus. Nat Genet 2008; 40:152–154.

Nath SK, Harley JB, Lee YH. Polymorphisms of complement receptor 1 and interleukin-10 genes and systemic lupus erythematosus: a meta-analysis. Hum Genet 2005;118(2):225–234

Nguyen KB, Watford WT, Salomon R et al. Critical role for STAT4 activation by type 1 interferons in the interferon-gamma response to viral infection. Science 2002;297:2063-6.

Niewold TB, Kelly JA, Flesch MH, Espinoza LR, Harley JB, Crow MK. Association of the IRF5 risk haplotype with high serum interferon-alpha activity in systemic lupus erythematosus patients. Arthritis Rheum. 2008;58(8):2481-7.

Nimmerjahn F, Ravetch J Fcgamma receptors as regulators of immune responses. Nat Rev Immunol. 2008;8(1):34-47.

Nishikomori R, Usui T, Wu CY, Morinobu A, O'Shea JJ, Strober W. Activated STAT4 has an essential role in Th1 differentiation and proliferation that is independent of its role in the maintenance of IL-12R beta 2 chain expression and signaling. J Immunol 2002;169:4388–98.

O. Avni and A. Rao, T cell differentiation: a mechanistic view. Curr Opin Immunol 12 (2000), pp. 654–659.

O'Connell RM, Rao DS, Chaudhuri AA, Baltimore D. Physiological and pathological roles for microRNAs in the immune system. Nat Rev Immunol 2010;10:111–22.

Oei SL, Shi Y. Poly(ADP-ribosyl)ation of transcription factor Yin Yang 1 under conditions of DNA damage. Biochem Biophys Res Commun 2001;285:27–31

Ogden CA, deCathelineau A, Hoffmann PR, Bratton D, Ghebrehiwet B, Fadok VA, et al. C1q and mannose binding lectin engagement of cell surface calreticulin and CD91 initiates macropinocytosis and uptake of apoptotic cells. J Exp Med 2001;194:781–95.

Okada M, Ogasawara H, Kaneko H, Hishikawa T, Sekigawa I, Hashimoto H, et al. Role of DNA methylation in transcription of human endogenous retrovirus in the pathogenesis of systemic lupus erythematosus. J Rheumatol 2002;29:1678–82.

Oliver FJ, Menissier-de Murcia J, de Murcia G. Poly(ADPribose) polymerase in the cellular response to DNA damage, apoptosis, and disease. Am J Hum Genet 1999;64:1282–1288

Orozco G, Sánchez E, González-Gay MA, López-Nevot MA, Torres B, Cáliz R, Ortego-Centeno N, Jiménez-Alonso J, Pascual-Salcedo D, Balsa A, de Pablo R, Nuñez-Roldan A, González-Escribano MF, Martín J. Association of a functional single-nucleotide polymorphism of PTPN22, encoding lymphoid protein phosphatase, with rheumatoid arthritis and systemic lupus erythematosus. Arthritis Rheum. 2005;52(1):219-24.

Orru V, Tsai SJ, Rueda B, Fiorillo E, Stanford SM, Dasgupta J. A loss-of-function variant of PTPN22 is associated with reduced risk of systemic lupus erythematosus. Hum. Mol. Genet. 2009;18, 569–579.

Oshima S, Turer EE, Callahan JA, Chai S, Advincula R, Barrera J, Shifrin N, Lee B, Benedict Yen TS, Woo T, Malynn BA, Ma A: ABIN-1 is a ubiquitin sensor that restricts cell death and sustains embryonic development. Nature 2009; 457:906-909.

Pan F, Tang X, Zhang K, Li X, Xu J, Chen H, Ye DQ. Genetic susceptibility and haplotype analysis between Fcgamma receptor IIB and IIIA gene with systemic lupus erythematosus in Chinese population. Lupus. 2008;17(8):733-8.

Pan HF, Leng RX, Wang C, Qin WZ, Chen LL, Zha ZQ, Tao JH, Ye DQ. Association of TNF-α promoter-308 A/G polymorphism with susceptibility to systemic lupus erythematosus: a meta-analysis. Rheumatol Int. 2011 Apr 16 [Epub ahead of print].

Pan Y, Sawalha AH. Epigenetic regulation and the pathogenesis of systemic lupus erythematosus. Transl Res 2009;153:4–10 .

Parren PW, Warmerdam PA, Boeije LC, et al. On the interaction of IgG subclasses with the low affinity Fc gamma RIIa (CD32) on human monocytes, neutrophils, and platelets. Analysis of a functional polymorphism to human IgG2. J Clin Invest 1992a;90 (4), 1537–46.

Parren PW, PA, Boeije LC, Capel PJ, van de Winkel JG, Aarden LA. Characterization of IgG FcR-mediated proliferation of human T cells induced by mouse and human anti-

CD3 monoclonal antibodies. Identification of a functional polymorphism to human IgG2 anti-CD3. J Immunol 1992b;148 (3), 695–701.

Pauley KM, Cha S, Chan EK. microRNA in autoimmunity and autoimmune diseases. J Autoimmun 2009;32:189–94.

Perez, L., Orte, J. and Brieva, J. A. Terminal differentiation of spontaneous rheumatoid factor-secreting B cells from rheumatoid arthritis patients depends on endogenous interleukin-10. Arthritis Rheum. 1995;38, 1771–1776.

Plenge RM, et al. Two independent alleles at 6q23 associated with risk of rheumatoid arthritis. Nat Genet. 2007; 39:1477–82.

Plenge RM. Recent progress in rheumatoid arthritis genetics: one step towards improved patient care. Curr Opin Rheumatol 2009; 21:262–271.

Poo H, Krauss JC, Mayo-Bond L, Todd RF III, Petty HR. Interaction of Fc gamma receptor type IIIB with complement receptor type 3 in fibroblast transfectants: evidence from lateral diffusion and resonance energy transfer studies. J Mol Biol 1995;247:597–603.

Pradhan V, Surve P, Ghosh K.Mannose binding lectin (MBL) in autoimmunity and its role in systemic lupus erythematosus (SLE). J Assoc Physicians India. 2010;58:688-90.

Prokunina L, Castillejo-López C, Oberg F, Gunnarsson I, Berg L, Magnusson V, Brookes AJ, Tentler D, Kristjansdóttir H, Gröndal G, Bolstad AI, Svenungsson E, Lundberg I, Sturfelt G, Jönssen A, Truedsson L, Lima G, Alcocer-Varela J, Jonsson R, Gyllensten UB, Harley JB, Alarcón-Segovia D, Steinsson K, Alarcón-Riquelme ME. A regulatory polymorphism in PDCD1 is associated with susceptibility to systemic lupus erythematosus in humans. Nat Genet. 2002;32(4):666-9.

Qiao JY, Shao W, Wei HJ, Sun YM, Zhao YC and Xing WL et al., Novel high-throughput profiling of human transcription factors and its use for systematic pathway mapping, J Proteome Res 7 (2008), pp. 2769–2779.

Ramasawmy R, Spina GS, Fae KC, Pereira AC, Nisihara R, Reason IJM, Grinberg M, Tarasoutchi F, Kalil J, and Guilherme L. Association of Mannose-Binding Lectin Gene Polymorphism but Not of Mannose Binding Serine Protease 2 with Chronic Severe Aortic Regurgitation of Rheumatic Etiology. Clin and vacc Immunol 2008;932–936.

Ramos PS, Kelly JA, Gray-McGuire C et al. Familial aggregation and linkage analysis of autoantibody traits in pedigrees multiplex for systemic lupus erythematosus. Genes Immun 2006;7:417–32.

Remmers EF, Plenge RM, Lee AT et al. STAT4 and the risk of rheumatoid arthritis and systemic lupus erythematosus. N Engl J Med 2007;357:977–86.

Reth, M. & wienands, J. Initiation and processing of signals from the B cell antigen receptor. Annu Rev. Immunol. 1997;15, 453–479.

Richardson B. Primer: epigenetics of autoimmunity. Nat Clin Pract Rheumatol 2007;3:521-7.

Richardson BC, Liebling MR and Hudson JL, CD4+ cells treated with DNA methylation inhibitors induce autologous B cell differentiation, Clin Immunol Immunopathol 55 (1990), pp. 368–381.

Richter MF, Dumenil G, Uze G, Fellous M, Pellegrini S. Specific contribution of Tyk2 JH regions to the binding and the expression of the interferon alpha/beta receptor component IFNAR1. J Biol Chem 1998;273:24723–9.

Rodriguez W, Mold C, Kataranovski M, Hutt J, Marnell LL, Du Clos TW. Reversal of ongoing proteinuria in autoimmune mice by treatment with C-reactive protein. Arthritis Rheum 2005;52:642–650

Ronnblom L. Alm GV. Systemic lupus erythematosus and the type I interferon system. Arthritis Res Ther 2003;5:68–75.

Rovin BH and Phan LT, "Chemotactic factors and renal inflammation," American Journal of Kidney Diseases, vol. 31, no. 6, pp. 1065–1084, 1998.

Rovin BH, Doe N, and Tan LC, "Monocyte chemoattractant protein-1 levels in patients with glomerular disease," American Journal of Kidney Diseases, vol.27,no.5,(1996) pp. 640–646.

Rovin BH, Song H, Birmingham DJ, Hebert LA, Yu CY, Nagaraja HN: Urine chemokines as biomarkers of human systemic lupus erythematosus activity. J Am Soc Nephrol 2005;16(2):467-473.

Russell AI, Cunninghame Graham DS, Shepherd C, Roberton CA, Whittaker J, Meeks J, Powell RJ, Isenberg DA, Walport MJ, Vyse TJ. Polymorphism at the C-reactive protein locus influences gene expression and predisposes to systemic lupus erythematosus. Hum Mol Genet. 2004; 1;13(1):137-47.

Saitoh A, Suzuki Y, Takeda M, Kubota K, Itoh K, and Tomino Y, "Urinary levels of monocyte chemoattractant protein (MCP)-1 and disease activity in patients with IgA nephropathy," Journal of Clinical Laboratory Analysis, vol. 12, no. 1, (1998) pp. 1–5.

Salloum R, Franek B, Kariuki S, Utset T, Niewold T. Genetic Variation at the IRF7/KIAA1542 Locus is Associated with Autoantibody Profile and Serum Interferon Alpha Levels in Lupus Patients Clinical Immunology (2009), 131, Supplement, pg. S54-S54

Salmon JE, Millard S, Schachter LA, Arnett FC, Ginzler EM, Gourley MF, Ramsey-Goldman R, Peterson MG, Kimberly RP. Fcγ RIIA alleles are heritable risk factors for lupus nephritis in African Americans. J. Clin. Invest. 1996;97, 1348-1354.

Savarese E, Steinberg C, Pawar RD. et al., "Requirement of Toll-like receptor 7 for pristane-induced production of autoantibodies and development of murine lupus nephritis," Arthritis and Rheumatism, vol. 58, no. 4, (2008) pp. 1107–1115.

Schifferli JA, Steiger G, Paccaud JP, Sjoholm AG, Hauptmann G. Difference in the biological properties of the two forms of the fourth component of human complement (C4). Clin Exp Immunol 1986;63:473-7.

Sebat J, Lakshmi B, Malhotra D et al. Strong association of de novo copy number mutations with autism. Science 2007; 316: 445-9.

Selbach M, Schwanhausser B, Thierfelder N, Fang Z, Khanin R, Rajewsky N. Widespread changes in protein synthesis induced by microRNAs. Nature 2008;455:58–63.

Sestak AL, Fürnrohr BG, Harley JB, Merrill JT, Namjou B. The genetics of systemic lupus erythematosus and implications for targeted therapy. Ann Rheum Dis. 2011;70 Suppl 1:I37-43.

Shimaoka M and Springer TA. Therapeutic antagonists and conformational regulation of integrin function, Nat Rev Drug Discov 2 (2003), pp. 703–716.

Shimizu S, Nakashima H, Masutani K, et al. Anti-monocyte chemoattractant protein-1 gene therapy attenuates nephritis in MRL/lpr mice. Rheumatology (Oxford). 2004;43(9):1121-8.

Shin HD, Park BL, Kim LH, Lee HS, Kim TY, Bae SC. Common DNase I polymorphism associated with autoantibody production among systemic lupus erythematosus patients. Hum Mol Genet 2004;13:2343–50.

Sigurdsson S, Göring HH, Kristjansdottir G, Milani L, Nordmark G, Sandling JK, Eloranta ML, Feng D, Sangster-Guity N, Gunnarsson I, Svenungsson E, Sturfelt G, Jönsen A, Truedsson L, Barnes BJ, Alm G, Rönnblom L, Syvänen AC. Comprehensive evaluation of the genetic variants of interferon regulatory factor 5 (IRF5) reveals a novel 5 bp length polymorphism as strong risk factor for systemic lupus erythematosus. Hum Mol Genet. 2008;17(6):872-81.

Sigurdsson S, Nordmark G, Göring HH, Lindroos K, Wiman AC, Sturfelt G, Jönsen A, Rantapää-Dahlqvist S, Möller B, Kere J, Koskenmies S, Widén E, Eloranta ML, Julkunen H, Kristjansdottir H, Steinsson K, Alm G, Rönnblom L, Syvänen AC: Polymorphisms in the tyrosine kinase 2 and interferon regulatory factor 5 genes are associated with systemic lupus erythematosus. Am J Hum Genet 2005;76:528-537.

Sigurdsson, S. et al. A risk haplotype of STAT4 for systemic lupus erythematosus is overexpressed, correlates with anti-dsDNA and shows additive effects with two risk alleles of IRF5. Hum. Mol. Genet. 2008;17, 2868–2876.

Siriboonrit U, Tsuchiya N, Sirikong M, Kyogoku C, Bejrachandra S, Suthipinittharm P, Luangtrakool K, Srinak D, Thongpradit R, Fujiwara K, Chandanayingyong D, Tokunaga K. Association of Fcgamma receptor IIb and IIIb polymorphisms with susceptibility to systemic lupus erythematosus in Thais. Tissue Antigens. 2003;61(5):374-83.

Song Y, Han CW, Kang SW, Baek HJ, Lee EB, Shin CH, Hahn BH, Tsao BP. Abnormal distribution of Fcγ receptor type IIa polymorphisms in Korean patients with systemic lupus erythematous. Arthritis Rheum. 1998;41(3):421-6.

Sonkoly E, Stahle M, Pivarcsi A. microRNAs and immunity: novel players in the regulation of normal immune function and inflammation. Semin Cancer Biol 2008;18:131–40.

Stahl RA, Thaiss F, Disser M, Helmchen U, Hora K, and Schl"ondorff D, "Increased expression of monocyte chemoattractant protein-1 in anti-thymocyte antibodyinduced glomerulonephriti," Kidney International, vol. 44, no. 5, (1993) pp. 1036–1047,.

Stockl J, Majdic O, Pickl WF et al. Granulocyte activation via a binding site near the C-terminal region of complement receptor type 3 alpha-chain (CD11b) potentially involved in intramembrane complex formation with glycosylphosphatidylinositolanchored Fc gamma RIIIB (CD16) molecules. J Immunol 1995;154:5452–63.

Stuber E, Neurath M, Calderhead D, Fell HP, Strober W. Cross-linking of OX40 ligand, a member of the TNF/NGF cytokine family, induces proliferation and differentiation in murine splenic B cells. Immunity 1995;2:507–21.

Stuber E, Strober W. The T cell-B cell interaction via OX40-OX40L is necessary for the T cell-dependent humoral immune response. J Exp Med 1996;183:979–89.

Su K, Wu J, Edberg JC et al. A promoter haplotype of the immunoreceptor tyrosine-based inhibitory motif-bearing FcgammaRIIb alters receptor expression and associates with autoimmunity. I. Regulatory FCGR2B polymorphisms and their association with systemic lupus erythematosus. J Immunol 2004;172:7186–7191

Suarez-Gestal M, Calaza M, Endreffy E, Pullmann R, Ordi-Ros J, Sebastiani GD, Ruzickova S, Jose Santos M, Papasteriades C, Marchini M, Skopouli FN, Suarez A, Blanco FJ, D'Alfonso S, Bijl M, Carreira P, Witte T, Migliaresi S, Gomez-Reino JJ, Gonzalez A. Replication of recently identified systemic lupus erythematosus genetic associations: a case-control study.European Consortium of SLE DNA Collections. Arthritis Res Ther. 2009;11(3): R69.

Sullivan, K. E. et al. Analysis of polymorphisms affecting immune complex handling in systemic lupus erythematosus. Rheumatology (Oxford) 2003;42, 446–452 ().

Suzuki T, Tahara H, Narula S, Moore KW, Robbins PD and Lotze MT. Viral interleukin 10 (IL-10), the human herpes virus 4 cellular IL-10 homologue, induces local anergy to allogeneic and syngeneic tumors. J. Exp. Med. 1995;182, 447–486.

Taganov KD, Boldin MP, Baltimore D. microRNAs and immunity:tiny players in a big field. Immunity 2007;26:133–7.

Takahashi R, Tsutsumi A, Ohtani K, Muraki Y, Goto D, Matsumoto I, Wakamiya N, Sumida T Association of mannose binding lectin (MBL) gene polymorphism and serum MBL concentration with characteristics and progression of systemic lupus erythematosus Ann Rheum Dis 2005;64:311–314

Takaoka A, Yanai H, Kondo S et al. Integral role of IRF-5 in the gene induction programme activated by Toll-like receptors. Nature 2005;434:243–249

Tan, E. M. Cohen AS, Fries JF, Masi AT, McShane DJ, Rothfield NF, Schaller JG, Talal N, Winchester RJ. The 1982 revised criteria for the classification of systemic lupus erythematosus. Arthritis Rheum. 1982;25,1271–1277.

Tang Y, Luo X, Cui H, Ni X, Yuan M, Guo Y, et al. MicroRNA-146a contributes to abnormal activation of the type I interferon pathway in human lupus by targeting the key signaling proteins. Arthritis Rheum 2009;60:1065–75.

Taylor, K. E. et al. Specificity of the STAT4 genetic association for severe disease manifestations of systemic lupus erythematosus. PLoS Genet. 2008;4(5):e1000084.

Tesar V, Masek Z, Rychlik I, et al. Cytokines and adhesion molecules in renal vasculitis and lupus nephritis. Nephrol Dial Transplant. 1998;13(7):1662-7.

Thomson W, et al. Rheumatoid arthritis association at 6q23. Nat Genet. 2007; 39:1431–3.

Tian C, Gregersen PK, Seldin MF. Accounting for ancestry: population substructure and genome-wide association studies. Hum Mol Genet 2008;17: R143–R150.

Tsao BP, Cantor RM, Grossman JM et al. PARP alleles within the linked chromosomal region are associated with systemic lupus erythematosus. J Clin Invest 1999;103:1135–1140

Tsao BP, Cantor RM, Grossman JM, Shen N, Teophilov NT, Wallace DJ, Arnett FC, Hartung K, Goldstein R, Kalunian KC, Hahn BH, Rotter JI. PARP alleles within the linked chromosomal region are associated with systemic lupus erythematosus. J Clin Invest 1999;103:1135–1140

Tsao BP, Cantor RM, Kalunian KC et al. Evidence for linkage of a candidate chromosome 1 region to human systemic lupus erythematosus. J Clin Invest 1997;99:725–731.

Tsao BP. Genetic susceptibility to lupus nephritis Lupus 1998;7, 585-590

Tsao BP. Lupus susceptibility genes on human chromosome 1. Int Rev Immunol. 2000;19(4-5):319-34.

Tsao BP. Update on human systemic lupus erythematosus genetics. Curr Opin Rheumatol 2004;16:513–521

Tsao, BP.; Wu, H. The genetics of human lupus. In: Wallace, LC.; Hahn, BH., editors. Dubois' Lupus Erythematosus. Vol. Seventh ed.. Philadeiphia: Lippincott Williams & Wilkins; 2008. p. 54-81.

Tsokos GC (2001; Dec) Systemic lupus erythematosus. A disease with a complex pathogenesis. Lancet 358 (Suppl),S65.

Tsuchiya N, Kyogoku C. Role of Fc gamma receptor IIb polymorphism in the genetic background of systemic lupus erythematosus: insights from Asia. Autoimmunity. 2005;38(5):347-52.

Tucci M, Barnes E.V, Sobel ES, et al., "Strong association of a functional polymorphism in the monocyte chemoattractant protein 1 promoter gene with lupus nephritis," Arthritis and Rheumatism, vol. 50, no. 6, (2004) pp. 1842-1849,.

Turner DM, Williams DM, Sankaran D, Lazarus M, Sinnott PJ, Hutchinson IV. An investigation of polymorphism in the interleukin-10 gene promoter. Eur J Immunogenet 1997;24:1-8

Ueda H, Howson JM, Esposito L et al. Association of the T-cell regulatory gene CTLA4 with susceptibility to autoimmune disease. Nature 2003;423:506-511

van der Linden MW, van der Slik AR, Zanelli E et al. Six microsatellite markers on the short arm of chromosome 6 in relation to HLA-DR3 and TNF-308A in systemic lupus erythematosus. Genes Immun 2001;2:373-380

Vang T, Congia M, Macis MD et al. Autoimmune-associated lymphoid tyrosine phosphatase is a gain-of-function variant. Nat Genet 2005;37:1317-9.

Vang T, Miletic AV, Arimura Y, Tautz L, Rickert RC, Mustelin T. Protein tyrosine phosphatases in autoimmunity. Annu Rev Immunol 2008;26:29–55.

Verstrepen L, Carpentier I, Verhelst K, Beyaert R: ABINs: A20 binding inhibitors of NF-_B and apoptosis signaling. Biochem Pharmacol 2009, 78:105-114.

Vollmer J, Tluk S, Schmitz C, Hamm S, Jurk M, Forsbach A, Akira S, Kelly KM, Reeves WH, Bauer S, and Krieg AM. Immune stimulation mediated by autoantigen binding sites within small nuclear RNAs involves Toll-like receptors 7 and 8. J. Exp. Med. 2005;202: 1575–1585.

Warmerdam PA, van de Winkel JG, Vlug A, Westerdaal NA, Capel PJ. A single amino acid in the second Ig-like domain of the human Fc gamma receptor II is critical for human IgG2 binding. J Immunol 1991;147 (4),n1338–43.

Watford WT, Hissong BD, Bream JH, Kanno Y, Muul L, O'Shea JJ. Signaling by IL-12 and IL-23 and the immunoregulatory roles of STAT4. Immunol Rev 2004;202:139-56.

Webb R, Wren JD, Jeffries M, et al. Variants within MECP2, a key transcription regulator, are associated with increased susceptibility to lupus and differential gene expression in patients with systemic lupus erythematosus. Arthritis Rheum 2009; 60: 1076 – 84 .

Westendorp RG, Langermans JA, Huizinga TW, Verweij CL, Sturk A. Genetic influence on cytokine production in meningococcal disease. Lancet. 1997;349(9069):1912-3.

Wilson JG, Murphy EE, Wong WW, Klickstein LB, Weis JH, Fearon DT. Identification of a restriction fragment length polymorphism by a CR1 cDNA that correlates with the number of CR1 on erythrocytes. J Exp Med. 1986 Jul 1;164(1):50-9.

Wojcik H, GriYths E, Staggs S, Hagman J, Winandy S. Expression of a non-DNA-binding Ikaros isoform exclusively in B cells leads to autoimmunity but not leukemogenesis. Eur J Immunol 2007;37:1022-1032.

Wong WW, Cahill JM, Rosen MD, Kennedy CA, Bonaccio ET, Morris MJ, Wilson JG, Klickstein LB, Fearon DT. Structure of the human CR1 gene. Molecular basis of the structural and quantitative polymorphisms and identification of a new CR1-like allele. J Exp Med 1989;169:847–863

Wong WW, Wilson JG, Fearon DT. Genetic regulation of a structural polymorphism of human C3b receptor. J Clin Invest 1983;72:685–693

Wu J et al. OR A novel polymorphism of FcγRIIIa (CD16) alters receptor function and predisposes to autoimmune disease. J Clin Invest 1997; 100: 1059-1070.

Xiao C, Rajewsky K. microRNA control in the immune system:basic principles. Cell 2009;136:26–36.

Xu AP, Yin PD, Su XY. [Association of CTLA-4 promoter -1722 polymorphism with systemic lupus erythematosus in Chinese]. Di Yi Jun Yi Da Xue Xue Bao 2004; 24: 1107–1112.

Y. Agata, A. Kawasaki, H. Nishimura, Y. Ishida, T. Tsubata, H. Yagita et al., Expression of the PD-1 antigen on the surface of stimulated mouse T and B lymphocytes. Int Immunol 8 (1996) pp. 765–772.

Yang W, Ng P, Zhao M, Hirankarn N, Lau CS, Mok CC, Chan TM, Wong RW, Lee KW, Mok MY, Wong SN, Avihingsanon Y, Lee TL, Ho MH, Lee PP, Wong WH, Lau YL. Population differences in SLE susceptibility genes: STAT4 and BLK, but not PXK, are associated with systemic lupus erythematosus in Hong Kong Chinese. Genes Immun. 2009;10(3):219-26.

Yang W, Zhao M, Hirankarn N, et al. ITGAM is associated with disease susceptibility and renal nephritis of systemic lupus erythematosus in Hong Kong Chinese and Thai. Hum Mol Genet 2009;18:2063–2070.

Yang Y, Chung EK, Wu YL et al. Gene copy-number variation and associated polymorphisms of complement component C4 in human systemic lupus erythematosus (SLE): low copy number is a risk factor for and high copy number is a protective factor against SLE susceptibility in European Americans. Am J Hum Genet 2007; 80: 1037–54.

Yang Z, Mendoza AR, Welch TR, Zipf WB, Yu CY. Modular variations of HLA class III genes for serine/threonine kinase RP, complement C4, steroid 21-hydroxylase CYP21 and tenascin TNX (RCCX): a mechanism for gene deletions and disease associations. J Biol Chem 1999;274:12147–12156.

Yang, W. Yang W, Ng P, Zhao M, Hirankarn N, Lau CS, Mok CC, Chan TM, Wong RW, Lee KW, Mok MY, Wong SN, Avihingsanon Y, Lee TL, Ho MH, Lee PP, Wong WH, Lau YL. Population differences in SLE susceptibility genes: STAT4 and BLK, but not PXK, are associated with systemic lupus erythematosus in Hong Kong Chinese. Genes Immun. 2009;10, 219–226.

Yap SN, Phipps ME, Manivasagar M, Tan SY and Bosco JJ. Human Fcγ receptor IIA (FcγRIIA) genotyping and association with systemic lupus erythematosus (SLE) in Chinese and Malays in Malaysia. 1999;Lupus 8, 305–310.

Yap WH, Yeoh E, Tay A, Brenner S, Venkatesh B. STAT4 is a target of the hematopoietic zinc-finger transcription factor Ikaros in T cells. FEBS Lett 2005; 579: 4470–4478.

Ye D, Pan F, Zhang K, Li X, Xu J, Hao J. A novel single-nucleotide polymorphism of the Fcgamma receptor IIIa gene is associated with genetic susceptibility to systemic lupus erythematosus in Chinese populations: a family-based association study. Clin Exp Dermatol. 2006;31(4):553-7.

Ye DQ, Hu YS, Li XP, et al., "The correlation between monocytes chemoattractant protein-1 and the arthritis of sytemic lupus erythematosus among Chinese," Archives of Dermatological Research, vol. 296, no. 8, (2005) pp. 366–371.

Yokoyama K, Su Ih IH, Tezuka T, Yasuda T, Mikoshiba K, Tarakhovsky A et al. BANK regulates BCR-induced calcium mobilization by promoting tyrosine phosphorylation of IP(3) receptor. EMBO J 2002; 21: 83–92.

Yu B, Shao Y, Li P, Zhang J, Zhong Q, Yang H, Hu X, Chen B, Peng X, Wu Q, Chen Y, Guan M, Wan J, Zhang W.Copy number variations of the human histamine H4 receptor gene are associated with systemic lupus erythematosus. Br J Dermatol. 2010;163(5):935-40.

Yu B, Wu Q, Chen Y, Li P, Shao Y, Zhang J, Zhong Q, Peng X, Yang H, Hu X, Chen B, Guan M, Zhang W, Wan J. Polymorphisms of PXK are associated with autoantibody production, but not disease risk, of systemic lupus erythematosus in Chinese mainland population. Lupus. 2011;20(1):23-7

Yu, CY.; Hauptmann, G.; Yang, Y.; Wu, YL.; Birmingham, DJ.; Rovin, BH., et al. Complement deficiencies in human systemic lupus erythematosus (SLE) and SLE nephritis: epidemiology and pathogenesis. In: Tsokos, GC., editor. Systemic Lupus Erythematosus: A Companion to Rheumatology. Philadelphia: Elsevier; 2007. p. 203-213.

Yung R, Chang S, Hemati N, Johnson K and Richardson B, Mechanisms of drug-induced lupus. IV. Comparison of procainamide and hydralazine with analogs in vitro and in vivo, Arthritis Rheum 40 (1997), pp. 1436–1443.

Yung R, Powers D, Johnson K, Ameto E, Carr D, Laing T, et al. Mechanisms of drug-induced lupus II. T cells overexpressing lymphocyte functionassociated antigen 1 become autoreactive and cause a lupus-like disease in systemic mice. J Clin Invest 1996;97:2866-71.

Zhang Z, Zhu KJ, Xu Q, Zhang XJ, Sun LD, Zheng HF, Han JW, Quan C, Zhang SQ, Cai LQ, Xu SX, Zuo XB, Cheng H, Yang S. The association of the BLK gene with SLE was replicated in Chinese Han. Arch Dermatol Res. 2010;302(8):619-24.

Zhao M, Sun Y, Gao F, Wu X, Tang J, Yin H, Luo Y, Richardson B, Lu Q. Epigenetics and SLE: RFX1 downregulation causes CD11a and CD70 overexpression by altering epigenetic modifications in lupus CD4+ T cells. J Autoimmun. 2010;35(1):58-69.

Zhou XJ, Lu XL, Lv JC, Yang HZ, Qin LX, Zhao MH, Su Y, Li ZG, Zhang H. Genetic association of PRDM1-ATG5 intergenic region and autophagy with systemic lupus erythematosus in a Chinese population. Ann Rheum Dis. 2011;70(7):1330-7.

3

Interferon and Apoptosis in Systemic Lupus Erythematosus

Daniel N. Clark and Brian D. Poole
Brigham Young University
USA

1. Introduction

Systemic lupus erythematosus (SLE) is generally diagnosed long after the disease begins. This means that the cause of the disease is hard to find, buried in the past. In the search for the elusive causal agents for SLE, one candidate is the immune signaling molecule, interferon (IFN). Interferon is a secreted signaling protein, or cytokine, which is expressed at higher levels in SLE patients and has been associated with incidence and severity of the disease.

A combination of environmental triggers and genetic susceptibility combine to initiate SLE. Although there are many etiological components, they usually converge on a heightened state of activation for the immune system, with resultant increases in interferon production and interferon signaling. That is to say that interferon could be thought of as either a causative agent, a result of the disease, or both.

This chapter will discuss the basics of interferon function and how de-regulation of apoptosis can lead to interferon production due to immune complexes. We will then discuss how the functioning of the immune system changes in someone with SLE, the genes which are associated with risk for SLE, and clinical manifestations of interferon in SLE.

2. How interferon works in the context of SLE

Interferon is a signaling protein which is secreted to activate neighboring cells in response to viruses or other infections. It is a cytokine, or immune signaling molecule which allows communication between cells. When a cell is infected with a virus, interferon is produced and secreted as a warning to other cells to prepare for an infection. Interferons alpha (IFNα) and beta (IFNβ) are the type I interferons, and interferon gamma (IFNγ) is the type II interferon. Most of the cells in the human body have receptors for type I IFN, whereas certain immune cells express the receptor for type II IFN (Su, et al., 2004). The proteins are made by many different cells, but generally speaking, IFNα is of leukocyte origin, IFNβ is of fibroblast origin, and IFNγ is made by lymphocytes (Lucero, et al., 1982). Other less studied interferons also exist, and interferons are conserved among many species. This chapter will talk mostly about type I interferons, which are IFNα and IFNβ.

The main purpose of interferon is to shut down a cell before a virus can take it over, although it has many other jobs (Niewold, et al., 2010). Interferon signaling leads to increased apoptosis, which is a normal response to control viral spread or to decrease the size of a tumor (Takaoka, et al., 2003). If one cell can undergo apoptosis before a virus can replicate and infect other cells, the infection is halted (Luker, et al., 2005).

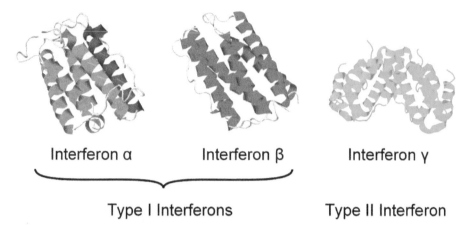

Fig. 1. Interferon protein structures. Interferons alpha and beta, the type I interferons, have a common structure composed mainly of five alpha helices (shown are IFNα2a and IFNβ1 based on PDB files 1itf and 1au1, respectively). Although the monomers of each are very similar in structure, the functional form of both is a dimer, and the two dimerize differently, IFNα2a along homologous surfaces and IFNβ1 on opposing sides of the protein (Karpusas, et al., 1997). IFNγ is show in its dimerized form, with the two colors representing two intertwined monomers (based on PDB file 1hig). Not shown to scale; figures drawn with Jmol (Jmol, 2011).

Interferon can be produced in response to infection, other cytokines, mitogens and several signaling pathways. Once produced it is secreted where it can be recognized by other cells, which is called paracrine signaling, or by the cell which produced it, called autocrine signaling. One type of cell, the plasmacytoid dendritic cell (pDC) is a natural IFN producer, and is able to make very large amounts of IFNα (Ronnblom & Alm, 2001).

When interferon ligates an interferon receptor, signaling pathways are activated. Interferon causes an increase in the expression of both major histocompatibility complexes (MHCI and MHCII) for presentation of viral peptides to T cells, which can then lead to activation of other cells in order to kill infected cells, and remove them (Fruh & Yang, 1999). Interferon also increases intracellular levels of protein kinase R (PKR) which recognizes viral nucleic acids and activates RNase L to degrade viral RNAs. PKR also slows protein synthesis by inactivating translational initiation factors, so that viral proteins synthesis is slowed (Pindel & Sadler, 2011). p53 is also activated, which is pro-apoptotic (Takaoka, 2003). Interferons activate immune cells, especially natural killer cells and macrophages (Murray, 1988). This activation cascade is normally "turned off" after an infection is cleared to prevent damage to uninfected cells. However this activation state is not reduced to the normal levels in individuals with SLE, where a higher level of interferon is present (T. Kim, et al., 1987; Ytterberg & Schnitzer, 1982). This higher amount of interferon is also measurable by an increase in the expression of interferon-stimulated genes seen in lupus patients, called the interferon response signature (Baechler, et al., 2003; Bennett, et al., 2003; Feng, et al., 2006).

This means that IFN is turned on and that it is actively affecting how other cells are functioning.

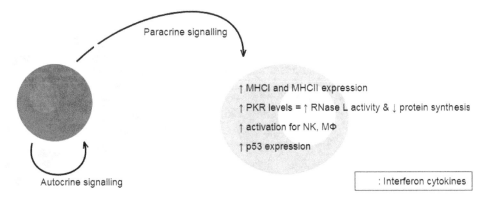

Fig. 2. Cell to cell IFN signaling and its effects. One cell produces interferon and either another cell (paracrine signaling) or the same cell (autocrine signaling) receives the signal. ↑: an increase, ↓: a decrease, MHC: major histocompatibility complex, PKR: protein kinase R, NK: natural killer cell, MΦ: macrophage

As a general feature of autoimmune diseases such as SLE, the immune system is in an "always on" state, which can lead to a breach in the body's natural tolerance to self. Once this self tolerance is lost, autoimmune disease can result. In addressing why the immune system generates an attack against one's own body, the over activation of the immune system, including the overproduction of interferon in SLE patients is a part of this picture.

3. Interferon leads to apoptosis, and the SLE-apoptosis connection

One effect of interferon production is the release of autoantigens due to increased cell death. This release is normally controlled by a process called efferocytosis, or apoptotic cell removal, where cell debris are processed by immune cells or neighboring cells which remove them by phagocytosis. Defects in apoptotic pathways have been noted in individuals with SLE (Gaipl, et al., 2006). Examples of why this occurs have been studied. For example, in SLE patients there is an overexpression of both soluble and membrane-bound Fas. Fas is a receptor which when ligated signals to a cell to undergo apoptosis. The levels of Fas also correlate with the amount of apoptotic lymphocytes and disease activity of SLE (Li, et al., 2009; Sahebari, et al., 2010). Mouse models of lupus commonly have genetic variations in apoptotic pathways such the Fas/Fas L pathway and interferon pathways.

Mouse as well as human SLE patients make antibodies to self antigens. This is likely because of over-exposure of potential autoantigens to the immune system. This could be due to an increased amount of apoptosis, or a decrease in the rate of clearance of apoptotic debris. Apoptosis, which can be induced by interferon, is also part of the natural cycle of cellular growth and death. Cells undergoing apoptosis are recognized as dead by other cells, so that they are cleared (Munoz, et al., 2010).

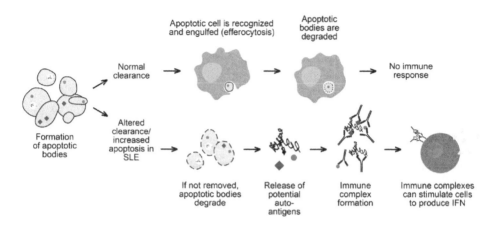

Fig. 3. Production of interferon can begin with defects in apoptosis. This can be due to either an increase in apoptosis or a decrease in clearance of apoptotic debris. If contents are released, they can form immune complexes with autoantibodies. These immune complexes can cause cells to produce interferon. Manipulating this pathway is also a common characteristic of mouse models of lupus.

3.1 Mouse models allow the study of IFN and apoptosis pathways

Mouse models have been very useful in understanding the etiology and pathogenesis of lupus. Two approaches to experimental mice have been used to generate information about the role of interferon in lupus. In the first approach, interferon-related genes are knocked out and the resulting effects on lupus are studied. For the second, established lupus mouse models are studied on a molecular level for differences in interferon pathways or interferon-related effects. These two approaches often overlap, as in cases where interferon-related genes are knocked out in lupus-prone mice. Several established lupus mouse models include the MRL/lpr mice, NZW/NZB, and others. These are mice that spontaneously develop lupus, and several of them have been investigated to understand the role of interferon in their pathogenesis. Although a complete description of the mouse models for lupus is beyond the scope of this or any one publication, a few illustrative examples represent the power of these model systems.

One mouse model that is especially relevant for the study of interferon in lupus is the BXSB/MpJ (BXSB) or Yaa mouse. These mice spontaneously develop lupus-like disease in a sex-linked fashion because of a duplication of the Toll-like receptor 7 (TLR7) gene on the Y chromosome (Izui, et al., 1994). TLR7 is responsible for inducing interferon in response to viral infection or autoantibody production.

Another interesting mouse for the study of interferon is the NZB/NZW mouse. These mice spontaneously develop a lupus-like autoimmune disease. They have been used to investigate the role of several interferon-related molecules and cells. For example, treating these mice with interferon accelerates disease in a T-cell like manner (Z. Liu, et al., 2010; Mathian, et al., 2005), while knocking out or inhibiting interferon-related genes slows or eliminates the development of lupus-like symptoms (Jorgensen, et al., 2007; Sharma, et al., 2005). These mice have been used to clarify the interactions between sex hormones and interferon in lupus etiology (Bynote, et al., 2008; Panchanathan, et al., 2009; Panchanathan, et al., 2010), and they serve as an excellent all-around model for spontaneous development of lupus.

The role of several interferon-related molecules has been examined using a combination of mouse models. As an example, consider the gene interferon regulatory factor five (IRF5). This gene is an interferon-regulating gene which will be described in section 5.2 below. It was discovered that knockout of IRF5 prevents or inhibits the development of lupus in MRL/lpr mice, Fcγ-/- Yaa mice, and pristine-injected mice (Richez, et al., 2010; Savitsky, et al., 2010; Tada, et al., 2011).

Mouse models for lupus represent a powerful and flexible mechanism for investigating the role of multiple aspects of lupus. However, it must be remembered that the mutations or disease manifestations in these mice are not necessarily related to those seen in human lupus, and therefore the results observed must be interpreted with caution.

4. A cycle of autoantibody production

When it comes to SLE we may think of interferon production as a cycle, which begins when an environmental trigger, such as a viral infection, UV light damage or medical treatment activates the immune system to produce interferon.

Normally B cells which produce antibodies to self-antigens undergo negative selection, where they receive signals to die off or become inactivated if they make antibody against a self-antigen. This self-tolerance is breached in SLE (Cancro, et al., 2009), and the self-antigens released from damaged or apoptotic cells during or after initial triggering events become the targets of autoantibodies. When autoantibodies are produced, they are made by B cells as well as plasma cells, which are a mature differentiated form of B cells.

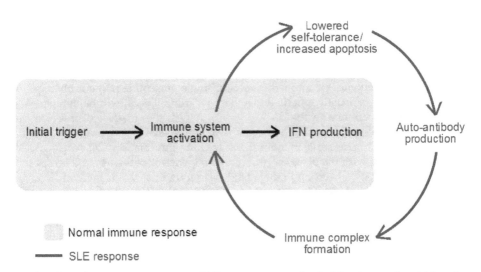

Fig. 4. The altered immune response in SLE generates a cycle. In blue is a cycle which exists in SLE, amplifying the amount of IFN present. This cycle needs a trigger, but once it begins, it can leave the immune system in an "always on" state.

Autoantibodies lead to the production of interferon by forming immune complexes which are immunostimulatory (Ronnblom, et al., 2011). Immune complexes are composed of aggregates of antibody and antigen molecules which are processed by the body. These immune complexes are a main source of SLE pathology, as they obstruct small passages in areas of the body such as the kidneys and joints (Crispin, et al., 2010).

Immune complexes may include the common SLE autoantigens such as RNA-containing protein complexes like Sm, RNPs, Ro, and La. Having a combination of both nucleic acids and protein complexed with antibody means many pathways can be turned on. For example, antibody can stimulate an immune cell through an Fc receptor, nucleic acids can stimulate cells through Toll-like receptors (TLRs), and proteins can be recognized by other antibodies.

Immune cells are activated by immune complexes and the cycle continues. Interferon production is instigated by immune cells which recognize part of the complex, be it the antibody, the antigen, or other associated molecules.

5. SLE genetic risk screens identify genes in interferon signaling pathways

We have looked at the disease state of SLE, and how the immune system functions improperly to instigate disease. Things begin when an environmental trigger works on the genetic background of varying degrees of susceptibility. Genetic susceptibility is thought to account for at least 20% of the risk for SLE (Deapen, et al., 1992). To find the actual genes involved, studies are performed to determine the linkage or association of a variation in the genome to a particular disease.

One important method is called a genome wide association study (GWAS). These GWA studies genotype thousands of individuals, grouped into SLE patients and non-patients comparing them at thousands of single nucleotide polymorphisms (SNPs). These studies reveal the genomic regions which contain disease-associated genes, because the variations are more common in people with the disease. Individual genes or gene pathways are pinpointed, and can ultimately lead to treatment strategies. Many genes have been identified that contain SNPs which confer risk to SLE.

These studies are especially useful for diseases with unknown or complex genetic components. The genome is examined for sets of single nucleotide polymorphisms (SNPs). When sets of SNPs are usually inherited together in a group it is called a haplotype. When a haplotype is more common in the disease group than in the unaffected group, it can be assumed that it is associated with the disease. Although specific genes are sometimes found which may predict a disease, it is more likely that the information will reveal molecular pathways associated with the disease. Association of genes or pathways to diseases such as heart disease, asthma, diabetes and others have been found using this method (Stranger, et al., 2011). The amount of effect is measured as an odds ratio (OR), which is a measure of the strength of association of the disease with a haplotype. A median OR value is around 1.3, with some genes having much higher association ORs. For example, one of the lupus-associated haplotypes TREX1, has a published OR of 25 (Lee-Kirsch, et al., 2007). In such cases, the genetic risk is almost certainly associated with the disease.

An important caveat to these tests is that they answer the question, "What?" but not the question, "How?" That is, they identify genetic loci which confer risk to SLE, but then further studies are needed to show what functional changes affect people with a risk haplotype. For most of the genes, we do not know what functional role they play. However it is promising to note that the genes are within certain pathways, some of which are already associated with lupus.

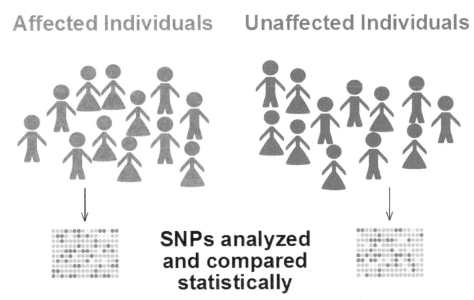

Fig. 5. Genome wide association studies (GWAS). Genome-wide association studies aim to discover the genetic risk component of a disease by finding differences in a group with the disease compared to a group of unaffected control individuals.

Several review articles have reviewed the findings of many lupus GWAS with varying degrees of certainty (R.R. Graham, et al., 2009; I.T.W. Harley, et al., 2009; Moser, et al., 2009; Rhodes & Vyse, 2008; Sebastiani & Galeazzi, 2009). In some cases the indicated susceptibility genes are common in many ethnicities and populations, while others are specific to certain groups. The statistical significance of many of these genes is well established, while others are novel and need to be replicated by other groups. An important finding is that most of the genes that have been identified in GWA studies can be grouped into several functional pathways. We will focus on the genes in the IFN pathway and the pathways involving clearing of apoptotic cells and immune complexes.

5.1 Interferon production pathways
Intracellular signaling pathways which control interferon production include the production of type I interferons by interferon regulatory factors (IRFs), and the production of type II interferon by STAT4. IRFs are activated by TLRs, which are extracellular or endosomal pattern recognition molecules. TLRs 7, 8, and 9 recognize nucleic acids and are endosomal. Maintaining these TLRs in the endosome instead of the cell surface is an important barrier to too frequent TLR activation. Once the nucleic acids are brought into the cells through endocytosis, the TLRs become activated to turn on IRFs. TLR 8 and TLR 9 have both been identified as lupus risk genes (Armstrong, et al., 2009; Xu, et al., 2009).

TLRs begin a signaling cascade through a MyD88 signaling complex. MyD88 activates another confirmed locus of SLE risk, the gene which encodes IL1 receptor-associated kinase 1

(IRAK1). In Sle1 and Sle3 mouse models of lupus, IRAK deficiency eliminated most lupus symptoms (Jacob, et al., 2009), which highlights the importance of IRAK1. Since this gene is on the X chromosome, it could help explain why lupus is more common among women. The MyD88 complex can be affected by osteopontin (OPN). It regulates IFNα production in plasmacytoid dendritic cells, which are the body's main IFNα producer cell (Cao & Liu, 2006). The lupus-risk variant of OPN was tied to high IFNα levels in certain lupus patients (Kariuki, et al., 2009b).

Two interacting proteins involved in inflammation, TNFα-induced protein 3 (TNFAIP3) and TNFAIP3-interacting protein 1 (TNIP1), are also lupus risk loci (Gateva, et al., 2009; Musone, et al., 2008). TNFAIP3 encodes the protein A20, which abrogates NFκB after an inflammatory response, and lupus-risk variants of this gene are associated with blood and kidney manifestations (Bates, et al., 2009). TNIP1 interacts with TNFAIP3 as well as affecting several other signal transduction pathways.

Interferon regulatory factors are activated next, downstream of TLRs; they are transcription factors which travel to the nucleus to bind DNA to initiate transcription. IRF5 binds to a sequence-specific region of DNA to induce IFN production. It has been confirmed as a risk factor for SLE in among several ethnicities (Kawasaki, et al., 2008; Kelly, et al., 2008; Lee & Song, 2009; Reddy, et al., 2007; Shimane, et al., 2009). There are three main genetic variants within IRF5, one copy number variant with either two or four copies of a 30-bp sequence, and two SNPs (R.R. Graham, et al., 2007b). The rs2004640 SNP changes the first exon, although this exon does not encode protein. The other SNP, rs10954213, creates an early polyadenylation sequence, which yields shorter more stable mRNA (D.S.C. Graham, et al., 2007a). Work has shown that these variants increase the amount of IFN in the presence of SLE autoantibodies (Niewold, et al., 2008; Salloum, et al., 2009).

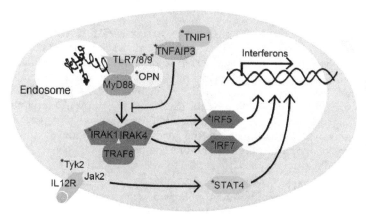

Fig. 6. Interferon production pathways are affected by lupus-risk genes. The * represents genes which have been identified as having risk for lupus. The endosomal TLRs (7, 8, and 9) can bind to autoantigenic nucleic acids and signal through a MyD88 complex which can be affected by association with osteopontin (OPN). If it is not blocked by TNFAIP3, this activates an IRAK signaling complex to phosphorylate the IRF5 and IRF7 transcription factors to produce type I IFN. IL-12 or IL-23 signal through Tyk2/Jak2 to activate the STAT4 transcription factor to produce type II IFN, commonly in T helper cells (Watford, et al., 2004).

IRF7 is associated with SLE risk by its proximity to SNPs in the IRF7/KIAA1542 locus (J.B. Harley, et al., 2008; Suarez-Gestal, et al., 2009). IRF7 SNPs have been shown to lead to increased IFNα levels and alter of which autoantibodies are made (Salloum, et al., 2009).

Signal transducer and activator of transcription 4 (STAT4) is also associated with risk for SLE. It is a transcription factor which activates genes in proliferation, differentiation and apoptosis pathways. Two STAT4 SNPs have been examined, rs7574865 increases sensitivity to IFNα (Kariuki, et al., 2009a), and rs3821236 causes STAT4 to be transcribed at higher levels and is additive with IRF5 risk loci so that when both are present, the risk to SLE is multiplied (Abelson, et al., 2009; Sigurdsson, et al., 2008).

5.2 Genes associated with apoptosis and immune complexes

Another set of risk genes can be placed into a functional group of apoptosis-associated genes. As we read earlier in the chapter, defects in apoptosis can lead to the presence of potential autoantigens. For example, a cell undergoes apoptosis and instead of being cleared by other cells, its contents are released. The cellular contents can contain things like nucleic acids, RNA binding proteins, and others which are common lupus autoantigens. If antibodies bind to these antigens, a complex of multiple antibodies and multiple antigens can aggregate. The resultant immune complexes can be broken down through reactions with complement components, which are commonly found at low levels in SLE patients (C.C. Liu & Ahearn, 2009). If they are not broken down, they reach areas such as the kidneys or joints, which can be damaged by these immune complexes. This is how organ damage usually occurs in lupus patients.

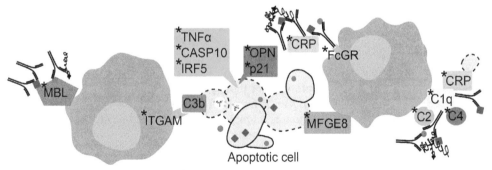

Fig. 7. Genes associated with risk for lupus in the apoptosis pathway. The * represents genes which have been identified as having risk for lupus. TNFα, CASP10 and IRF5 are pro-apoptotic whereas OPN and p21 are anti-apoptotic. These genes all have a role in how much apoptosis is occurring. Once apoptosis has transpired, the cell must be cleared. Parts of apoptotic cells or immune complexes can be recognized by other cells to facilitate their removal. This is aided by recognition molecules such as the complement components shown here.

The problem of creating autoantibodies could stem from too much apoptosis or too little clearance of apoptotic debris. Genes identified in GWA studies that could alter the amount of apoptosis include TNFα, caspase 10, IRF5, osteopontin and p21.

TNFα was identified as a risk factor for lupus in certain ethnicities (Jimenez-Morales, et al., 2009; Lin, et al., 2009). TNFα is a cytokine which is produced and secreted to signal to other cells and is found at high levels in the serum of lupus patients (Davas, et al., 1999; Emilie, et al., 1996; Sabry, et al., 2006). Part of its function is to induce apoptosis – when a cell binds TNFα, it activates the caspase cascade. Caspases are proteases which are activated under certain conditions and are a hallmark of apoptosis. They cleave other caspases as well, and the combined proteolytic activity of several different activated caspases breaks down cellular components as the cell prepares to die. Caspase 10 is part of this cascade and is another lupus susceptibility gene (Armstrong, et al., 2009). Caspase 8, is activated by TNF signaling, and cleaves caspase 10, which then cleaves caspases 3 and 7. IRF5, as well as being a transcription factor which helps produce IFN, is also a tumor suppressor gene which is commonly inactivated in cancers. This is because of IRF5's pro-apoptotic function.

Osteopontin (OPN) and p21 are also lupus risk genes, both anti-apoptotic. OPN promotes proliferation, as well as prevention of death under apoptotic stimuli (Standal, et al., 2004). A mimic of p21 was used in the treatment of murine lupus in the NZB/NZW mouse, and it was found to dramatically reduce the disease (Goulvestre, et al., 2005).

So, there are genes which dysregulate the amount of apoptosis, and they are associated with risk for lupus. But this is only half of the picture; the other part is the clearance of apoptotic cells or immune complexes. Several SLE susceptibility genes in this pathway have been identified as well. Active SLE can be assessed when low levels of complement proteins are found in circulation. Complement can function against microbes during an infection, but can also help to degrade immune complexes. Once attached, they can help cells recognize and degrade them. Other proteins function to bind apoptotic cells or immune complexes to facilitate their uptake by other cells.

Integrin αM (ITGAM) has been convincingly associated to SLE (Nath, et al., 2008). Risk variants of ITGAM have been associated with certain clinical manifestations of lupus (Kim-Howard, et al., 2010). It is a cell receptor which binds to OPN or to complement C3b. C3b binds to apoptotic cells or immune complexes.

SLE association with complement components C1q, C2, C4a and C4b have large OR values, meaning that the risk haplotypes of these genes are causing a large effect. When C1q is expressed at low levels it can lead to lupus, and it was shown to increase the amount the of IFN produced due to immune complexes (Lood, et al., 2009). Complement components function by binding immune complexes by the Fc region of antibody or by binding to other parts of apoptotic cells, which can opsonize them for easier uptake by other cells. Cells can then remove the immune complex or apoptotic debris by endocytosis. Receptors for the Fc region of antibody have also been implicated in SLE risk (Lee-Kirsch, et al., 2007). These receptors can bind to antibody within an immune complex.

Other proteins such as milk fat globule EGF factor 8 (MFG-E8) and C-reactive protein (CRP) can bind to apoptotic cells by recognizing phospholipids on their membranes. MFG-E8 binds to phosphatidylserine, an "eat me" signal which is expressed on apoptotic cells. The MFG-E8 knockout mouse gets SLE because of failure to remove apoptotic cells (Yamaguchi, et al., 2010). CRP binds to phosphocholine, which is present on dying or damaged cells. Both MFG-E8 and CRP are lupus risk genes (Batuca & Alves, 2009; Hu, et al., 2009; H.A. Kim, et al., 2009). Low mannose-binding lectin (MBL) levels can lead to higher levels of apoptosis is this lupus-risk associated gene (Pradhan, et al., 2010).

The number of genes associated with risk for SLE will likely increase, though we have an interesting pool of genes already that point to certain pathways associated with the disease. The interferon and apoptosis pathways are certainly important in SLE etiopathogenesis.

6. Clinical component of interferon and SLE

Many researchers have sought to determine if higher levels of IFN, which is common in lupus patients, is a cause of lupus or an effect of lupus. An interesting occurrence can happen when someone undergoes treatment with IFNα. The presence of increased levels of IFN leads to lupus or a lupus-like syndrome (Gota & Calabrese, 2003; Ioannou & Isenberg, 2000; Niewold & Swedler, 2005). Because the lupus symptoms usually disappear after IFN treatment ends, this connection suggests that IFN may be more of a cause than an effect. In a small number of cases, some patients also develop SLE as a result of these IFN treatments. Furthermore, within a family, the levels of interferon among all members correlate, suggesting that this is a heritable trait (Niewold, et al., 2007). That is, even the siblings of a lupus patient with high IFN levels are more likely to have higher IFN levels. This also supports a causal role for IFN.

Clinically, disease activity can be measured and correlated to other observations to determine the cause of the different levels of activity. One item linked to SLE activity is interferon, where higher levels of IFN in the serum correlated with more severe disease in most cases (Bauer, et al., 2009; Dall'Era, et al., 2005; Feng, et al., 2006; Landolt-Marticorena, et al., 2009; Petri, et al., 2009; Zhuang, et al., 2005).

Common autoantibodies also correlate with IFN levels. A very strong correlation is consistently observed between IFNα levels and the presence of antibodies to common SLE autoantigens like Ro, La, Sm, RNP, and dsDNA (Kirou, et al., 2005).

Another set of findings has to do with properties of main producer of IFNα, the plasmacytoid dendritic cells (pDCs). High numbers of IFN-producing pDCs have been observed in lupus skin lesions (Blomberg, et al., 2001; Farkas, et al., 2001). Since the cells are present at the scene of the crime, the increased interferon could have to do with the pathology in these cases.

At the time of writing, two clinical drug trials for SLE are being conducted, Sifalimumab is in Phase II, and Rontalizumab is in Phase I. Both are antibodies, designed to block interferon alpha signaling by binding it to prevent its recognition by neighboring cells (Clinical Trials, 2011). If these drugs are found to be effective, it will show that IFN plays a critical role in the pathogenesis of lupus. In addition, the United States Food and Drug Administration recently approved an antibody to B lymphocyte stimulator (BLyS) to treat SLE called Belimumab (Sanz, et al., 2011). This should help control the selective apoptosis and autoantibody production to some degree.

7. Conclusions

Several themes have been examined in this chapter. Specifically that the production of interferon is tied to lupus and that apoptosis, clearance of apoptotic cells, and the formation of immune complexes are events that can augment the production of interferon. Exciting findings about the actual genetic causes of SLE are being examined which will lead to better treatments for this complex disease. Although most of the data discussed in this chapter are inferential, there is a large body of evidence in support of the hypothesis that increased interferon signaling promotes an autoimmune state in those genetically prone to SLE.

8. References

Abelson, A.K.; Delgado-Vega, A.M.; Kozyrev, S.V.; Sanchez, E.; Velazquez-Cruz, R.; Eriksson, N.; Wojcik, J.; Reddy, M.; Lima, G.; D'Alfonso, S.; Migliaresi, S.; Baca, V.; Orozco, L.; Witte, T.; Ortego-Centeno, N.; Abderrahim, H.; Pons-Estel, B.A.; Gutierrez, C.; Suarez, A.; Gonzalez-Escribano, M.F.; Martin, J.; Alarcon-Riquelme, M.E. & Grp, A. (2009). STAT4 associates with systemic lupus erythematosus through two independent effects that correlate with gene expression and act additively with IRF5 to increase risk. *Annals of the Rheumatic Diseases*, 68 pp. 1746-1753

Armstrong, D.L.; Reiff, A.; Myones, B.L.; Quismorio, F.P.; Klein-Gitelman, M.; McCurdy, D.; Wagner-Weiner, L.; Silverman, E.; Ojwang, J.O.; Kaufman, K.M.; Kelly, J.A.; Merrill, J.T.; Harley, J.B.; Bae, S.C.; Vyse, T.J.; Gilkeson, G.S.; Gaffney, P.M.; Moser, K.L.; Putterman, C.; Edberg, J.C.; Brown, E.E.; Ziegler, J.; Langefeld, C.D.; Zidovetzki, R. & Jacob, C.O. (2009). Identification of new SLE-associated genes with a two-step Bayesian study design. *Genes and Immunity*, 10 pp. 446-456

Baechler, E.C.; Batliwalla, F.M.; Karypis, G.; Gaffney, P.M.; Ortmann, W.A.; Espe, K.J.; Shark, K.B.; Grande, W.J.; Hughes, K.M.; Kapur, V.; Gregersen, P.K. & Behrens, T.W. (2003). Interferon-inducible gene expression signature in peripheral blood cells of patients with severe lupus. *Proceedings of the National Academy of Sciences of the United States of America*, 100 pp. 2610-2615

Bates, J.S.; Lessard, C.J.; Leon, J.M.; Nguyen, T.; Battiest, L.J.; Rodgers, J.; Kaufman, K.M.; James, J.A.; Gilkeson, G.S.; Kelly, J.A.; Humphrey, M.B.; Harley, J.B.; Gray-McGuire, C.; Moser, K.L. & Gaffney, P.M. (2009). Meta-analysis and imputation identifies a 109 kb risk haplotype spanning TNFAIP3 associated with lupus nephritis and hematologic manifestations. *Genes and Immunity*, 10 pp. 470-477

Batuca, J. & Alves, J.D. (2009). C-reactive protein in systemic lupus erythematosus. *Autoimmunity*, 42 pp. 282-285

Bauer, J.W.; Petri, M.; Batliwalla, F.M.; Koeuth, T.; Wilson, J.; Slattery, C.; Panoskaltsis-Mortari, A.; Gregersen, P.K.; Behrens, T.W. & Baechler, E.C. (2009). Interferon-Regulated Chemokines as Biomarkers of Systemic Lupus Erythematosus Disease Activity A Validation Study. *Arthritis and Rheumatism*, 60 pp. 3098-3107

Bennett, L.; Palucka, A.K.; Arce, E.; Cantrell, V.; Borvak, J.; Banchereau, J. & Pascual, V. (2003). Interferon and granulopoiesis signatures in systemic lupus erythematosus blood. *Journal of Experimental Medicine*, 197 pp. 711-723

Blomberg, S.; Eloranta, M.L.; Cederblad, B.; Nordlind, K.; Alm, G.V. & Ronnblom, L. (2001). Presence of cutaneous interferon-alpha producing cells in patients with systemic lupus erythematosus. *Lupus*, 10 pp. 484-490

Bynote, K.K.; Hackenberg, J.M.; Korach, K.S.; Lubahn, D.B.; Lane, P.H. & Gould, K.A. (2008). Estrogen receptor-alpha deficiency attenuates autoimmune disease in (NZB x NZW)F1 mice. *Genes Immun*, 9 pp. 137-152

Cancro, M.P.; D'Cruz, D.P. & Khamashta, M.A. (2009). The role of B lymphocyte stimulator (BLyS) in systemic lupus erythematosus. *Journal of Clinical Investigation*, 119 pp. 1066-1073

Cao, W. & Liu, Y.J. (2006). Opn: key regulator of pDC interferon production. *Nature Immunology*, 7 pp. 441-443

ClinicalTrials.gov. (2011) http://www.clinicaltrials.gov

Crispin, J.C.; Liossis, S.N.C.; Kis-Toth, K.; Lieberman, L.A.; Kyttaris, V.C.; Juang, Y.T. & Tsokos, G.C. Pathogenesis of human systemic lupus erythematosus: recent advances. *Trends in Molecular Medicine*, 16 pp. 47-57

Dall'Era, M.C.; Cardarelli, P.M.; Preston, B.T.; Witte, A. & Davis, J.C. (2005). Type I interferon correlates with serological and clinical manifestations of SLE. *Annals of the Rheumatic Diseases*, 64 pp. 1692-1697

Davas, E.M.; Tsirogianni, A.; Kappou, I.; Karamitsos, D.; Economidou, I. & Dantis, P.C. (1999). Serum IL-6, TNF alpha, p55 srTNF alpha, p75 srTNF alpha, srIL-2 alpha levels and disease acitivity in systemic lupus erythematosus. *Clinical Rheumatology*, 18 pp. 17-22

Deapen, D.; Escalante, A.; Weinrib, L.; Horwitz, D.; Bachman, B.; Royburman, P.; Walker, A. & Mack, T.M. (1992). A revised estimate of twin concordance in systemic lupus erythematosus. *Arthritis and Rheumatism*, 35 pp. 311-318

Emilie, D.; Llorente, L. & Galanaud, P. (1996). Cytokines and systemic lupus erythematosus. *Annales De Medecine Interne*, 147 pp. 480-484

Farkas, L.; Beiske, K.; Lund-Johansen, F.; Brandtzaeg, P. & Jahnsen, F.L. (2001). Plasmacytoid dendritic cells (natural interferon-alpha/beta-producing cells) accumulate in cutaneous lupus erythematosus lesions. *American Journal of Pathology*, 159 pp. 237-243

Feng, X.B.; Wu, H.; Grossman, J.M.; Hanvivadhanakul, P.; FitzGerald, J.D.; Park, G.S.; Dong, X.; Chen, W.L.; Kim, M.H.; Weng, H.H.; Furst, D.E.; Gorn, A.; McMahon, M.; Taylor, M.; Brahn, E.; Hahn, B.H. & Tsao, B.P. (2006). Association of increased interferon-inducible gene expression with disease activity and lupus nephritis in patients with systemic lupus erythematosus. *Arthritis and Rheumatism*, 54 pp. 2951-2962

Fruh, K. & Yang, Y. (1999). Antigen presentation by MHC class I and its regulation by interferon gamma. *Current Opinion in Immunology*, 11 pp. 76-81

Gaipl, U.S.; Sheriff, A.; Franz, S.; Munoz, L.E.; Voll, R.E.; Kalden, J.R. & Herrmann, M. (2006). Inefficient clearance of dying cells and autoreactivity. *Current Concepts in Autoimmunity and Chronic Inflamation*, 305 pp. 161-176

Gateva, V.; Sandling, J.K.; Hom, G.; Taylor, K.E.; Chung, S.A.; Sun, X.; Ortmann, W.; Kosoy, R.; Ferreira, R.C.; Nordmark, G.; Gunnarsson, I.; Svenungsson, E.; Padyukov, L.; Sturfelt, G.; Jonsen, A.; Bengtsson, A.A.; Rantapaa-Dahlqvist, S.; Baechler, E.C.; Brown, E.E.; Alarcon, G.S.; Edberg, J.C.; Ramsey-Goldman, R.; McGwin, G.; Reveille, J.D.; Vila, L.M.; Kimberly, R.P.; Manzi, S.; Petri, M.A.; Lee, A.; Gregersen, P.K.; Seldin, M.F.; Ronnblom, L.; Criswell, L.A.; Syvanen, A.C.; Behrens, T.W. & Graham, R.R. (2009). A large-scale replication study identifies TNIP1, PRDM1, JAZF1, UHRF1BP1 and IL10 as risk loci for systemic lupus erythematosus. *Nature Genetics*, 41 pp. 1228-U1293

Gota, C. & Calabrese, L. (2003). Induction of clinical autoimmune disease by therapeutic interferon-alpha. *Autoimmunity*, 36 pp. 511-518

Goulvestre, C.; Chereau, C.; Nicco, C.; Mouthon, L.; Weill, B. & Batteux, F. (2005). A mimic of p21(WAF1)/(CIP1) ameliorates murine lupus. *Journal of Immunology*, 175 pp. 6959-6967

Graham, D.S.C.; Manku, H.; Wagner, S.; Reid, J.; Timms, K.; Gutin, A.; Lanchbury, J.S. & Vyse, T.J. (2007a). Association of IRF5 in UK SLE families identifies a variant involved in polyadenylation. *Human Molecular Genetics*, 16 pp. 579-591

Graham, R.R.; Hom, G.; Ortmann, W. & Behrens, T.W. (2009). Review of recent genome-wide association scans in lupus. *Journal of Internal Medicine*, 265 pp. 680-688

Graham, R.R.; Kyogoku, C.; Sigurdsson, S.; Vlasova, I.A.; Davies, L.R.; Baechler, E.C.; Plenge, R.M.; Koeuth, T.; Ortmann, W.A.; Hom, G.; Bauer, J.W.; Gillett, C.; Burtt, N.; Cunninghame Graham, D.S.; Onofrio, R.; Petri, M.; Gunnarsson, I.; Svenungsson, E.; Ronnblom, L.; Nordmark, G.; Gregersen, P.K.; Moser, K.; Gaffney, P.M.; Criswell, L.A.; Vyse, T.J.; Syvanen, A.C.; Bohjanen, P.R.; Daly, M.J.; Behrens, T.W. & Altshuler, D. (2007b). Three functional variants of IFN regulatory factor 5 (IRF5) define risk and protective haplotypes for human lupus. *Proc Natl Acad Sci U S A*, 104 pp. 6758-6763

Harley, I.T.W.; Kaufman, K.M.; Langefeld, C.D.; Harley, J.B. & Kelly, J.A. (2009). Genetic susceptibility to SLE: new insights from fine mapping and genome-wide association studies. *Nature Reviews Genetics*, 10 pp. 285-290

Harley, J.B.; Alarcon-Riquelme, M.E.; Criswell, L.A.; Jacob, C.O.; Kimberly, R.P.; Moser, K.L.; Tsao, B.P.; Vyse, T.J.; Langefeld, C.D. & Int Consortium Systemic Lupus, E. (2008). Genome-wide association scan in women with systemic lupus erythematosus identifies susceptibility variants in ITGAM, PXK, KIAA1542 and other loci. *Nature Genetics*, 40 pp. 204-210

Hu, C.Y.; Wu, C.S.; Tsai, H.F.; Chang, S.K.; Tsai, W.I. & Hsu, P.N. (2009). Genetic polymorphism in milk fat globule-EGF factor 8 (MFG-E8) is associated with systemic lupus erythematosus in human. *Lupus*, 18 pp. 676-681

Ioannou, Y. & Isenberg, D.A. (2000). Current evidence for the induction of autoimmune rheumatic manifestations by cytokine therapy. *Arthritis and Rheumatism*, 43 pp. 1431-1442

Izui, S.; Merino, R.; Fossati, L. & Iwamoto, M. (1994). The role of the Yaa gene in lupus syndrome. *Int Rev Immunol*, 11 pp. 211-230

Jacob, C.O.; Zhu, J.K.; Armstrong, D.L.; Yan, M.; Han, J.; Zhou, X.J.; Thomas, J.A.; Reiff, A.; Myones, B.L.; Ojwang, J.O.; Kaufman, K.M.; Klein-Gitelman, M.; McCurdy, D.; Wagner-Weiner, L.; Silverman, E.; Ziegler, J.; Kelly, J.A.; Merrill, J.T.; Harley, J.B.; Ramsey-Goldman, R.; Vila, L.M.; Bae, S.C.; Vyse, T.J.; Gilkeson, G.S.; Gaffney, P.M.; Moser, K.L.; Langefeld, C.D.; Zidovetzki, R. & Mohan, C. (2009). Identification of IRAK1 as a risk gene with critical role in the pathogenesis of systemic lupus erythematosus. *Proceedings of the National Academy of Sciences of the United States of America*, 106 pp. 6256-6261

Jimenez-Morales, S.; Velazquez-Cruz, R.; Ramirez-Bello, J.; Bonilla-Gonzalez, E.; Romero-Hidalgo, S.; Escamilla-Guerrero, G.; Cuevas, F.; Espinosa-Rosales, F.; Martinez-Aguilar, N.E.; Gomez-Vera, J.; Baca, V. & Orozco, L. (2009). Tumor necrosis factor-alpha is a common genetic risk factor for asthma, juvenile rheumatoid arthritis, and systemic lupus erythematosus in a Mexican pediatric population. *Human Immunology*, 70 pp. 251-256

Jmol: an open-source Java viewer for chemical structures in 3D. http://www.jmol.org

Jorgensen, T.N.; Roper, E.; Thurman, J.M.; Marrack, P. & Kotzin, B.L. (2007). Type I interferon signaling is involved in the spontaneous development of lupus-like disease in B6.Nba2 and (B6.Nba2 x NZW)F(1) mice. *Genes Immun*, 8 pp. 653-662

Kariuki, S.N.; Kirou, K.A.; MacDermott, E.J.; Barillas-Arias, L.; Crow, M.K. & Niewold, T.B. (2009a). Cutting Edge: Autoimmune Disease Risk Variant of STAT4 Confers increased Sensitivity to IFN-alpha in Lupus Patients In Vivo. *Journal of Immunology*, 182 pp. 34-38

Kariuki, S.N.; Moore, J.G.; Kirou, K.A.; Crow, M.K.; Utset, T.O. & Niewold, T.B. (2009b). Age- and gender-specific modulation of serum osteopontin and interferon-alpha by osteopontin genotype in systemic lupus erythematosus. *Genes and Immunity*, 10 pp. 487-494

Karpusas, M.; Nolte, M.; Benton, C.B.; Meier, W.; Lipscomb, W.N. & Goelz, S. (1997). The crystal structure of human interferon beta at 2.2-angstrom resolution. *Proceedings of the National Academy of Sciences of the United States of America*, 94 pp. 11813-11818

Kawasaki, A.; Kyogoku, C.; Ohashi, J.; Miyashita, R.; Hikami, K.; Kusaoi, M.; Tokunaga, K.; Takasaki, Y.; Hashimoto, H.; Behrens, T.W. & Tsuchiya, N. (2008). Association of IRF5 polymorphisms with systemic lupus erythematosus in a Japanese population: support for a crucial role of intron 1 polymorphisms. *Arthritis Rheum*, 58 pp. 826-834

Kelly, J.A.; Kelley, J.M.; Kaufman, K.M.; Kilpatrick, J.; Bruner, G.R.; Merrill, J.T.; James, J.A.; Frank, S.G.; Reams, E.; Brown, E.E.; Gibson, A.W.; Marion, M.C.; Langefeld, C.D.; Li, Q.Z.; Karp, D.R.; Wakeland, E.K.; Petri, M.; Ramsey-Goldman, R.; Reveille, J.D.; Vila, L.M.; Alarcon, G.S.; Kimberly, R.P.; Harley, J.B. & Edberg, J.C. (2008). Interferon regulatory factor-5 is genetically associated with systemic lupus erythematosus in African Americans. *Genes Immun*, 9 pp. 187-194

Kim-Howard, X.; Maiti, A.K.; Anaya, J.M.; Bruner, G.R.; Brown, E.; Merrill, J.T.; Edberg, J.C.; Petri, M.A.; Reveille, J.D.; Ramsey-Goldman, R.; Alarcon, G.S.; Vyse, T.J.; Gilkeson, G.; Kimberly, R.P.; James, J.A.; Guthridge, J.M.; Harley, J.B. & Nath, S.K. ITGAM coding variant (rs1143679) influences the risk of renal disease, discoid rash and immunological manifestations in patients with systemic lupus erythematosus with European ancestry. *Annals of the Rheumatic Diseases*, 69 pp. 1329-1332

Kim, H.A.; Chun, H.Y.; Kim, S.H.; Park, H.S. & Suh, C.H. (2009). C-Reactive Protein Gene Polymorphisms in Disease Susceptibility and Clinical Manifestations of Korean Systemic Lupus Erythematosus. *Journal of Rheumatology*, 36 pp. 2238-2243

Kim, T.; Kanayama, Y.; Negoro, N.; Okamura, M.; Takeda, T. & Inoue, T. (1987). Serum
    levels of interferons in patients with systemic lupus-erythematosus. *Clinical and
    Experimental Immunology*, 70 pp. 562-569
Kirou, K.A.; Lee, C.; George, S.; Louca, K.; Peterson, M.G.E. & Crow, M.K. (2005). Activation
    of the interferon-alpha pathway identifies a subgroup of systemic lupus
    erythematosus patients with distinct serologic features and active disease. *Arthritis
    and Rheumatism*, 52 pp. 1491-1503
Landolt-Marticorena, C.; Bonventi, G.; Lubovich, A.; Ferguson, C.; Unnithan, T.; Su,
    J.; Gladman, D.D.; Urowitz, M.; Fortin, P.R. & Wither, J. (2009). Lack of association
    between the interferon-alpha signature and longitudinal changes in disease activity
    in systemic lupus erythematosus. *Annals of the Rheumatic Diseases*, 68 pp. 1440-
    1446
Lee-Kirsch, M.A.; Gong, M.; Chowdhury, D.; Senenko, L.; Engel, K.; Lee, Y.A.; de Silva, U.;
    Bailey, S.L.; Witte, T.; Vyse, T.J.; Kere, J.; Pfeiffer, C.; Harvey, S.; Wong, A.;
    Koskenmies, S.; Hummel, O.; Rohde, K.; Schmidt, R.E.; Dominiczak, A.F.; Gahr, M.;
    Hollis, T.; Perrino, F.W.; Lieberman, J. & Hubner, N. (2007). Mutations in the gene
    encoding the 3 '-5 ' DNA exonuclease TREX1 are associated with systemic lupus
    erythematosus. *Nature Genetics*, 39 pp. 1065-1067
Lee, Y.H. & Song, G.G. (2009). Association between the rs2004640 functional polymorphism
    of interferon regulatory factor 5 and systemic lupus erythematosus: a meta-
    analysis. *Rheumatology International*, 29 pp. 1137-1142
Li, L.H.; Li, W.X.; Wu, O.; Zhang, G.Q.; Pan, H.F.; Li, X.P.; Xu, J.H.; Dai, H. & Ye, D.Q.
    (2009). Fas expression on peripheral blood lymphocytes in systemic lupus
    erythematosus: relation to the organ damage and lymphocytes apoptosis. *Molecular
    Biology Reports*, 36 pp. 2047-2052
Lin, Y.J.; Chen, R.H.; Wan, L.; Sheu, J.J.C.; Huang, C.M.; Lin, C.W.; Chen, S.Y.; Lai, C.H.; Lan,
    Y.C.; Hsueh, K.C.; Tsai, C.H.; Lin, T.H.; Huang, Y.M.; Chao, K.; Chen, D.Y. & Tsai,
    F.J. (2009). Association of TNF-alpha gene polymorphisms with systemic lupus
    erythematosus in Taiwanese patients. *Lupus*, 18 pp. 974-979
Liu, C.C. & Ahearn, J.M. (2009). The search for lupus biomarkers. *Best Practice & Research in
    Clinical Rheumatology*, 23 pp. 507-523
Liu, Z.; Bethunaickan, R.; Huang, W.; Lodhi, U.; Solano, I.; Madaio, M.P. & Davidson, A.
    (2011). Interferon-alpha accelerates murine systemic lupus erythematosus in a T
    cell-dependent manner. *Arthritis Rheum*, 63 pp. 219-229
Lood, C.; Gullstrand, B.; Truedsson, L.; Olin, A.I.; Alm, G.V.; Ronnblom, L.; Sturfelt, G.;
    Eloranta, M.L. & Bengtsson, A.A. (2009). C1q Inhibits Immune Complex-Induced
    Interferon-alpha Production in Plasmacytoid Dendritic Cells A Novel Link
    Between C1q Deficiency and Systemic Lupus Erythematosus Pathogenesis. *Arthritis
    and Rheumatism*, 60 pp. 3081-3090
Lucero, M.A.; Magdelenat, H.; Fridman, W.H.; Pouillart, P.; Billardon, C.; Billiau, A.; Cantell,
    K. & Falcoff, E. (1982). Comparison of effects of leukocyte and fibroblast interferon
    on immunological parameters in cancer-patients. *European Journal of Cancer &
    Clinical Oncology*, 18 pp. 243-251

Luker, K.E.; Hutchens, M.; Schultz, T.; Pekosz, A. & Luker, G.D. (2005). Bioluminescence imaging of vaccinia virus: Effects of interferon on viral replication and spread. *Virology*, 341 pp. 284-300

Mathian, A.; Weinberg, A.; Gallegos, M.; Banchereau, J. & Koutouzov, S. (2005). IFN-alpha induces early lethal lupus in preautoimmune (New Zealand Black x New Zealand White) F1 but not in BALB/c mice. *J Immunol*, 174 pp. 2499-2506

Moser, K.L.; Kelly, J.A.; Lessard, C.J. & Harley, J.B. (2009). Recent insights into the genetic basis of systemic lupus erythematosus. *Genes and Immunity*, 10 pp. 373-379

Munoz, L.E.; Lauber, K.; Schiller, M.; Manfredi, A.A. & Herrmann, M. (2010). The role of defective clearance of apoptotic cells in systemic autoimmunity. *Nature Reviews Rheumatology*, 6 pp. 280-289

Murray, H.W. (1988). Interferon-gamma, the activated macrophage, and host defense against microbial challenge. *Annals of Internal Medicine*, 108 pp. 595-608

Musone, S.L.; Taylor, K.E.; Lu, T.T.; Nititham, J.; Ferreira, R.C.; Ortmann, W.; Shifrin, N.; Petri, M.A.; Kamboh, M.I.; Manzi, S.; Seldin, M.F.; Gregersen, P.K.; Behrens, T.W.; Ma, A.; Kwok, P.Y. & Criswell, L.A. (2008). Multiple polymorphisms in the TNFAIP3 region are independently associated with systemic lupus erythematosus. *Nature Genetics*, 40 pp. 1062-1064

Nath, S.K.; Han, S.Z.; Kim-Howard, X.; Kelly, J.A.; Viswanathan, P.; Gilkeson, G.S.; Chen, W.; Zhu, C.; McEver, R.P.; Kimberly, R.P.; Alarcon-Riquelme, M.E.; Vyse, T.J.; Li, Q.Z.; Wakeland, E.K.; Merrill, J.T.; James, J.A.; Kaufman, K.M.; Guthridge, J.M. & Harley, J.B. (2008). A nonsynonymous functional variant in integrin-alpha M (encoded by ITGAM) is associated with systemic lupus erythematosus. *Nature Genetics*, 40 pp. 152-154

Niewold, T.B.; Clark, D.N.; Salloum, R. & Poole, B.D. Interferon Alpha in Systemic Lupus Erythematosus. *Journal of Biomedicine and Biotechnology*, pp. 8

Niewold, T.B.; Hua, J.; Lehman, T.J.A.; Harley, J.B. & Crow, M.K. (2007). High serum IFN-alpha activity is a heritable risk factor for systemic lupus erythematosus. *Genes and Immunity*, 8 pp. 492-502

Niewold, T.B.; Kelly, J.A.; Flesch, M.H.; Espinoza, L.R.; Harley, J.B. & Crow, M.K. (2008). Association of the IRF5 risk haplotype with high serum interferon-alpha activity in systemic lupus erythematosus patients. *Arthritis and Rheumatism*, 58 pp. 2481-2487

Niewold, T.B. & Swedler, W.I. (2005). Systemic lupus erythematosus arising during interferon-alpha therapy for cryoglobulinemic vasculitis associated with hepatitis C. *Clinical Rheumatology*, 24 pp. 178-181

Panchanathan, R.; Shen, H.; Bupp, M.G.; Gould, K.A. & Choubey, D. (2009). Female and male sex hormones differentially regulate expression of Ifi202, an interferon-inducible lupus susceptibility gene within the Nba2 interval. *J Immunol*, 183 pp. 7031-7038

Panchanathan, R.; Shen, H.; Zhang, X.; Ho, S.M. & Choubey, D. (2010). Mutually positive regulatory feedback loop between interferons and estrogen receptor-alpha in mice: implications for sex bias in autoimmunity. *PLoS ONE*, 5 pp. e10868

Petri, M.; Singh, S.; Tesfasyone, H.; Dedrick, R.; Fry, K.; Lal, P.G.; Williams, G.; Bauer, J.W.; Gregersen, P.K.; Behrens, T.W. & Baechler, E.C. (2009). Longitudinal expression of type I interferon responsive genes in systemic lupus erythematosus. *Lupus*, 18 pp. 980-989

Pindel, A. & Sadler, A. The Role of Protein Kinase R in the Interferon Response. *Journal of Interferon and Cytokine Research*, 31 pp. 59-70

Pradhan, V.; Surve, P. & Ghosh, K. Mannose binding lectin (MBL) in autoimmunity and its role in systemic lupus erythematosus (SLE). *J Assoc Physicians India*, 58 pp. 688-690

Reddy, M.V.; Velazquez-Cruz, R.; Baca, V.; Lima, G.; Granados, J.; Orozco, L. & Alarcon-Riquelme, M.E. (2007). Genetic association of IRF5 with SLE in Mexicans: higher frequency of the risk haplotype and its homozygozity than Europeans. *Hum Genet*, 121 pp. 721-727

Rhodes, B. & Vyse, T.J. (2008). The genetics of SLE: an update in the light of genome-wide association studies. *Rheumatology*, 47 pp. 1603-1611

Richez, C.; Yasuda, K.; Bonegio, R.G.; Watkins, A.A.; Aprahamian, T.; Busto, P.; Richards, R.J.; Liu, C.L.; Cheung, R.; Utz, P.J.; Marshak-Rothstein, A. & Rifkin, I.R., (2010) IFN regulatory factor 5 is required for disease development in the FcγRIIB-/- Yaa and FcγRIIB-/- mouse models of systemic lupus erythematosus. *J Immunol*, 184 pp. 796-806

Ronnblom, L. & Alm, G.V. (2001). A pivotal role for the natural interferon alpha-producing cells (plasmacytoid dendritic cells) in the pathogenesis of lupus. *Journal of Experimental Medicine*, 194 pp. F59-F63

Ronnblom, L.; Alm, G.V. & Eloranta, M.L. The type I interferon system in the development of lupus. *Seminars in Immunology*, 23 pp. 113-121

Sabry, A.; Sheashaa, H.; El-husseini, A.; Mahmoud, K.; Eldahshan, K.F.; George, S.K.; Abdel-Khalek, E.; El-Shafey, E.M. & Abo-Zenah, H. (2006). Proinflammatory cytokines (TNF-alpha and IL-6) in Egyptian patients with SLE: Its correlation with disease activity. *Cytokine*, 35 pp. 148-153

Sahebari, M.; Hatef, M.R.; Rezaieyazdi, Z.; Abbasi, M.; Abbasi, B. & Mahmoudi, M. Correlation between Serum Levels of Soluble Fas (CD95/Apo-1) with Disease Activity in Systemic Lupus Erythematosus Patients in Khorasan, Iran. *Archives of Iranian Medicine*, 13 pp. 135-142

Salloum, R.; Franek, B.; Kariuki, S.; Utset, T. & Niewold, T. (2009). T.16. Genetic Variation at the IRF7/KIAA1542 Locus is Associated with Autoantibody Profile and Serum Interferon Alpha Levels in Lupus Patients. *Clinical Immunology*, 131 pp. S54-S54

Sanz, I.; Yasothan, U. & Kirkpatrick, P. Belimumab. *Nature Reviews Drug Discovery*, 10 pp. 335-336

Savitsky, D.A.; Yanai, H.; Tamura, T.; Taniguchi, T. & Honda, K. (2010). Contribution of IRF5 in B cells to the development of murine SLE-like disease through its transcriptional control of the IgG2a locus. *Proc Natl Acad Sci U S A*, 107 pp. 10154-10159

Sebastiani, G.D. & Galeazzi, M. (2009). Immunogenetic studies on systemic lupus erythematosus. *Lupus*, 18 pp. 878-883

Sharma, R.P.; He, Q. & Riley, R.T. (2005). Lupus-prone NZBWF1/J mice, defective in cytokine signaling, are resistant to fumonisin hepatotoxicity despite accumulation of liver sphinganine. *Toxicology*, 216 pp. 59-71

Shimane, K.; Kochi, Y.; Yamada, R.; Okada, Y.; Suzuki, A.; Miyatake, A.; Kubo, M.; Nakamura, Y. & Yamamoto, K. (2009). A single nucleotide polymorphism in the IRF5 promoter region is associated with susceptibility to rheumatoid arthritis in the Japanese population. *Annals of the Rheumatic Diseases*, 68 pp. 377-383

Sigurdsson, S.; Nordmark, G.; Garnier, S.; Grundberg, E.; Kwan, T.; Nilsson, O.; Eloranta, M.L.; Gunnarsson, I.; Svenungsson, E.; Sturfelt, G.; Bengtsson, A.A.; Jonsen, A.; Truedsson, L.; Rantapaa-Dahlqvist, S.; Eriksson, C.; Alm, G.; Goring, H.H.H.; Pastinen, T.; Syvanen, A.C. & Ronnblom, L. (2008). A risk haplotype of STAT4 for systemic lupus erythematosus is over-expressed, correlates with anti-dsDNA and shows additive effects with two risk alleles of IRF5. *Human Molecular Genetics*, 17 pp. 2868-2876

Standal, T.; Borset, M. & Sundan, A. (2004). Role of osteopontin in adhesion, migration, cell survival and bone remodeling. *Experimental Oncology*, 26 pp. 179-184

Stranger, B.E.; Stahl, E.A. & Raj, T. Progress and Promise of Genome-Wide Association Studies for Human Complex Trait Genetics. *Genetics*, 187 pp. 367-383

Su, A.I.; Wiltshire, T.; Batalov, S.; Lapp, H.; Ching, K.A.; Block, D.; Zhang, J.; Soden, R.; Hayakawa, M.; Kreiman, G.; Cooke, M.P.; Walker, J.R. & Hogenesch, J.B. (2004). A gene atlas of the mouse and human protein-encoding transcriptomes. *Proceedings of the National Academy of Sciences of the United States of America*, 101 pp. 6062-6067

Suarez-Gestal, M.; Calaza, M.; Endreffy, E.; Pullmann, R.; Ordi-Ros, J.; Sebastiani, G.D.; Ruzickova, S.; Santos, M.J.; Papasteriades, C.; Marchini, M.; Skopouli, F.N.; Suarez, A.; Blanco, F.J.; D'Alfonso, S.; Bijl, M.; Carreira, P.; Witte, T.; Migliaresi, S.; Gomez-Reino, J.J.; Gonzalez, A. & European Consortium, S.D. (2009). Replication of recently identified systemic lupus erythematosus genetic associations: a case-control study. *Arthritis Research & Therapy*, 11 pp.

Tada, Y.; Kondo, S.; Aoki, S.; Koarada, S.; Inoue, H.; Suematsu, R.; Ohta, A.; Mak, T.W. & Nagasawa, K. (2011). Interferon regulatory factor 5 is critical for the development of lupus in MRL/lpr mice. *Arthritis Rheum*, 63 pp. 738-748

Takaoka, A.; Hayakawa, S.; Yanai, H.; Stoiber, D.; Negishi, H.; Kikuchi, H.; Sasaki, S.; Imai, K.; Shibue, T.; Honda, K. & Taniguchi, T. (2003). Integration of interferon-alpha/beta signalling to p53 responses in tumour suppression and antiviral defence. *Nature*, 424 pp. 516-523

Watford, W.T.; Hissong, B.D.; Bream, J.H.; Kanno, Y.; Muul, L. & O'Shea, J.J. (2004). Signaling by IL-12 and IL-23 and the immunoregulatory roles of STAT4. *Immunological Reviews*, 202 pp. 139-156

Xu, C.J.; Zhang, W.H.; Pan, H.F.; Li, X.P.; Xu, J.H. & Ye, D.Q. (2009). Association study of a single nucleotide polymorphism in the exon 2 region of toll-like receptor 9 (TLR9) gene with susceptibility to systemic lupus erythematosus among Chinese. *Molecular Biology Reports*, 36 pp. 2245-2248

Yamaguchi, H.; Fujimoto, T.; Nakamura, S.; Ohmura, K.; Mimori, T.; Matsuda, F. & Nagata,
        S. Aberrant splicing of the milk fat globule-EGF factor 8 (MFG-E8) gene in human
        systemic lupus erythematosus. *European Journal of Immunology*, 40 pp. 1778-1785

Ytterberg, S.R. & Schnitzer, T.J. (1982). Serum interferon levels in patients with systemic
        lupus-erythematosus. *Arthritis and Rheumatism*, 25 pp. 401-406

Zhuang, H.Y.; Narain, S.; Sobel, E.; Lee, P.Y.; Naconales, D.C.; Kelly, K.M.; Richards, H.B.;
        Segal, M.; Stewart, C.; Satoh, M. & Reeves, W.H. (2005). Association of anti-
        nucleoprotein autoantibodies with upregulation of Type I interferon-inducible gene
        transcripts and dendritic cell maturation in systemic lupus erythematosus. *Clinical
        Immunology*, 117 pp. 238-250

4

Regulation of Nucleic Acid Sensing Toll-Like Receptors in Systemic Lupus Erythematosus

Cynthia A. Leifer and James C. Brooks
College of Veterinary Medicine, Cornell University
USA

1. Introduction

Autoimmune disease is an aberrant response of the immune system to self. Unlike the adaptive immune system, the innate immune system is not selected during development and was originally thought to inherently discriminate between host and foreign molecular structures (Janeway, 1989). This is true for many innate immune receptor ligands including lipopolysaccharide, which is only synthesized by Gram-negative bacteria. However, some innate immune receptors detect nucleic acids that are shared between microbes and the host. Immune complexes containing nucleic acids are a hallmark of Systemic Lupus Erythematosus (SLE), and the nucleic acid sensing Toll-like receptors (TLRs) respond to the DNA and RNA within these complexes thereby contributing to disease. Defects in regulation of this class of innate immune receptors likely play a key role in precipitation of disease. Here we review nucleic acid sensing TLRs in SLE and recent advances in our understanding of the regulatory mechanisms governing TLR activity. Since breakdown of regulatory mechanisms controlling response of nucleic acid-sensing TLRs likely contributes to development of SLE, targeting specific proteins in these regulatory pathways has the potential to block nucleic acid-driven autoimmune inflammation.

2. Nucleic acid sensing toll-like receptors in SLE

2.1 Toll-like receptors

Toll-like receptors (TLRs) are a family of innate immune receptors that directly detect molecular structures and initiate signaling. Engagement of TLRs initiates innate immune responses that promote microbial killing and antigen presentation to educate T cells and B cells. At least 10 different TLRs recognize various microbial structures such as lipopeptides (TLR1, TLR2, and TLR6), lipopolysaccharide (TLR4), bacterial flagellin (TLR5), double stranded RNA (dsRNA, TLR3), single stranded RNA (ssRNA, TLR7, TLR8), and single stranded DNA (ssDNA, TLR9) (Takeda, et al. 2003).

TLRs are type 1 transmembrane receptors with C-termini facing the cytoplasm of the cell and ectodomains either at the cell surface or in the lumen of intracellular compartments. The cytoplasmic domain has homology with the IL-1 and IL-18 receptors and has been called the Toll/IL-1-like receptor domain (TIR). The three-dimensional structures of two TLR cytoplasmic TIR domains have been solved and are globular with many surfaces for protein-protein interactions (Xu, et al. 2000). The TIR domain associates with several adapter proteins that initiate signal transduction. These adapters include myeloid differentiation factor 88 (MyD88), and TIR-domain-containing adapter-inducing interferon-β (TRIF, also known as MyD88 adapter-like, MAL), which promote production of proinflammatory cytokines and type I interferons. The ectodomain is composed of a series of leucine rich repeats that form a curved solenoid. Alignment studies predicted a model structure for the ectodomains of TLRs (Bell, et al. 2003), which was supported by crystallographic studies (Bell, et al. 2005; Choe, et al. 2005). TLRs are expressed on a wide variety of cell types including B cells, T cells, dendritic cells, macrophages, and intestinal epithelial cells, although different cell types have unique repertoires of TLR expression (Takeda, et al. 2003). For example, human plasmacytoid dendritic cells express the nucleic acid-sensing TLRs, TLR7 and TLR9. TLR7- and TLR9-dependent responses by both B cells and plasmacytoid dendritic cells have been proposed to contribute to SLE (Marshak-Rothstein, 2006).

2.2 Nucleic acids as TLR ligands

Multiple nucleic acids, including ssRNA, dsRNA, and DNA, induce inflammatory responses. For DNA, the response is dependent on a 5'- cytosine-guanosine-3' dinucleotide (CpG). The central cytosine must be unmethylated, and is active when surrounded by specific bases, which together form the CpG motif (Krieg, 2002). These CpG motifs are rare in vertebrate DNA due to reduced frequency of the CG dinucleotide (CpG suppression) and increased frequency of cytosine methylation (Cardon, et al. 1994; Klinman, et al. 1996; Krieg, et al. 1995). However, CpG motifs are present and functional in bacterial DNA, in plasmid DNA produced in bacteria, and in synthetic DNA. Variation of sequence and physical structure of synthetic DNAs have resulted in characterization of at least four types of CpG oligodeoxynucleotides each with different activity on cells. Three are stimulatory, and one is inhibitory (Gursel, et al. 2003; Verthelyi, et al. 2001). Inhibitory DNAs do not require a CpG motif and the mechanism of inhibition has not been clearly defined (Gursel, et al. 2003; Krieg, et al. 1998; Lenert, et al. 2003). Type A CpG DNAs (also called D) induce robust type I interferon production, while type B CpG DNAs (also called K) induce B cell proliferation and proinflammatory cytokine production (Verthelyi, et al. 2001). The last class type C CpG DNAs have properties of both type A and type B CpG DNAs and thus induces both types of cellular responses (Vollmer, et al. 2004).

Regardless of their class, CpG DNAs require endocytosis and acidification of endosomes for activity (Figure 1). Blockade of uptake by immobilization of the CpG DNA on beads inhibits the B cell proliferative activity of synthetic CpG DNAs (Manzel & Macfarlane, 1999). Inhibition of endosomal acidification blocks CpG DNA-induced cytokine release by macrophages (Hacker, et al. 1998). Furthermore, cellular activation by CpG DNA initiates on endosomes (Ahmad-Nejad, et al. 2002). Vertebrate DNAs are poorly internalized, which contributes to their poor stimulatory activity. However, vertebrate DNA is stimulatory when in complex with proteins such as high mobility group box 1 (HMGB1), the antimicrobial peptide LL37, or anti-DNA antibodies (Lande, et al. 2007; Leadbetter, et al. 2002; Tian, et al. 2007). Whether the CpG DNA induces proinflammatory cytokines or type I interferon also depends on the endosomal compartment where the DNA is retained (Honda, et al. 2005). Honda and colleagues demonstrated that different types of DNA were trafficked to and retained within different endosomal compartments. For example, the type I interferon inducing CpG DNAs (type A) rapidly co-localized with FITC-dextran, a marker for early endosomes, but failed to co-localize with lysosomal markers. In contrast, rapid localization with lysosomal markers correlated with proinflammatory cytokine production induced by type B CpG DNAs. In another study the outcome of cellular responses to the DNA types could be swapped by changing the physical and chemical properties of the DNA (Guiducci, et al. 2006). Multimerization of type B CpG DNAs, so that their physical structure resembled type A CpG DNAs, caused them to be retained in early endosomes and induce A-type responses. Response of B cells was also dependent on CpG DNA type and delivery mechanism (Avalos, et al. 2009). These studies strongly correlated location of DNA detection with cellular outcome and suggested that manipulation of localization and receptor recognition could change the outcome of cellular response.

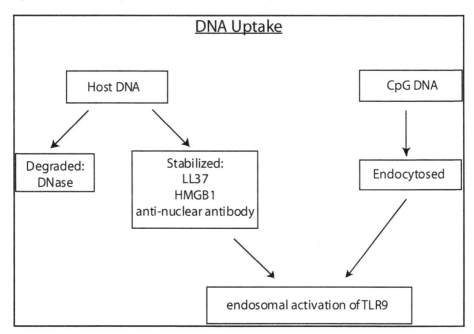

Fig. 1. DNA uptake into the cell. Host DNA is degraded in the extracellular space by DNase and does not normally induce inflammatory responses. However, several host proteins including LL37, HMGB1, and anti-nuclear antibodies stabilize host DNA and facilitate uptake into the endosomal compartment. Endocytosed host DNA activates TLR9. Unlike host DNA, synthetic CpG DNAs, or bacterial DNA, are efficeintly endocytosed and activate TLR9.

At concentrations of CpG DNA used by many investigators, uptake occurs by fluid phase endocytosis. Uptake of CpG DNA reached a plateau at 2 hours, was slowed at low temperature and was inhibited by known endocytosis inhibitors such as sodium azide and cytochalasin B (Yakubov, et al. 1989). Yet, at lower concentrations, uptake was significantly more efficient, which indicated that the CpG DNA was internalized by receptor-mediated endocytosis. Using radiolabeled cells, multiple groups demonstrated specific DNA binding proteins that likely assisted in internalization and trafficking of CpG DNA to the correct endosomal compartment where it encountered TLR9 (Beltinger, et al. 1995; Yakubov, et al. 1989). However, the identity of these receptors remains unknown. During the internalization process, CpG DNA transits though both early and late endosomes, which is important because, as mentioned above, CpG DNAs trigger different cellular outcomes depending on the compartment where signaling initiates.

A hallmark of SLE is elevated serum antibodies to nuclear components, which enhance response to DNA (Leadbetter, et al. 2002). Immune complexes from SLE patient serum were enriched in CG content within the DNA, consistent with increased presence of potential stimulatory motifs (Sano & Morimoto, 1982). Complexes with DNA bound to anti-idiotype B cell receptors (rheumatoid factor) and to Fc receptors to mediate internalization (Boule, et al. 2004; Leadbetter, et al. 2002). By either mechanism the uptake was very efficient and delivered the complexes to the endosomal compartment. Synergistic cytokine production and autoantibody induction by enhanced uptake of DNA-containing immune complexes likely contributes to the induction and propagation of anti-nucleic acid antibody production so frequently observed in SLE.

Internalization of CpG DNA and host DNA is also facilitated by several other host proteins including high mobility group protein 1 (HMGB-1), and the antimicrobial peptide LL37. The cationic antimicrobial peptide LL37 was highly elevated in the skin of patients with psoriases (Lande, et al. 2007). LL37 formed a stable complex with host DNA, and induced a TLR9-dependent, DNase-sensitive, type I interferon response from human plasmacytoid dendritic cells. The nuclear factor HMGB1 is retained within cells under normal conditions, but cell death and inflammation releases HMGB1, which formed a stable complex with host DNA. Association of CpG DNA-A with HMGB1 dramatically enhanced production of type I interferon (Tian, et al. 2007). In fact, HMGB1 was found in immune complexes with host DNA. Altogether, these studies demonstrate that while host DNA alone is not very immunostimulatory, association with a variety of different proteins, present in disease states, promote endosomal uptake where the DNA can associate with TLRs and induce pathologic interferon responses.

2.3 The role of TLRs in B cells and DC in SLE models

Mouse models have provided significant experimental evidence for the importance of TLRs in SLE. Deficiency in UNC93B1, a chaperone-like protein required for endocytic trafficking of nucleic acid-sensing TLRs, results in less severe disease in induced models of SLE in mice (Kono, et al. 2009). Furthermore, UNC93B1 protein is upregulated in SLE (Nakano, et al. 2010), underscoring the importance of TLRs in disease manifestations. The Y-linked autoimmune accelerator (Yaa) mutation, which accelerates and enhances spontaneous disease on the B6/FcRIIB -/- background, is due to TLR7 gene duplication (Pisitkun, et al. 2006), and disease in Fas-deficient MRL/lpr mice is dependent on TLR7 expression (Christensen, et al. 2006). Together these studies show that nucleic acid-sensing TLRs contribute to SLE.

The role for TLR9 in SLE-like disease in mice is less clear. TLR9 deficient mice have reduced anti-DNA antibodies, but enhanced disease (Christensen, et al. 2005). Despite these limitations, much is known about the regulation of TLR9, and TLR9 remains a good model to study the regulation of nucleic acid-sensing TLRs. A specific role for TLR9 in B cell responses to DNA containing immune complexes was supported by studies using a mouse expressing a transgenic "rheumatoid factor" receptor. In vitro stimulation with immune complexes that included DNA, such as anti-nucleosome complexes, induced proliferation of the transgenic B cells, but non-nucleic acid complexes, such as BSA-anti-BSA complexes did not. The response was DNase sensitive and dependent on MyD88 and uptake of the immune complexes into the endosomal compartment (Leadbetter, et al. 2002). Therefore, while TLR9 may not be a major contributor to disease in patients, defects in TLR9 regulation may have very specific functional consequences and a better understanding of the regulatory mechanisms may provide necessary information to therapeutically target TLR9 and other nucleic acid-sensing TLRs.

Patients with SLE have high levels of type I interferons in the blood and their peripheral blood mononuclear cells have a characteristic upregulation of interferon regulated genes (Bennett, et al. 2003). Plasmacytoid dendritic cells circulating in the blood are a major source of type I interferons and were originally called natural interferon producing cells (NIPCs). In humans, this subset of dendritic cells expresses predominantly TLR7 and TLR9 (Hornung, et al. 2002; Krug, et al. 2004). Production of type I interferons by plasmacytoid dendritic cells can be induced by immune complexes produced in abundance in patients with SLE (Ronnblom & Alm, 2001). Dendritic cells have Fc receptors on their cell surface that capture and internalize immune complexes, which induces interferon in a CpG motif- and TLR9-dependent manner (Boule, et al. 2004; Yasuda, et al. 2009). High circulating type I interferon correlates with immune pathology and disease severity in SLE. Therefore, TLR9 contributes to interferon production, and interferon can in turn augment TLR9-dependent responses.

2.4 Nucleic acid-sensing TLRs detection of self-ligands

When the stimulatory activity of CpG DNA was first described, it was thought to represent microbial DNA and that self-DNA was non-stimulatory. This was due to the requirement for the central CG dinucleotide, unmethylation of the C, and for selectivity for surrounding bases. These arguments held for many years, but it was known, even then, that the mammalian genome had the potential to induce TLR9-mediated responses (Ishii, et al. 2001; Yasuda, et al. 2005). Many studies, including the ones reviewed below, have been focussed on understanding what regulates TLR9 mediated responses and why self-DNA is not normally detected. However, recent studies suggest that TLR9 signaling is important for normal responses like wound repair.

Cells go to great lengths to assure DNA is not released into the extracellular milieu when they die by condensing and digesting their DNA during apoptosis. However, necrosis and neutrophil extracellular trap (NET) formation intentionally releases DNA that can induce inflammatory responses (Garcia-Romo, et al. 2011; Lande, et al. 2011; Villanueva, et al. 2011). Interestingly, SLE neutrophils were primed by high type I interferon levels in vivo, and in response to immune complexes, the neutrophils from SLE patients generated NETs that had a high content of DNA, LL37 and HMGB1. These proteins protected the DNA from degradation and facilitated internalization, and thereby increased the inflammatory potential of the host DNA. Therefore, since it is purposefully released under certain conditions, there must be other regulatory mechanisms to avoid response to host DNA. DNase is present in serum and in the extracellular environment and degrades potentially stimulatory host DNA. DNase deficient mice were born healthy but develop lupus like disease around six months of age (Napirei, et al. 2000). Heterozygous mice had increased serum concentrations of anti-nuclear antibodies, and more glomerulonephritis. However, in homozygous DNase deficient mice these SLE parameters were even higher. Mutations in DNase have been identified in SLE patients (Yasutomo, et al. 2001), and together these studies suggest that DNase is an important mechanism to prevent response to host DNA.

Interestingly, recent studies have shown that detection of self-DNA may be a normal biological process, and is, in fact, critical for wound healing (Gregorio, et al. 2010; Sato, et al. 2010). In the absence of TLR9, full thickness biopsy wound healing was delayed, and application of CpG DNA enhanced healing in a TLR9 dependent manner (Sato, et al. 2010). These data suggest that TLR9 plays an important role in wound healing. In a different model, tape stripping-induced epidermal injury induced plasmacytoid dendritic cell and neutrophil infiltration (Guiducci, et al. 2010). This response was accompanied by production of type I interferon, and was dependent on the signaling adapter molecule MyD88. Treatment of wild-type mice with a TLR7-TLR9 inhibitor inhibited the response, implicating these TLRs in the process. In lupus-prone mice, the same tape-stripping procedure led to chronic wounds with a type I interferon signature that resembled SLE skin lesions. Therefore, detection of DNA and RNA by TLR9 and TLR7 is important for normal wound healing. Dysregulation of this pathway in SLE likely contributes to autoimmune inflammation, especially in the skin, and is a potential target for therapeutic intervention.

3. Regulation of TLR9

3.1 Compartmentalization of TLR9

Infectious agents replicate in various locations outside and inside cells. Bacteria and viruses are internalized into endosomes, and some can escape into the cytoplasm. Therefore, positioning of TLRs is important for detecting components of microbes in the varied locations where they can reside. Some TLRs, such as TLR2, TLR4, and TLR5, are expressed at the cell surface to detect ligands expressed on the surface of bacteria (lipopolysaccharide, TLR4; lipopeptides, TLR2; and flagellin, TLR5). However, nucleic acids, such as DNA and RNA, are encapsulated within bacteria and viruses, and are only released upon internalization into endosomes. To accommodate this, nucleic acid sensing TLRs are localized intracellularly. For example, TLR9 is primarily found in the endoplasmic reticulum (ER) of resting cells (Latz, et al. 2004; Leifer, et al. 2004) where it colocalizes with ER, and not endosomal, markers. Since detection of DNA occurs in endosomes, these data suggest that that there is an induced trafficking event that leads to TLR9 entry into this compartment (Leifer, et al. 2004). The unique compartmentalization of nucleic acid-sensing TLRs has been proposed as a major regulatory mechanism to prevent response to host DNA (Barton, et al. 2006). Fusion of the ectodomain of TLR9 with the transmembrane domain and cytoplasmic tail of TLR4 created a protein that localized to the cell surface. This change in localization endowed the TLR9 ectodomain with the ability to respond to host DNA (Barton, et al. 2006). These data support a model where TLR9 is specifically trafficked intracellularly to avoid access to the extracellular milieu, thereby preventing recognition of host DNA.

3.2 Trafficking of TLR9 through the Golgi to localize in the endolysosomes

While TLR9 predominantly resides in the ER it must traffic to the endosomal compartment where it encounters endocytosed CpG DNA (Latz, et al. 2004; Leifer, et al. 2004) (Figure 2). Normally, transmembrane or secreted proteins synthesized in the ER traffic through the Golgi to access the cell surface or intracellular endosomes. However, TLR9 was sensitive to endoglycosidase H (endo H) treatment, which indicated that TLR9 had not reached the

Golgi (Latz, et al. 2004). In 2009 Chockalingam et al., showed that Brefeldin A inhibited TLR9 response to CpG DNA (Chockalingam, et al. 2009). Since Brefeldin A is a small molecule that inhibits transport of proteins from ER to Golgi, TLR9 signaling appeared to be dependent on Golgi trafficking.

When proteins traffic through the Golgi, the high mannose glycans are processed to hybrid forms that are still cleaved by Endo H; therefore, highly specific lectins were used to determine whether TLR9 had glycan modifications indicative of Golgi transit (Chockalingam, et al. 2009). Lectins are plant proteins that selectively recognize carbohydrate structures. For example, *Datura stramonium* (DS) lectin specifically recognizes "Galβ1→4GlcNac" structures present only on proteins that have been processed by Golgi resident enzymes. DS lectin bound to TLR9, which confirmed that TLR9 trafficked through the Golgi during synthesis (Chockalingam, et al. 2009). TLR9 immunoprecipitated from the lysosomal compartment of HEK293 cells also bound DS lectin, and co-immunoprecipitated with the signaling adapter MyD88 (Chockalingam, et al. 2009). These data indicated that lysosomal TLR9 had transited through the Golgi and contributed to signaling.

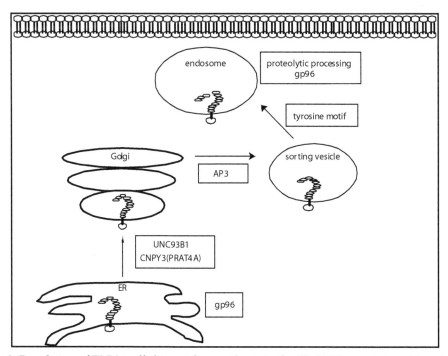

Fig. 2. Regulation of TLR9 trafficking. After synthesis in the ER TLR9 associates with gp96. TLR9 traffics out of the ER to the Golgi in a manner dependent on gp96, PRAT4A, and UNC93B1. TLR9 traffics from the Golgi to a sorting vesicle in an AP3 dependent manner where it is then sorted to the endosomal compartment via a cytoplasmic tyrosine motif. In the endosomal compartment TLR9 is proteolytically processed either active or negative regulatory forms that modulate TLR9 signaling. Lack of gp96 prevents TLR9 proteolytic processing.

3.3 Proteins that regulate intracellular localization and trafficking

Several proteins are critical for TLR9 trafficking both out of the ER and to the endosomal compartment (Figure 2): UNC93B1, adapter protein 3 (AP3), a protein associated with TLR4 (PRAT4A), Slc15a4, and glycoprotein 96 (gp96, also known as glucose regulated protein 94 (gp94). Recessive N-ethyl-N-nitrosourea-induced mutagenesis revealed a mouse line that lacked response to TLR3, TLR7, and TLR9 ligands. These mice had a single point mutation (H412R) in UNC93B1 (Tabeta, et al. 2006). In dendritic cells from these mice, TLR7 and TLR9 did not localize to the endosomal compartment (Kim, et al. 2008). Interestingly, UNC93B1 seems to play opposing roles in regulation of TLR7 and TLR9 (Fukui, et al. 2009). Reconstitution of UNC93B1 deficient cells with UNC93B1 containing a single point mutation (D34A) resulted in hyperresponsivenss to TLR7, yet hyporesponsiveness to TLR9, ligands. Therefore, the role of UNC93B1 in regulation of nucleic acid sensing TLRs is clearly important and interfering with UNC93B1 function has different effects on signaling by different TLRs.

Two ER luminal proteins, gp96 and PRAT4A, are essential for TLR9 exit from the ER. PRAT4A, also known as CNPY3, bound to TLR9, which depended on methionine 145 of PRAT4A (Kiyokawa, et al. 2008). In the absence of PRAT4A, TLR9 did not access endosomes, and PRAT4A deficient cells lacked response through all TLRs, except TLR3 (Takahashi, et al. 2007). The heat shock protein gp96 also bound to TLR9 and was required for B cell and macrophage response to CpG DNA (Randow & Seed, 2001; Yang, et al. 2007). A pre-B cell line with a frame-shift mutation in gp96 was 10,000 times less sensitive to LPS then the non-mutant line, which was due to a lack of TLR4 on the cell surface (Randow & Seed, 2001). This study suggested that gp96 regulated trafficking of TLRs. Further studies using a mouse with macrophage specific knockout of gp96 showed that gp96 is essential for TLR9 trafficking and signaling, and was in fact a chaperone for all TLRs except TLR3 (Liu, et al. 2010; Yang, et al. 2007). In 2011 Liu et al., demonstrated that gp96 and PRAT4A directly interacted to form a multimeric complex with TLR9 (Liu, et al. 2010). Very recent studies using gp96 specific inhibitors have examined the role of gp96 after TLR9 synthesis and trafficking is complete. These studies show that gp96 remains associated with TLR9 in the endosomal compartment and that specific inhibitors block CpG DNA signaling and cause a loss of TLR9 protein (JC Brooks and CA Leifer unpublished observations). This suggests that gp96 has an additional function in regulating the conformational stability of TLR9 in the endosomal compartment.

Cytoplasmic proteins are also important for TLR9 trafficking. Plasmacytoid DCs from adapter protein 3 (AP3) deficient mice failed to induce a type I interferon response after CpG DNA stimulation despite normal IL-12 production (Sasai, et al. 2010). AP3 is a cytosolic protein that associates with endosomes and sorts transmembrane proteins from the endosomal compartment to lysosome-related organelles (Bonifacino & Traub, 2003). In the absence of AP3, TLR9 did not colocalize with markers for lysosome-related organelles (Sasai, et al. 2010). This group suggested that it was these lysosome-related organelles that were critical for induction of type I interferons (Sasai, et al. 2010). However, this conclusion contradicts previously published studies showing that initiation of signaling that results in type I interferon production occurs on early endosomes (Guiducci, et al. 2006; Honda, et al. 2005). In a separate study using the same AP3 deficient mice, both proinflammatory and type I interferon production were lost. Therefore, AP3 is important for TLR9-induced cytokine production, but its exact role in TLR9 biology remains unclear.

Recent data have shown that TLR9 signaling also depends on Slc15a4, a twelve-spanning transmembrane oligopeptide transporter that localizes to the endolysosomal compartment (Blasius, et al. 2010; Yamashita, et al. 1997). Cells from Slc15a4 deficient mice lack response to nucleic acid sensing TLRs (Blasius, et al. 2010). Again, the specific role of Slc15a4 remains unknown, but may involve endolysosomal transport of TLR9 or a TLR9-associated protein required for TLR9 function.

3.4 Specific motifs in TLR9 that regulate localization and trafficking

Localization of TLRs is regulated by sequences in their transmembrane domains and cytoplasmic tails. Fusion of TLR4 to the transmembrane and cytoplasmic tail of various TLRs resulted in distinct localizations of the chimeric proteins (Nishiya & DeFranco, 2004). For example, TLR4 by itself localized to the cell surface, and fusion of TLR4's ectodomain with the transmembrane and cytoplasmic tail of TLR1, TLR2, TLR5, or TLR6 resulted in similar localization. In contrast, when TLR4 was fused to the transmembrane and cytoplasmic tail of any of the nucleic acid-sensing TLRs, the resulting chimeric receptor was not detected at the cell surface. Further studies using different approaches identified different motifs in TLR9 responsible for this localization (Barton, et al. 2006; Leifer, et al. 2006). TLR9's ectodomain fused to TLR4's transmembrane and cytoplasmic domains localized to the cell surface (Barton, et al. 2006). The chimera retained the ability to respond to CpG DNA, yet was resistant to endosomal acidification inhibitors. Interestingly, TLR9 associates with UNC93B1 via the transmembrane domain and this may explain, in part, the requirement for this association in TLR9 signaling.

The cytoplasmic tail of TLR9 also contains a specific localization motif (Leifer, et al. 2006). In this study, the ectodomain of the IL-2 receptor alpha chain, which normally localized to cell surface, was fused to the transmembrane and cytoplasmic tail of different TLRs (Leifer, et al. 2006). A fusion with the TLR4 transmembrane and cytoplasmic tail localized to the cell surface; however, a fusion with the same regions of TLR9 was not. Truncation analysis revealed that deletion of all but four amino acids of the cytoplasmic tail generated a protein that was robustly expressed at the cell surface, ruling out a contribution of the transmembrane domain to intracellular localization. It is unclear why these two studies showed opposite requirements for TLR9 transmembrane domain. Regardless, additional truncations and mapping identified a 14 amino acid motif that was important for TLR9 intracellular localization. Follow-up studies showed that mutation of a critical tyrosine (888) within this motif abolished proinflammatory cytokine production. Interestingly, this mutant maintained normal interferon responses suggesting that this motif was required for trafficking TLR9 to the compartment selectively required for induction of proinflammatory cytokines (A Chockalingam and CA Leifer unpublished observations). It remains to be determined if this motif is necessary for association with AP3 or other regulatory proteins.

3.5 Proteolytic regulation of TLR9

In addition to trafficking to specific endocytic compartments, several recent studies have demonstrated that TLR9 is proteolytically processed in endosomes and that this processing regulates TLR9 function (Chockalingam, et al. 2011; Ewald, et al. 2011; Ewald, et al. 2008; Park, et al. 2008; Sepulveda, et al. 2009). The ectodomain of TLR9 contains 25 leucine rich repeats. The first 14 and the second 15 leucine-rich repeats are interrupted by a region predicted to have very little secondary structure, often referred to as the hinge (Bell, et al.

2003). The first described proteolytic event was mapped to this hinge region through a mass spectrometric approach (Park, et al. 2008). The form of TLR9 generated encompasses one-half of the ectodomain and all of the transmembrane and cytoplasmic tail (Figure 3). This proteolytic event is inhibited by endosomal acidification inhibitors and by broad-spectrum cathepsin inhibitors (Ewald, et al. 2008; Park, et al. 2008). Additional studies with specific cathepsin inhibitors, and in cathepsin deficient mice, did not reveal a unique cathepsin responsible for the cleavage. An independent study, showed an additional proteolytic event (Sepulveda, et al. 2009). While this study did not reveal the precise location of the proteolysis, a specific enzyme, asaparagine endopeptidase was shown to be important. A more recent study suggested that stepwise processing of TLR9 is required to attain fully functional proteolytically processed TLR9 (Ewald, et al. 2011). Interestingly, knockdown of either PRAT4A (CNPY3) or gp96 by shRNA targeting resulted in a loss of proteolytic processing of TLR9, and suggested that these chaperones were required for TLR9 to access endosomes (Liu, et al. 2010).

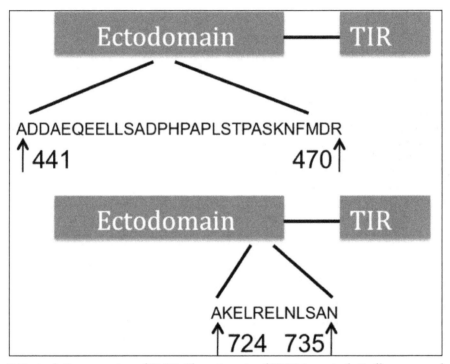

Fig. 3. Proteolytic processing of TLR9. The ectomain of TLR9 is proteolytically processed into two forms. The first form is active and consists of one half of the ectodomain of TLR9 and the transmembrane and cytoplasmic tail (amino acids 471-1032) The second form is a negative regulator of TLR9 signaling and consists of almost the entire ectodomain with no transmembrane or cytoplasmic tail. This form, called soluble TLR9, is released into endosomes, but is not secreted. By binding to internalized DNA, and to full-length TLR9, this form blocks signaling. The relative ratio of these two fragments likely determines the cellular response upon exposure to DNA.

TLR9 is also proteolytically processed at a completely different position to generate a negative regulator of TLR9 signaling (Chockalingam, et al. 2011). This proteolytic event resulted in generation of an intact ectodomain separated from the transmembrane domain and cytoplasmic tail (Figure 2). This soluble form of TLR9 bound to CpG DNA, associated with full length TLR9, and dominant negatively inhibited responses by the full-length receptor (Chockalingam, et al. 2011). In contrast to the other proteolytic cleavage events, generation of soluble TLR9 occurred in cells expressing endogenous TLR9 (Chockalingam, et al. 2011). Soluble TLR9 is likely important in regulating TLR9 responses since intestinal epithelial cells poorly responded to CpG DNA, and abundantly generated soluble TLR9 (Chockalingam, et al. 2011). Therefore, correlative studies on TLR9 in different pathological conditions must account for the complexity of TLR9 post-translational modification.

4. Conclusion

In this review we have highlighted recent studies describing regulatory mechanisms governing nucleic acid-sensing TLRs. While TLRs are critical for host defence against infection, some TLRs recognize ligands shared between infectious agents and the host (Marshak-Rothstein & Rifkin, 2007). Despite complex regulatory mechanisms, these TLRs do contribute to autoimmune disease (Marshak-Rothstein, 2006). Recent studies have revealed multiple post-translational mechanisms that regulate this family of TLRs, and if dysregulated could also contribute to the development of autoimmune disease. By exploiting mechanisms that control nucleic acid sensing TLRs we will relieve TLR-mediate autoimmune inflammation.

Host DNA and RNA are not typically inflammatory since there are several regulatory mechanisms to prevent availability of host DNA. These include preventing its release (apoptosis), and degrading it once it is released (DNase). Association with various host proteins such as HMGB1, LL37, and autoantibodies stabilize host DNA and enhance its uptake where it gains access to intracellular nucleic acid sensing TLRs (Lande, et al. 2007; Leadbetter, et al. 2002; Tian, et al. 2007). When this occurs, especially by anti-nuclear antibodies, host DNA and RNA enhance type I interferon production from dendritic cells and promote proliferation and antibody production from B cells. Defects in expression of the nucleic acid stabilizing proteins changes susceptibility to autoimmunity in mouse models. Development of drugs that block stabilization of DNA by these host proteins, and thereby block proinflammatory or interferon responses, will reduce autoinflammation and offer new ways to treat SLE.

The nucleic acid-sensing TLRs are also carefully regulated to avoid response to host DNA. To avoid detection of host DNAs and RNAs, nucleic acid-sensing TLRs are excluded from the cell surface (Latz, et al. 2004; Leifer, et al. 2004). Several proteins including UNC93B1, and gp96 regulate nucleic acid-sensing TLR access to endosomes (Kim, et al. 2008; Yang, et al. 2007). Specific parts of TLR9 have been found to be important for this regulation and may interact with some of the localization regulators (Barton, et al. 2006; Leifer, et al. 2006). Development of drugs that affect the activity of these proteins would change the intracellular distribution of TLRs, thereby affecting the ability of these receptors to detect and respond to nucleic acids.

Once nucleic acid-sensing TLRs do reach endosomes, they are proteolytically processed (Chockalingam, et al. 2011; Ewald, et al. 2008; Park, et al. 2008), which modifies their function. Cleavage at two different locations within the ectodomain leads to either activation (Ewald, et al. 2008; Park, et al. 2008), or inhibition (Chockalingam, et al. 2011), of TLR9 activity. Specific identification of the enzymes responsible for these proteolytic events will provide new targets for drug development to interfere with TLR signaling and response to host DNA.

When host DNA, or RNA, does activate a TLR, it induces robust inflammation and production of pathologic levels of cytokines such as type I interferon. While several contributing factors to the development of SLE have been found, new data on post-translational regulation of nucleic acid-sensing TLRs show that we still have much to learn. Dysregulation in any of these regulatory proteins will change the intracellular localization of TLR9 and could potentially lead to aberrant response to host nucleic acids. Identifying these regulatory pathways is the first step to understanding how defects in these pathways lead to disease. Specifically targeting these regulatory proteins within these pathways will reduce, or restore, function as necessary to return the regulatory networks to the non-disease state. Therefore, future studies should be focused on improving our understanding of the basic regulatory networks for nucleic acid-sensing TLRs so that we may determine which are defective in SLE. Our hope is that these studies will lead to novel drug development, and improve our repertoire of options to treat autoimmune disease.

5. Acknowledgments

Studies from the Leifer lab described in this review were supported by awards to CAL (NCI K22CA113705, and NIAID AI076588). The authors would like to thank A Chockalingam for helpful suggestions.

6. References

Ahmad-Nejad, P, Hacker, H, Rutz, M, Bauer, S, Vabulas, RM, & Wagner, H. (2002) Bacterial CpG-DNA and lipopolysaccharides activate Toll-like receptors at distinct cellular compartments. European Journal of Immunolology 32:1958-1968.

Avalos, AM, Latz, E, Mousseau, B, Christensen, SR, Shlomchik, MJ, Lund, F, & Marshak-Rothstein, A. (2009) Differential cytokine production and bystander activation of autoreactive B cells in response to CpG-A and CpG-B oligonucleotides. Journal of Immunology 183:6262-6268.

Barton, GM, Kagan, JC, & Medzhitov, R. (2006) Intracellular localization of Toll-like receptor 9 prevents recognition of self DNA but facilitates access to viral DNA. Nature Immunology 7:49-56.

Bell, JK, Botos, I, Hall, PR, Askins, J, Shiloach, J, Segal, DM, & Davies, DR. (2005) The molecular structure of the Toll-like receptor 3 ligand-binding domain. Procedings of the National Academy of Science U S A 102:10976-10980.

Bell, JK, Mullen, GE, Leifer, CA, Mazzoni, A, Davies, DR, & Segal, DM. (2003) Leucine-rich repeats and pathogen recognition in Toll-like receptors. Trendsin Immunol 24:528-533.

Beltinger, C, Saragovi, HU, Smith, RM, LeSauteur, L, Shah, N, DeDionisio, L, Christensen, L, Raible, A, Jarett, L, & Gewirtz, AM. (1995) Binding, uptake, and intracellular trafficking of phosphorothioate-modified oligodeoxynucleotides. Journal of Clinical Investigation 95:1814-1823.

Bennett, L, Palucka, AK, Arce, E, Cantrell, V, Borvak, J, Banchereau, J, & Pascual, V. (2003) Interferon and granulopoiesis signatures in systemic lupus erythematosus blood. Journal of Experimental Medicine 197:711-723.

Blasius, AL, Arnold, CN, Georgel, P, Rutschmann, S, Xia, Y, Lin, P, Ross, C, Li, X, Smart, NG, & Beutler, B. (2010) Slc15a4, AP-3, and hermansky-pudlak syndrome proteins are required for Toll-like receptor signaling in plasmacytoid dendritic cells. Procedings of the National Academy of Science U S A 107:19973-19978.

Bonifacino, JS, & Traub, LM. (2003) Signals for sorting of transmembrane proteins to endosomes and lysosomes. Annual Review of Biochemistry 72:395-447.

Boule, MW, Broughton, C, Mackay, F, Akira, S, Marshak-Rothstein, A, & Rifkin, IR. (2004) Toll-like receptor 9-dependent and -independent dendritic cell activation by chromatin-immunoglobulin G complexes. Journal of Experimental Medicine 199:1631-1640.

Cardon, LR, Burge, C, Clayton, DA, & Karlin, S. (1994) Pervasive CpG suppression in animal mitochondrial genomes. Procedings of the National Academy of Science U S A 91:3799-3803.

Chockalingam, A, Brooks, JC, Cameron, JL, Blum, LK, & Leifer, CA. (2009) TLR9 traffics through the Golgi complex to localize to endolysosomes and respond to CpG DNA. Immunology and Cell Biology 87:209-217.

Chockalingam, A, Cameron, JL, Brooks, JC, & Leifer, CA. (2011) Negative regulation of signaling by a soluble form of Toll-like receptor 9. European Journal of Immunology DOI: 10.1002/eji.201041034

Choe, J, Kelker, MS, & Wilson, IA. (2005) Crystal structure of human Toll-like receptor 3 (TLR3) ectodomain. Science 309:581-585.

Christensen, SR, Kashgarian, M, Alexopoulou, L, Flavell, RA, Akira, S, & Shlomchik, MJ. (2005) Toll-like receptor 9 controls anti-DNA autoantibody production in murine lupus. Journal of Experimental Medicine 202:321-331.

Christensen, SR, Shupe, J, Nickerson, K, Kashgarian, M, Flavell, RA, & Shlomchik, MJ. (2006) Toll-like receptor 7 and TLR9 dictate autoantibody specificity and have opposing inflammatory and regulatory roles in a murine model of lupus. Immunity 25:417-428.

Ewald, SE, Engel, A, Lee, J, Wang, M, Bogyo, M, & Barton, GM. (2011) Nucleic acid recognition by Toll-like receptors is coupled to stepwise processing by cathepsins and asparagine endopeptidase. Journal of Experimental Medicine 208:643-651.

Ewald, SE, Lee, BL, Lau, L, Wickliffe, KE, Shi, GP, Chapman, HA, & Barton, GM. (2008) The ectodomain of Toll-like receptor 9 is cleaved to generate a functional receptor. Nature 456:658-662.

Fukui, R, Saitoh, S, Matsumoto, F, Kozuka-Hata, H, Oyama, M, Tabeta, K, Beutler, B, & Miyake, K. (2009) Unc93B1 biases Toll-like receptor responses to nucleic acid in dendritic cells toward DNA- but against RNA-sensing. Journal of Experimental Medicine 206:1339-1350.

Garcia-Romo, GS, Caielli, S, Vega, B, Connolly, J, Allantaz, F, Xu, Z, Punaro, M, Baisch, J, Guiducci, C, Coffman, RL, Barrat, FJ, Banchereau, J, & Pascual, V. (2011) Netting neutrophils are major inducers of type I IFN production in pediatric Systemic Lupus Erythematosus. Science Translational Medicine 3:73ra20.

Gregorio, J, Meller, S, Conrad, C, Di Nardo, A, Homey, B, Lauerma, A, Arai, N, Gallo, RL, Digiovanni, J, & Gilliet, M. (2010) Plasmacytoid dendritic cells sense skin injury and promote wound healing through type I interferons. Journal of Experimental Medicine 207:2921-2930.

Guiducci, C, Ott, G, Chan, JH, Damon, E, Calacsan, C, Matray, T, Lee, KD, Coffman, RL, & Barrat, FJ. (2006) Properties regulating the nature of the plasmacytoid dendritic cell response to Toll-like receptor 9 activation. Journal of Experimental Medicine 203:1999-2008.

Guiducci, C, Tripodo, C, Gong, M, Sangaletti, S, Colombo, MP, Coffman, RL, & Barrat, FJ. (2010) Autoimmune skin inflammation is dependent on plasmacytoid dendritic cell activation by nucleic acids via TLR7 and TLR9. Journal of Experimental Medicine 207:2931-2942.

Gursel, I, Gursel, M, Yamada, H, Ishii, KJ, Takeshita, F, & Klinman, DM. (2003) Repetitive elements in mammalian telomeres suppress bacterial DNA-induced immune activation. Journal of Immunology 171:1393-1400.

Hacker, H, Mischak, H, Miethke, T, Liptay, S, Schmid, R, Sparwasser, T, Heeg, K, Lipford, GB, & Wagner, H. (1998) CpG-DNA-specific activation of antigen-presenting cells requires stress kinase activity and is preceded by non-specific endocytosis and endosomal maturation. EMBO Journal 17:6230-6240.

Honda, K, Ohba, Y, Yanai, H, Negishi, H, Mizutani, T, Takaoka, A, Taya, C, & Taniguchi, T. (2005) Spatiotemporal regulation of MyD88-IRF-7 signalling for robust type-I interferon induction. Nature 434:1035-1040.

Hornung, V, Rothenfusser, S, Britsch, S, Krug, A, Jahrsdorfer, B, Giese, T, Endres, S, & Hartmann, G. (2002) Quantitative expression of Toll-like receptor 1-10 mRNA in cellular subsets of human peripheral blood mononuclear cells and sensitivity to CpG oligodeoxynucleotides. Journal of Immunology 168:4531-4537.

Ishii, KJ, Suzuki, K, Coban, C, Takeshita, F, Itoh, Y, Matoba, H, Kohn, LD, & Klinman, DM. (2001) Genomic DNA released by dying cells induces the maturation of apcs. Journal of Immunology 167:2602-2607.

Janeway, CA, Jr. (1989) Approaching the asymptote? Evolution and revolution in immunology. Cold Spring Harorb Symposium on Quantative Biology 54 Pt 1:1-13.

Kim, YM, Brinkmann, MM, Paquet, ME, & Ploegh, HL. (2008) UNC93B1 delivers nucleotide-sensing Toll-like receptors to endolysosomes. Nature 452:234-238.

Kiyokawa, T, Akashi-Takamura, S, Shibata, T, Matsumoto, F, Nishitani, C, Kuroki, Y, Seto, Y, & Miyake, K. (2008) A single base mutation in the PRAT4A gene reveals differential interaction of PRAT4A with Toll-like receptors. International Immunology 20:1407-1415.

Klinman, DM, Yi, AK, Beaucage, SL, Conover, J, & Krieg, AM. (1996) CpG motifs present in bacteria DNA rapidly induce lymphocytes to secrete interleukin 6, interleukin 12, and interferon gamma. Proceedings of the National Academy of Science U S A 93:2879-2883.

Kono, DH, Haraldsson, MK, Lawson, BR, Pollard, KM, Koh, YT, Du, X, Arnold, CN, Baccala, R, Silverman, GJ, Beutler, BA, & Theofilopoulos, AN. (2009) Endosomal TLR signaling is required for anti-nucleic acid and rheumatoid factor autoantibodies in lupus. Proceedings of the National Academy of Science U S A   106:12061-12066.

Krieg, AM. (2002) CpG motifs in bacterial DNA and their immune effects. Annual Review of Immunology 20:709-760.

Krieg, AM, Wu, T, Weeratna, R, Efler, SM, Love-Homan, L, Yang, L, Yi, AK, Short, D, & Davis, HL. (1998) Sequence motifs in adenoviral DNA block immune activation by stimulatory CpG motifs. Proceedings of the National Academy of Science U S A 95:12631-12636.

Krieg, AM, Yi, AK, Matson, S, Waldschmidt, TJ, Bishop, GA, Teasdale, R, Koretzky, GA, & Klinman, DM. (1995) CpG motifs in bacterial DNA trigger direct B-cell activation. Nature 374:546-549.

Krug, A, French, AR, Barchet, W, Fischer, JA, Dzionek, A, Pingel, JT, Orihuela, MM, Akira, S, Yokoyama, WM, & Colonna, M. (2004) TLR9-dependent recognition of MCMV by iPC and DC generates coordinated cytokine responses that activate antiviral NK cell function. Immunity 21:107-119.

Lande, R, Ganguly, D, Facchinetti, V, Frasca, L, Conrad, C, Gregorio, J, Meller, S, Chamilos, G, Sebasigari, R, Riccieri, V, Bassett, R, Amuro, H, Fukuhara, S, Ito, T, Liu, YJ, & Gilliet, M. (2011) Neutrophils activate plasmacytoid dendritic cells by releasing self-DNA-peptide complexes in Systemic Lupus Erythematosus. Science Translational Medicine 3:73ra19.

Lande, R, Gregorio, J, Facchinetti, V, Chatterjee, B, Wang, YH, Homey, B, Cao, W, Wang, YH, Su, B, Nestle, FO, Zal, T, Mellman, I, Schroder, JM, Liu, YJ, & Gilliet, M. (2007) Plasmacytoid dendritic cells sense self-DNA coupled with antimicrobial peptide. Nature 449:564-569.

Latz, E, Schoenemeyer, A, Visintin, A, Fitzgerald, KA, Monks, BG, Knetter, CF, Lien, E, Nilsen, NJ, Espevik, T, & Golenbock, DT. (2004) TLR9 signals after translocating from the ER to CpG DNA in the lysosome. Nature Immunology 5:190-198.

Leadbetter, EA, Rifkin, IR, Hohlbaum, AM, Beaudette, BC, Shlomchik, MJ, & Marshak-Rothstein, A. (2002) Chromatin-IgG complexes activate B cells by dual engagement of IgM and Toll-like receptors. Nature 416:603-607.

Leifer, CA, Brooks, JC, Hoelzer, K, Lopez, JL, Kennedy, MN, Mazzoni, A, & Segal, DM. (2006) Cytoplasmic targeting motifs control localization of Toll-like receptor 9. Journal of Biological Chemistry 281:35585-35592.

Leifer, CA, Kennedy, MN, Mazzoni, A, Lee, C, Kruhlak, MJ, & Segal, DM. (2004) TLR9 is localized in the endoplasmic reticulum prior to stimulation. Journal of Immunology 173:1179-1183.

Lenert, P, Rasmussen, W, Ashman, RF, & Ballas, ZK. (2003) Structural characterization of the inhibitory DNA motif for the type A (D)-CpG-induced cytokine secretion and NK-cell lytic activity in mouse spleen cells. DNA Cell Biology 22:621-631.

Liu, B, Yang, Y, Qiu, Z, Staron, M, Hong, F, Li, Y, Wu, S, Hao, B, Bona, R, Han, D, & Li, Z. (2010) Folding of Toll-like receptors by the hsp90 paralogue gp96 requires a substrate-specific cochaperone. Nature Communications 1:79.

Manzel, L, & Macfarlane, DE. (1999) Lack of immune stimulation by immobilized CpG-oligodeoxynucleotide. Antisense Nucleic Acid Drug Development 9:459-464.

Marshak-Rothstein, A. (2006) Toll-like receptors in systemic autoimmune disease. Nature Reviews Immunology 6:823-835.

Marshak-Rothstein, A, & Rifkin, IR. (2007) Immunologically active autoantigens: The role of Toll-like receptors in the development of chronic inflammatory disease. Annual Review of Immunology 25:419-441.

Nakano, S, Morimoto, S, Suzuki, S, Watanabe, T, Amano, H, & Takasaki, Y. (2010) Up-regulation of the endoplasmic reticulum transmembrane protein UNC93b in the B cells of patients with active Systemic Lupus Erythematosus. Rheumatology (Oxford) 49:876-881.

Napirei, M, Karsunky, H, Zevnik, B, Stephan, H, Mannherz, HG, & Moroy, T. (2000) Features of Systemic Lupus Erythematosus in DNase1-deficient mice. Nature Genetics 25:177-181.

Nishiya, T, & DeFranco, AL. (2004) Ligand-regulated chimeric receptor approach reveals distinctive subcellular localization and signaling properties of the Toll-like receptors. Journal of Biological Chemistry 279:19008-19017.

Park, B, Brinkmann, MM, Spooner, E, Lee, CC, Kim, YM, & Ploegh, HL. (2008) Proteolytic cleavage in an endolysosomal compartment is required for activation of Toll-like receptor 9. Nature Immunology 9:1407-1414.

Pisitkun, P, Deane, JA, Difilippantonio, MJ, Tarasenko, T, Satterthwaite, AB, & Bolland, S. (2006) Autoreactive B cell responses to RNA-related antigens due to TLR7 gene duplication. Science 312:1669-1672.

Randow, F, & Seed, B. (2001) Endoplasmic reticulum chaperone gp96 is required for innate immunity but not cell viability. Nature Cell Biology 3:891-896.

Ronnblom, L, & Alm, GV. (2001) A pivotal role for the natural interferon alpha-producing cells (plasmacytoid dendritic cells) in the pathogenesis of lupus. Journal of Experimental Medicine 194:F59-63.

Sano, H, & Morimoto, C. (1982) DNA isolated from DNA/anti-DNA antibody immune complexes in Systemic Lupus Erythematosus is rich in guanine-cytosine content. Journal of Immunology 128:1341-1345.

Sasai, M, Linehan, MM, & Iwasaki, A. (2010) Bifurcation of Toll-like receptor 9 signaling by adaptor protein 3. Science 329:1530-1534.

Sato, T, Yamamoto, M, Shimosato, T, & Klinman, DM. (2010) Accelerated wound healing mediated by activation of Toll-like receptor 9. Wound Repair Regeneration 18:586-593.

Sepulveda, FE, Maschalidi, S, Colisson, R, Heslop, L, Ghirelli, C, Sakka, E, Lennon-Dumenil, AM, Amigorena, S, Cabanie, L, & Manoury, B. (2009) Critical role for asparagine endopeptidase in endocytic Toll-like receptor signaling in dendritic cells. Immunity 31:737-748.

Tabeta, K, Hoebe, K, Janssen, EM, Du, X, Georgel, P, Crozat, K, Mudd, S, Mann, N, Sovath, S, Goode, J, Shamel, L, Herskovits, AA, Portnoy, DA, Cooke, M, Tarantino, LM, Wiltshire, T, Steinberg, BE, Grinstein, S, & Beutler, B. (2006) The UNC93B1 mutation 3d disrupts exogenous antigen presentation and signaling via Toll-like receptors 3, 7 and 9. Nature Immunology 7:156-164.

Takahashi, K, Shibata, T, Akashi-Takamura, S, Kiyokawa, T, Wakabayashi, Y, Tanimura, N, Kobayashi, T, Matsumoto, F, Fukui, R, Kouro, T, Nagai, Y, Takatsu, K, Saitoh, S, & Miyake, K. (2007) A protein associated with Toll-like receptor (TLR) 4 (PRAT4A) is required for TLR-dependent immune responses. Journal of Experimental Medicine 204:2963-2976.

Takeda, K, Kaisho, T, & Akira, S. (2003) Toll-like receptors. Annual Review of Immunology 21:335-376.

Tian, J, Avalos, AM, Mao, SY, Chen, B, Senthil, K, Wu, H, Parroche, P, Drabic, S, Golenbock, D, Sirois, C, Hua, J, An, LL, Audoly, L, La Rosa, G, Bierhaus, A, Naworth, P, Marshak-Rothstein, A, Crow, MK, Fitzgerald, KA, Latz, E, Kiener, PA, & Coyle, AJ. (2007) Toll-like receptor 9-dependent activation by DNA-containing immune complexes is mediated by HMGB1 and rage. Nature Immunology 8:487-496.

Verthelyi, D, Ishii, KJ, Gursel, M, Takeshita, F, & Klinman, DM. (2001) Human peripheral blood cells differentially recognize and respond to two distinct CpG motifs. Journal of Immunology 166:2372-2377.

Villanueva, E, Yalavarthi, S, Berthier, CC, Hodgin, JB, Khandpur, R, Lin, AM, Rubin, CJ, Zhao, W, Olsen, SH, Klinker, M, Shealy, D, Denny, MF, Plumas, J, Chaperot, L, Kretzler, M, Bruce, AT, & Kaplan, MJ. (2011) Netting neutrophils induce endothelial damage, infiltrate tissues, and expose immunostimulatory molecules in Systemic Lupus Erythematosus. Journal of Immunology 187:538-552.

Vollmer, J, Weeratna, R, Payette, P, Jurk, M, Schetter, C, Laucht, M, Wader, T, Tluk, S, Liu, M, Davis, HL, & Krieg, AM. (2004) Characterization of three CpG oligodeoxynucleotide classes with distinct immunostimulatory activities. Euopeanr Journal of Immunology 34:251-262.

Xu, Y, Tao, X, Shen, B, Horng, T, Medzhitov, R, Manley, JL, & Tong, L. (2000) Structural basis for signal transduction by the Toll/interleukin-1 receptor domains. Nature 408:111-115.

Yakubov, LA, Deeva, EA, Zarytova, VF, Ivanova, EM, Ryte, AS, Yurchenko, LV, & Vlassov, VV. (1989) Mechanism of oligonucleotide uptake by cells: Involvement of specific receptors? Proceedings of the National Academy of Science U S A 86:6454-6458.

Yamashita, T, Shimada, S, Guo, W, Sato, K, Kohmura, E, Hayakawa, T, Takagi, T, & Tohyama, M. (1997) Cloning and functional expression of a brain peptide/histidine transporter. Journal of Biological Chemistry 272:10205-10211.

Yang, Y, Liu, B, Dai, J, Srivastava, PK, Zammit, DJ, Lefrancois, L, & Li, Z. (2007) Heat shock protein gp96 is a master chaperone for Toll-like receptors and is important in the innate function of macrophages. Immunity 26:215-226.

Yasuda, K, Richez, C, Uccellini, MB, Richards, RJ, Bonegio, RG, Akira, S, Monestier, M, Corley, RB, Viglianti, GA, Marshak-Rothstein, A, & Rifkin, IR. (2009) Requirement for DNA CpG content in TLR9-dependent dendritic cell activation induced by DNA-containing immune complexes. Journal of Immunology 183:3109-3117.

Yasuda, K, Yu, P, Kirschning, CJ, Schlatter, B, Schmitz, F, Heit, A, Bauer, S, Hochrein, H, & Wagner, H. (2005) Endosomal translocation of vertebrate DNA activates dendritic cells via TLR9-dependent and -independent pathways. Journal of Immunology 174:6129-6136.

Yasutomo, K, Horiuchi, T, Kagami, S, Tsukamoto, H, Hashimura, C, Urushihara, M, &
    Kuroda, Y. (2001) Mutation of DNase1 in people with systemic lupus
    erythematosus. Nature Genetics 28:313-314.

5

Fas Pathway of Cell Death and B Cell Dysregulation in SLE

Roberto Paganelli, Alessia Paganelli and Maria C. Turi
Department of Medicine and Sciences of Aging
University "G. d'Annunzio" of Chieti-Pescara
and Ce.S.I.- U.d'A. Foundation, Chieti scalo (CH)
Italy

1. Introduction

Systemic lupus erythematosus (SLE) is a generalized autoimmune disease affecting several organ systems, characterized by the presence of a vast array of autoantibodies, characteristically directed to nuclear antigens (ANA) (Arbuckle et al, 2003, Hahn, 1998, Rothman and Isenberg, 2008). Systemic lupus erythematosus (SLE) is the second most common human autoimmune disease affecting between 400 and 1000 per million people worldwide (Craft, 2011).

SLE is caused by the breakdown of tolerance to nuclear self-antigens, which leads to activation of autoreactive B cells that produce autoantibodies against self-nucleic acids and associated proteins (Lande et al, 2011). These autoantibodies bind self-nucleic acids released by dying cells, and form immune complexes that are deposited in different parts of the body, leading to detrimental inflammation and tissue damage. A key early event that triggers autoimmunity in SLE is the chronic innate activation of plasmacytoid dendritic cells (pDCs) to secrete type I interferons (IFNs) (Theofilopoulos et al, 2005; Ronnblom et al, 2006; Banchereau and Pascual, 2006). The high levels of type I IFNs induce an unabated differentiation of monocytes into dendritic cells that stimulate autoreactive B and T cells (Blanco et al, 2001), licensing T cells recognize autoantigens and lower the activation threshold of autoreactive B cells (LeBon et al, 2006), thereby promoting autoimmunity in SLE.

Analysis of genes encoding components of the interferon pathway has led to extensive support for an association of polymorphic variants of interferon regulatory factor 5 (*IRF5*) with SLE (Bennett et al, 2003; Crow, 2008; Niewold et al,2007;). Recent genomewide association studies confirm associations of HLA and *STAT4* variants with SLE and also the role of *PTPN22* (International Consortium, 2008; Rieck et al, 2007; Remmers et al, 2007). New reports of genetic SNPs associations include the B-cell-receptor–signaling pathway and the mechanisms of adhesion of inflammatory cells to the vasculature (Hom et al, 2008; Kozyrev et al, 2008).

The heterogeneity of clinical manifestations and the disease's unpredictable course (Tan et al, 1982) characterized by flares and remissions are very likely a reflection of heterogeneity at the origin of disease, with a final common pathway leading to loss of tolerance to nuclear antigens. Impaired clearance of immune complexes and apoptotic material and production of autoantibodies have long been recognized as major pathogenic events (Arbuckle et al, 2003; Rothman and Isenberg, 2008). Apoptotic defects underlie some models of autoimmune diseases, and they have been proposed in the pathogenesis of SLE, a prototypic autoimmune disorder.

SLE disease activity can be difficult to monitor, and flares are unpredictable in both frequency and severity. Certain clinical laboratory tests, including anti-double-stranded DNA antibodies (anti-dsDNA), complement factor levels, and the erythrocyte sedimentation rate (ESR) are often measured as potential indicators of disease activity (Ippolito et al, 2011).

Neutrophils are part of the innate immune response and they have long been suspected to play a role in SLE pathogenesis. Nevertheless, their role has not been elucidated until very recently.

In 1948, Hargraves et al. described mature bone marrow neutrophils containing intracytoplasmic nuclear material in 25 SLE patients at the Mayo Clinic (Hargraves, 1948). This phenomenon, which they called the "LE cell," helped develop the first diagnostic test for this disease (Haserick and Bortz, 1949a). In 1949, Haserick and Bortz found that plasma from 50 to 75% of patients with SLE reproduced the LE cell phenomenon in vitro, with the formation of clumps of neutrophils around amorphous masses of nuclear material (Haserick and Borts, 1949b). Subsequent reports described the LE factor binding to nuclear components, including RNPs and histones. The identification of anti-nuclear antibodies (Baugh et al, 1960; Hahn, 1998) later replaced the LE cell as a diagnostic test, and switched the focus of lupus research from neutrophils to B cells, which now seems to switch back again (see below, NETosis).

2. Types of cell death

In human adults, billions of cells die every day as part of the body's natural processes. Cells that become damaged by microbial infection or mechanical stress also die. The cell death that occurs in the physiological setting is programmed (Nagata et al, 2010).

Four different cell-death processes (apoptosis, cornification, necrosis, and autophagy) have been officially proposed (Kroemer et al., 2009). In apoptosis, the cell and nuclei condense and become fragmented and are engulfed by phagocytes (Kerr et al., 1972). Apoptosis is the major death process, but necrosis and autophagic cell death have also been proposed to play roles in programmed cell death (Kroemer et al., 2009). Dying cells secrete a "find me" signal, and they expose an "eat me" signal on their surface. In response to the "find me" signal, macrophages approach the dead cells; they then recognize the "eat me" signal (Ravichandran and Lorenz, 2007).

The machinery used for the engulfment and degradation of the extruded nuclei appears similar to that used for the removal of apoptotic cells. Mice deficient in the engulfment of apoptotic cells develop SLE-type autoimmune diseases (Hanayama et al., 2004). A defect in the degradation of the chromosomal DNA from engulfed cells in mice activates macrophages, leading to lethal anemia in embryos and chronic arthritis in adults (Kawane et al., 2001; Kawane et al., 2006). These observations indicate that dead cells and the nuclei expelled from erythroid precursor cells need to be swiftly cleared for animals to maintain homeostasis.

2.1 High mobility group box 1 (HMGB1)

In 1999, K.J. Tracey and colleagues discovered that the abundant chromatin-associated protein HMGB1 is secreted by activated macrophages during inflammation, and plays a critical role as a late mediator of lethal endotoxemia and sepsis (Wang et al, 1999). Since this initial report, the cytokine activity of HMGB1 has been confirmed by many groups and HMGB1 has now been proposed to be a crucial mediator in the pathogenesis of many diseases including sepsis, arthritis, and cancer (Erlandsson Harris and Andersson, 2004; Dumitriu et al, 2005; Ulloa and Messmer, 2006).

HMGB1 is an intracellular protein that when present in the extracellular milieu acts as a "necrotic marker" for the immune system. Recent studies indicate that damaged or necrotic cells can release HMGB1 into the extracellular milieu, where it triggers inflammatory responses. In contrast to necrosis, cells undergoing programmed cell death or apoptosis induce negligible inflammation in the surrounding tissue (Yang et al, 2004), which is attributed in part, to the retention of HMGB1 within the apoptotic cells (Kokkola, 2003). Indeed, there are two mechanisms for cells to liberate HMGB1 into the extracellular milieu . The first mechanism is a "passive release" of HMGB1 from damaged or necrotic cells: extracellular HMGB1 acts as an immune-stimulatory signal that indicates the extent of tissue injury (Wang et al, 2004; Yang, 2004), promotes the recruitment of mononuclear cells to clear cellular debris and protects against possible infection that often follows trauma (Carriere et al, 2007). The second mechanism is an "active secretion" of HMGB1 from immune cells to act as a pro-inflammatory cytokine during an immunological challenge.

IL-33, the most recent addition to the IL-1 family, is a potent proinflammatory cytokine that induces production of Th2-associated cytokines IL-4, IL-5, and IL-13, both in vitro and in vivo (Schmitz, 2005). Surprisingly, IL-33 has also been described as an abundant chromatin associated nuclear factor, which associates with mitotic chromosomes in living cells and with interphase chromatin in the nucleus of endothelial cells in vivo (Baekkevold, 2003). IL-33 therefore constitutes a second example of a chromatin associated cytokine (Yamada, 2007).

2.2 NETosis

Neutrophils in circulation are directed by cytokines into infected tissues, where they encounter invading microbes. This encounter leads to the activation of neutrophils and the engulfment of the pathogen into a phagosome. In the phagosome, two events are required for antimicrobial activity. First, the presynthesized subunits of the NADPH oxidase assemble at the phagosomal membrane and transfer electrons to oxygen to form superoxide anions. Second, the granules fuse with the phagosome, discharging antimicrobial peptides and enzymes. Together, they are responsible for microbial killing (Klebanoff, 1999). Patients with mutations in the NADPH oxidase suffer from chronic granulomatous disease (CGD; Heyworth et al., 2003).

Upon activation, neutrophils release extra cellular traps (neutrophil extracellular traps [NETs]; Brinkmann et al., 2004). NETs are composed of chromatin decorated with granular proteins, including LL-37, antibiotic peptides, neutrophil peptides and nuclear proteins, e.g. histones and HMGB1. These structures bind Gram-positive and -negative bacteria. Activated neutrophils initiate a process where first the classical lobulated nuclear morphology and the distinction between eu- and hetero-chromatin are lost. Later, all the internal membranes disappear, allowing NET components to mix. Finally, NETs emerge from the cell as the cytoplasmic membrane is ruptured by a process that is distinct from necrosis or apoptosis. This active process is dependent on the generation of ROS by NADPH oxidase (Fuchs et al., 2007). With the loss of nuclear and granular membranes, the decondensed chromatin comes into direct contact with cytoplasmic and granular components. 120 min after activation the granular marker neutrophil elastase colocalizes with chromatin. NETs were detected after PMA activation, but not after incubation with Fas antibody (inducing apoptosis) or treatment with *S. aureus* toxins (inducing necrosis).

Together, these data indicate that neither apoptosis nor necrosis lead to NET formation, and that NET-inducing cell death is different from both apoptosis and necrosis by morphological and molecular criteria. A hitherto unknown form of active cell death apparently evolved to allow neutrophils to kill microbes post mortem. In this form of cell death, the potent cationic antimicrobial peptides and proteins of neutrophils are mixed with chromatin and released to form NETs. Interestingly, the generation of ROS by NADPH oxidase is required for efficient phagocytic killing, and ROS act as a second messenger to trigger NET formation (Lande et al, 2011).

Importantly, in this form of cell death DNA fragmentation is not activated, allowing the chromatin to unfold in the extracellular space. NETs can bind and kill microbes by providing a high local concentration of antimicrobial peptides and, at the same time, minimize tissue damage by sequestering the noxious granule enzymes (Fuchs et al, 2007). Therefore, intact nucleosomes decorated with antimicrobial peptides and nuclear proteins may be released in NETosis, whose dysregulation has been postulated to represent a critical event in SLE pathogenesis (Craft, 2011).

3. Cell death as driving force for autoantibodies production

Phagocytes engulf dead cells, which are recognized as dead by virtue of a characteristic "eat me" signal exposed on their surface. Inefficient engulfment of dead cells activates the immune system, causing disease (such as SLE). The molecular details of these processes have been recently superbly reviewed in Cell (Nagata, 2010).

During apoptosis, the asymmetric distribution of phospholipids of the plasma membrane gets lost and phosphatidylserine (PS) is translocated to the outer leaflet of the plasma membrane. There, PS acts as one major "eat me" signal that ensures efficient recognition and uptake of apoptotic cells by phagocytes. PS recognition of activated phagocytes induces the secretion of anti-inflammatory cytokines like interleukin-10 (Fadok, 2001). Accumulation of dead cells containing nuclear autoantigens in sites of immune selection may provide survival signals for autoreactive B-cells.

The production of antibodies against nuclear structures determines the initiation of chronic autoimmunity in systemic lupus erythematosus. Various soluble molecules and biophysical properties of the surface of apoptotic cells play significant roles in the appropriate recognition and further processing of dying and dead cells. High mobility group box 1 (HMGB1), C-reactive protein (CRP), and anti-nuclear autoantibodies may contribute to the etiopathogenesis of the disease (Craft, 2011).

3.1 Autoantibodies in SLE

Patients with SLE have autoantibodies in their sera against nuclear components (anti-ribonucleoprotein and anti-DNA antibodies) and sometimes exhibit circulating DNA or nucleosomes (Rumore and Steinman, 1990). As unengulfed apoptotic cells are present in the germinal centers of the lymph nodes of some SLE patients and macrophages from these patients often show a reduced ability to engulf apoptotic cells, a deficiency in the clearance of apoptotic cells is proposed to be one of the causes of SLE (Gaipl et al., 2006). Apoptotic corps are disposed by phagocytes (Savill, 1994) and show immunosuppressive activity (Voll,

1997) and recently are reported to be conducive to generation of B regulatory cells (see below) (Gray 2007).

There is increasing evidence that in systemic lupus erythematosus, nucleosomes, the basic chromatin component, represent both a driving immunogen and a major in vivo target for antibodies (Casciola-Rosen, 1994; Huggins et al, 1999). Either a disturbed apoptosis or a reduced clearance of apoptotic cells by phagocytes may lead to an increased exposure of apoptotic nucleosomes protected by HMGB1, to the immune system (Urbonaviciute et al., 2008). One possible new source of HMGB1-nucleosome complexes is thought to derive from NETosis (Lande, 2011; Garcia-Romo, 2011).

3.2 The Fas/FasL pathway of apoptosis in SLE

Apoptosis is activated by two pathways, the intrinsic and extrinsic pathways (Ow et al., 2008). Fas ligand (FasL), tumor necrosis factor (TNF), and TRAIL (TNF-related apoptosis-inducing ligand) are type II membrane proteins that can activate the extrinsic death pathway (Krammer, 2000; Nagata, 1997; Strasser et al., 2009). The binding of FasL to its receptor (Fas) induces the formation of the death inducing signaling complex (DISC), consisting of Fas, an adaptor protein (FADD), and procaspase 8. Formation of the DISC leads to the processing and activation of caspase 8. In both the intrinsic and extrinsic pathways, apoptosis is completed by the cleavage of a set of cellular proteins (more than 500 substrates) by effector caspases (caspases 3 and 7) (Lüthi and Martin, 2007; Timmer and Salvesen, 2007).

Fas is a 43 kDa glycoprotein molecule which is involved in inducing apoptosis in both B and T lymphocytes (Singh, 1995). In the murine MRL/lpr/lpr model of systemic lupus erythematosus (SLE), the lymphoproliferation (lpr) mutation results in defective transcription of the gene that codes for the Fas protein. MRL mice which carry the homozygous recessive lpr mutation develop a severe early-onset genetically predetermined autoimmune syndrome. Susceptibility to SLE is found to be associated with many genes (see Table 1), one of which is APO-1/Fas gene, which is present on chromosome 10 in humans (Singh et al, 2009). The APO-1/Fas promoter contains consensus sequences for binding of several transcription factors that affect the intensity of Fas expression in cells. The mutations in the APO-1/Fas promoter are associated with risk and severity in various autoimmune diseases. A decreased rate of apoptosis may possibly be related also to elevated levels of soluble Fas (sFas) which can inhibit Fas mediated apoptosis of lymphocytes (Kruse et al, 2010).

GENETIC	TYPE I IFN (*Irf-5, etc*)	TLRs (7 to 9)	B cell R and activation	Apoptotic control and disposal
FACTORS	Complement factors (classical/alternate)	NETs control	CD4 activation	*ITGAM* *FcGRII*

Table 1. Possible genetic loci controlling SLE predisposition; they include antigen presentation, IFN type-I production by pDCs, activation of autoreactive T and B cells and neutrophils, complement cascade and nucleic acid sensing and antibody signalling.

In overwhelming majority of situations alterations in Fas and FasL expression are viewed in frames of Fas-mediated apoptosis (Tinazzi et al, 2009; Nozawa, 1997). Telegina et al. (2008) tested a possible involvement of Fas-ligand-mediated "reverse signaling" in the pathogenesis of autoimmune diseases such as rheumatoid arthritis (RA) and SLE. The results indicated that high level of sFas in RA patient blood correlates with a high activity of disease; in SLE patients with elevated sFas level there was a correlation between sFas concentration and tissue and organ damage. In serum sFas is present in oligomeric form (Tokano, 1996). Oligomeric sFas demonstrated cytotoxicity in lymphocyte primary culture and in transformed cells, while non-toxic recombinant Fas-ligand partially blocked this effect (Telegina, 2008). Levels of sFas correlated with the percentages of activated B cells defined as CD20(+)CD38(+) cells. Serum levels of sFas correlate with percentages of activated B cells but not with that of activated T cells (Bijl, 1998). There is a significant correlation between serum concentrations of sFas and serum IL-18 in SLE patients (Sahebari, 2010). sFas and TNFα serum levels are increased in SLE patients (Miret et al, 2001). sFas levels seems to be secondary to TNFα action, which is enhanced in inflammatory conditions such as SLE. Bcl-2 antigen expression and IL-10 serum levels are related to the maintenance of SLE activity. These alterations may interfere with the apoptotic process.

3.2.1 Role of Fas/FasL in SLE

Fas ligand (FasL), an apoptosis-inducing member of the TNF cytokine family, and its receptor Fas are critical for the shutdown of chronic immune responses and prevention of autoimmunity. Accordingly, mutations in their genes cause severe lymphadenopathy and autoimmune disease in mice and humans. FasL function is regulated by deposition in the plasma membrane and metalloprotease-mediated shedding. mFasL is essential for cytotoxic activity and constitutes the guardian against lymphadenopathy, autoimmunity and cancer, whereas excess sFasL appears to promote autoimmunity (O'Reilly et al., 2009). Lymphocytes from aged autoimmune MRL/lpr mice overexpress Fas ligand (FasL), and are cytotoxic against Fas+ target cells. This cytotoxic potential is only partly due to FasL, as wild-type MRL+/+ lymphocytes are not able to kill Fas+ targets after induction of FasL (Hadj-Slimane et al, 2004). IFN alpha, which is increased in SLE, induces overexpression of Fas on lymphocyte surface of lpr mice.

In healthy subjects, more memory than naive T lymphocytes undergo TNF alpha-induced apoptosis. By contrast, in patients with SLE, more naive T cells undergo apoptosis with TNFalpha (Habib et al, 2009). Enhanced apoptosis of T cells in SLE seems to be independent of disease activity or medication. Finally, inhibition experiments showed that apoptosis in the presence of TNFalpha was only partly blocked by anti-FasL antibody (Habib, 2009). Another study showed that mFas expression levels were significantly higher among SLE patients than in healthy controls, and the expression levels had a positive correlation with the early apoptosis rate of mononuclear cells in SLE patients (Li et al, 2009).

Data from several studies demonstrate increasing serum concentrations of the soluble molecules sFas and sFasL starting the first days after birth, indicating possibly a gradual decrease of apoptosis in early neonatal life (Telegina, 2009). In our study (Turi et al., 2009) SLE patients with lower ratios of sFas/sFasL in their sera were of younger age, and had a shorter disease duration (as calculated by the time from diagnosis) and also shorter duration of therapy and/or less organ damage. This pointed to the association of the index with age, which resulted to be strongly correlated with this parameter. Therefore the main variable associated with changes of the sFas/sFasL ratio is the age of the subjects.

Neutrophil apoptosis was significantly increased in patients with juvenile-onset SLE as compared with the noninflamed controls (Midgley et al, 2009). Concentrations of TRAIL and FasL were significantly increased in sera from patients with juvenile-onset SLE, but formation of NETs was not assessed in this study. Finally, it has been reported that SLE serum is capable of inducing apoptosis independent of Fas or TNF-R (Bengtsson et al, 2008).

3.3 Type I Interferons and apoptosis

Type I IFN (IFN-I) was firstly described in 1957 as a soluble factor responsible for viral resistance in vitro. IFN-I can be considered a "director" of protective immune responses (Sozzani et al, 2010). The recent finding of the so-called interferon signature in patients suffering from different autoimmune diseases has underlined its possible role in the pathogenesis of these diseases (Obermoser and Pascual, 2010). Type I IFN has immunoregulatory functions by affecting cell proliferation and by inducing antiinflammatory responses (Cantaert et al, 2010).

pDCs, specialized type I IFN producers, significantly enhance autoreactive B cell proliferation, autoantibody production, and survival in response to TLR and BCR stimulation (Thibault, 2009). IFNAR2-/- B cells fail to upregulate nucleic acid-sensing Toll-like receptors TLR7 as well as TLR9 expression in response to IFN-I (Ding et al, 2009). In addition, serum levels of IFN-alpha increase in parallel with the Fas-dependent cytotoxic potential of lymphocytes from MRL/lpr mice as they age (Hadj-Slimane, 2004). MRL/lpr lymphocytes overexpressed mRNA for the IFN-alpha receptor (IFNAR-1 and IFNAR-2) chains of the IFN-I receptor and exhibited high endogenous levels of phosphorylated Stat1. These data suggest that IFN-alpha plays an important role in the SLE-like syndrome occurring in MRL/lpr mice, and link aberrant apoptosis caused by FasL to high levels of IFN-I.

It has been found that type 1 IFNs protect human B cells in culture from spontaneous apoptosis and from apoptosis mediated by anti-CD95 agonist, in a dose- and time-dependant manner (Badr et al, 2010). Such effect on human B cells was totally abrogated by blockade of IFNR1 chain. PI3Kδ, Rho-A, NFκB and Bcl-2/Bcl$_{XL}$ are active downstream of IFN receptors and are the major effectors of IFN-I-rescued B cells from apoptosis. Furthermore, marked reduction in numbers of CD20 positive B cell in both spleen and Peyer's patches was seen in mice treated with anti-IFNR1. Type I IFNs can stimulate B-cell proliferation and differentiation into antibody-secreting plasma cells, and differentiation of immature monocytes into antigen presenting dendritic cells. These dendritic cells can activate autoreactive lymphocytes and promote autoantibody production (Ding, 2009). These functions of type I IFN, coupled with impaired clearance of apoptotic debris in SLE patients, promote formation of immune complexes, which are potent inducers of type I IFN (Craft, 2011). Inappropriate IFN production and/or an inability to dampen IFN responses thus may initiate a positive feedback loop, resulting in perpetuation of the autoimmune response.

4. B cell phenotypes in SLE

4.1 B lymphocytes development

Cells that have recently emerged from the bone marrow and have yet to acquire follicular markers such as IgD and CD23, but that express very low levels of CD21 and invariably express high levels of CD24 and AA4.1, are called T1 or newly formed (NF) B cells (Carsetti, 2004a). These cells do not require BAFF (B cell–activating factor of the TNF family) for their survival (Schneider, 2001), but like all B cells they depend on signals from the BCR for survival (Kraus, 2004; Hardy and Hayakawa, 2001). These cells, after emerging from the marginal sinus, mature and are drawn into follicles following a CXCL13 gradient (Pillai,

2008), initially become transitional follicular B cells, and eventually give rise to at least two lineages of B cells, mature FO B cells and MZ B cells. Transitional follicular B cells can be subdivided into two distinct categories. NF (newly formed)/T1 (transitional stage 1) B cells are believed to differentiate into T2-FP (transitional stage 2-follicular precursors), which may either differentiate into mature FO B cells or sequentially into T2-MZP (transitional stage 2-MZ B cell precursors) or MZ (marginal zone) B cells (Cariappa and Pillai, 2002).

Although MZ B cells are defined primarily on the basis of their anatomical localization (Martin and Kearney, 2002), the surface expression of a number of markers can also be used to characterize these cells. In rodents the only secondary lymphoid organ in which cells bearing surface markers characteristic of MZ B cells are normally found is the spleen. Unlike follicular B cells that express high levels of IgD and CD23, with either high or low levels of IgM, MZ B cells express high levels of IgM and very low levels of IgD and CD23 (Oliver, 1999). They also express higher levels of CD21 (complement receptor type II), CD1d (an MHC class Ib protein linked to the presentation of lipid antigens), CD38 (an ADP-ribosyl cyclase), CD9 (a scavenger receptor family protein), and CD25 (the α chain of the IL-2 receptor) than those on follicular B cells. MZ B cells also express higher levels of B7 proteins than do follicular B cells and overall are described as having an "activated" phenotype (Oliver, 1997).

4.1.1 Transitional B cells

To identify human transitional B cells, two developmentally regulated markers, CD24 and CD38, are used in combination with the B-lineage marker CD19. In the peripheral blood, all cells of the B lineage (CD19pos) coexpress CD24 and CD38, and, conversely, all non-B cells (CD19neg) lack CD24. (Carsetti, 2004b) Three populations of B cells can be discriminated based on the relative distribution of CD24 and CD38. The CD24brightCD38neg population includes 60% of all B cells and only 2% expressed high levels of both CD24 and CD38 (CD24brightCD38bright). To distinguish mature from memory B cells, the expression of CD27 (a marker of memory cells) can be studied in the three populations. Essentially all CD24brightCD38neg cells are memory B cells, and mature B cells correspond to the CD24dullCD38pos population. CD24brightCD38bright cells lack CD27 (Carsetti 2004 a, b). The analysis of IgM and IgD in the CD24brightCD38bright population shows that transitional B cells coexpress IgM and IgD. IL-10 produced by B cells can downregulate autoimmune disease in EAE (Fillatreau et al., 2002), collagen-induced arthritis (Mauri et al., 2003), and inflammatory bowel disease (Mizoguchi et al., 2002). IL-10-deficient (Il10-/-) mice also have enhanced hypersensitivity responses (Berg et al., 1995). Neutralizing IL-10 by monoclonal antibody (mAb) treatment also enhances these responses, whereas systemic IL-10 administration reduces them (Ferguson et al., 1994; Schwarz et al., 1994). IL-10 is secreted by multiple cell types, including T cells, monocytes, macrophages, mast cells, eosinophils, and keratinocytes, and can suppress both Th1 and Th2 polarization (Yanaba, 2008) and inhibit macrophage antigen presentation and proinflammatory cytokine production (Asadullah et al., 2003). Thus, B cells and IL-10 play important inhibitory roles during T cell-mediated inflammatory responses.

4.1.2 Negative regulation by B cells

B cells have been recently shown to negatively regulate autoimmunity and inflammation in numerous mouse models (Bouaziz, 2008). Mizoguchi and Bhan (2006) were the first to use the term 'regulatory B cells' to designate B cells with regulatory properties. Suppressor/regulatory B-cell populations have predominantly been identified using diverse mouse models of autoimmune diseases, suggesting that autoimmunity itself promotes the expansion of these cells as a compensatory mechanism to limit self-directed inflammation.

Immunological tolerance exemplifies the capacity of the immune system to downmodulate host immune responses (Shevach, 2000). Several regulatory T-cell subsets have been identified that contribute to immunological tolerance, including naturally arising CD4+CD25+Forkhead box protein 3 (FoxP3)+ regulatory T cells (Sakaguchi, 2004) and T-regulatory type 1 cells that produce high amounts of interleukin-10 (Groux, 1997). B cells are generally considered to be positive regulators of immune responses.

Whether negative regulation is a general property of B cells induced as a consequence of normal B-cell activation or whether only a specific subset of B cells posses this property has also been unknown. However, it has been recently shown that regulatory B cells are a phenotypically unique (CD1dhi CD5+) and rare subset of B cells in the spleens of naïve wildtype mice that can significantly influence T-cell activation and some inflammatory responses (Yanaba, 2008). This specific subset of regulatory B cells only produces IL-10 and is responsible for most IL-10 production by B cells. Other regulatory B-cell subsets that may also exist (Mauri and Ehrestein, 2008, Bouaziz, 2008).

Stimulation of arthritogenic B cells with an agonistic anti-CD40 and collagen generated a subset of B cells producing IL-10 (Mauri, 2007). Transfer of collagen and anti-CD40-stimulated Bcells to syngeneic immunized mice prevented the induction of arthritis and ameliorated established disease. This suppressive effect was associated with a downregulation of Th1 cytokines and was dependent upon the release of IL-10 because B cells isolated from IL-10- deficient mice stimulated with collagen and anti-CD40 failed to suppress disease (Mauri et al, 2007). The engagement of CD40 on B cells is also a principal requirement for the generation of Bregs in EAE. Additional in vivo results have shown that MZ B cells participate in the suppression of systemic lupus erythematosus (Lenert et al, 2005). After anti-CD40 treatment an increase of IL-10 production and a decrease of IFN-gamma release was observed (Mauri, 2000) so it was suggested that the therapeutic effect observed after administration of anti-CD40, could have been achieved by redirecting pathogenic Th1 type response toward the "protective" Th2 type (Harris et al, 2000). These data show that the dialogue between B and T cells during an (auto)-immune response is not one sided and demonstrate that B cells have a strong impact in conditioning T cell differentiation.

4.2 Breg phenotype(s)

Further phenotypical identification showed that the majority of CD19+CD38hiCD24hi B cells were also IgMhiIgDhiCD5+CD10+CD20+CD27-CD1dhi (Blair et al, 2010). Interestingly, the majority of the CD19+CD5+CD1dhiB cells (71%), previously reported to be regulatory in experimental models of inflammation (Matsushita et al., 2008; Yanaba et al., 2008a), are contained within the CD24hiCD38hi B cell subset. Co-culture of CD4+ T cells with CD19+CD24hiCD38hi B cells significantly suppressed the frequencies of CD4+IFN-γ+ and CD4+TNF-α+ T cells.

The group of Mauri evaluated whether there was a numerical deficit in CD19+CD38hiCD24hi B cells in patients with SLE (Blair et al, 2010). The absolute cell numbers were not statistically different from controls. In contrast, the numbers of both CD19+CD38intCD24int and CD19+CD24hiCD38- B cells were both significantly reduced in

SLE patients. These results suggest that the inability of SLE CD19+CD38hiCD24hi B cells to suppress the expression of proinflammatory cytokines by CD4+ T cells is unlikely to be due to a numerical deficiency. Depleting CD19+ CD38hiCD24hi B cells from PBMCs of healthy donors and SLE patients leads to an increased production of inflammatory cytokines such as IFN gamma and TNF alpha in healthy donors, suggesting an immunoregulatory effect, but this was not observed in SLE patients.

4.3 Other novel B cell subsets

A novel subset of circulating memory B cells with >2-fold higher levels of CD19 [CD19(hi) B cells] correlates with long-term adverse outcomes in SLE (Nicholas et al, 2008). These B cells do not appear anergic, as they exhibit high basal levels of phosphorylated Syk and ERK1/2, signal transduce in response to BCR crosslinking, and can become plasma cells in vitro. Autoreactive anti-Smith (Sm) B cells are enriched within this subset. Quantitative genetic variation in CD19 expression correlates with autoimmunity (Sato et al, 2000). CD19(hi) B cells have elevated CXCR3 levels and chemotax in response to its ligand CXCL9. Thus, CD19(hi) B cells are precursors to anti-self PCs, and identify an SLE patient subset likely to experience poor clinical outcomes (Nicholas, 2008). CD19(hi)CD21(lo/neg) B cells of uncertain origin are expanded also in common variable immunodeficiency patients with autoimmune features (Warnatz et al, 2002).

B cell functions are under the regulation of B cell antigen receptor (BCR)-induced signals and by specialized cell surface coreceptors, or "response regulators", which inform B cells of their microenvironment. These response regulators include CD19 and CD22 (Fujimoto and Sato, 2007). Importantly, this "CD19/CD22 loop" is significantly related to an autoimmune phenotype in mice. Thus, the CD19/CD22 loop may be a potential therapeutic target. Regulatory B cells that produce IL-10 are now recognized as an important component of the immune system .

4.4 Role of TLR 7 and 9

A previously uncharacterized population of B cells has been recently described in aged mice, called Age-associated B cells (ABCs), which express integrin α_X chain CD11c (Rubtsov et al, 2011). This subset is present also in young lupus-prone mice. Upon stimulation, CD11c+ B cells secrete autoantibodies and depletion of these cells in vivo leads to reduction of autoreactive antibodies. Toll-like receptor 7 (TLR7) is crucial for development of this B cell population. A similar population of B cells was observed in elderly women with autoimmune disease (Rubtsov et al, 2011). Age-associated mature B cells have been described also by Hao et al (2011): they are refractory to BCR and CD40 stimulation but respond to TLR9 or TLR7 stimulation and divide maximally upon combined BCR and TLR ligation, leading to Ig production and preferential secretion of IL-10. They derive from normal mature B cells but have lost the need of BLyS for survival. Finally, they present antigen effectively and favor polarization to a TH17 profile. It has been reported four years ago (Treml, 2007) that TLR9 stimulates TACI expression in all follicular and marginal zone B cells, but only BLyS enhances survival in TLR stimulated B cells. Following the exit from the bone marrow, peripheral B cells develop through transitional type 1 (T1) and transitional type 2 (T2) B-cell stages. Emerging data suggest that the T2 subset is the immediate precursor of the mature B-cell populations. T2 cells uniquely activate a proliferative, pro-survival, and differentiation program in response to B-cell antigen receptor (BCR) engagement. The type of signal(s) encountered by T2 cells lead to their differential maturation toward the follicular mature versus marginal zone mature B-cell populations (Su et al, 2004).

Among the principal targets of autoantibodies produced in murine SLE are nucleic acid–protein complexes, such as chromatin and ribonucleoproteins, and the envelope glycoprotein gp70 of endogenous retroviruses. The preferential production of these autoantibodies is apparently promoted by the presence of genetic abnormalities leading to defects in the elimination of apoptotic cells and to an enhanced expression of endogenous retroviruses. Moreover, recent studies revealed that the innate receptors TLR7 and TLR9 are critically involved in the activation of dendritic cells and autoreactive B cells through the recognition of endogenous DNA- or RNA-containing antigens and subsequent development of autoimmune responses against nuclear autoantigens (Santiago-Raber et al, 2009). Furthermore, the regulation of autoimmune responses against endogenous retroviral gp70 by TLR7 suggested the implication of endogenous retroviruses in this autoimmune response. Clearly, further elucidation of the precise molecular role of TLR7 and TLR9 in the development of autoimmune responses will help to develop novel therapeutic strategies and targets for SLE (Goeken et al, 2010).

4.5 Relationship of B1 to Breg cells

B1 cells constitute a specialized B cell lineage with remarkable properties that include spontaneous secretion of immunoglobulin, autoreactive repertoire skewing, focused memory characteristics, abnormal receptor signaling, induction of Th17 cell differentiation, and production of immunomodulatory IL-10. A particularly exciting issue is the relationship of B1 cells to regulatory B cells and the extent to which these cell types may be one and the same (Cancro, 2009).

Colonna-Romano et al (2009) describe the IgD$^-$CD27$^-$ double-negative B cell population which is increased in the elderly. Most of these cells are IgG$^+$. Evaluation of the telomere length and expression of the ABCB1 transporter and anti-apoptotic molecule, Bcl2, shows that they have the markers of memory B cells. These cells do not act as antigen presenting cells, as indicated by the low levels of CD80 and DR, nor do they express significant levels of the CD40 molecule necessary to interact with T lymphocytes through the ligand, CD154 (Duffau et al, 2010). The authors hypothesize that these expanded cells are late memory or exhausted cells that have down-modulated the expression of CD27.

It is interesting to note that platelets are the main source of circulating CD154, and they can stimulate IFN typeI production from pDCs as well as ligate CD40 on autoreactive B cells (Duffau et al, 2010; Craft, 2011).

5. SLE as the result of defects both in apoptosis control and B cell regulation

Recent data have emerged to support the role of IFN alpha in both control of cell death and regulation of B lymphocyte functions. Two papers (Lande, 2011; Garcia-Romo, 2011) have reported the induction of neutrophil changes due to autoantibodies to DNA or RNA in immune complexes interacting with FcγRIIa as well as TLRs in the presence of inflammatory cytokines and IFN type I, resulting in the formation of NETs which represent a type of cell death with DNA extrusion and release of antimicrobial peptides and cytolytic enzymes that is very effective in defence against bacteria.

5.1 Neutrophils, NETosis and B cells

SLE neutrophils undergo accelerated spontaneous apoptosis in vitro, and SLE sera induce the apoptosis of healthy neutrophils, and nuclear material such as DNA and histones, which comprises the major structural components of NETs, is released in immunogenic form. The inappropriate amplification of this phenomenon in SLE perpetuates B cell stimulation to produce anti-DNA and –RNA antibodies, as well as autoantibodies to antibiotic peptides, and also, via TLR 7 and 9 interactions, IFN alpha production by pDC (Craft, 2011). IFNα in turn primes neutrophils for death with NET formation, which makes more immunogenic DNA and RNA available to the immune system. Both IFN-α and SLE serum up-regulate neutrophil TLR7 expression. In addition, sera from ~40% of SLE patients contain TLR7 ligands in the form of ICs derived from antibodies recognizing small nuclear RNA/RNA binding protein complexes. These ICs have been shown to activate pDCs and induce type I IFN secretion. Anti-RNP antibodies are not efficient activators of pDCs in vitro, however, unless combined with dying cells, which provide the substrate to form ICs that might be internalized via FcγRIIa.

Anti-RNP Ig–induced SLE NETosis requires FcγRIIa and endosomal TLR7 signaling and depends on the formation of ROS. Furthermore, anti-RNP antibodies induce SLE but not healthy neutrophils to secrete high levels of LL37 and HMGB1, two endogenous proteins that contribute to increase the immunogenicity and uptake of mammalian DNA by pDCs. Therefore other sources of immunogenic nuclear material has to be present, and this is provided by increased apoptosis, mostly due to Fas/FasL dysregulation, and inefficient disposal of IC due to complement and reticulo-endothelial defects.

5.2 Fas/FasL dysregulation in SLE

The Fas(CD95) antigen and its ligand (FasL, CD95L) are members of the TNF/TNFR families, expressed on the surface of immune and other cell types. They regulate one important extrinsic apoptotic pathway, by higher or lower expression and by their splice or cleaved soluble variants, sFas and sFasL (Sheriff et al., 2004; Tinazzi et al., 2009). Peripheral T cell apoptosis is upregulated in active SLE, in parallel with high expression of both membrane-bound and soluble Fas (Silvestris et al., 2003; Hao et al., 2006). Previous studies postulated that sFas down-regulates apoptosis in vitro through its blockade of the FasL of cytotoxic cells. This paradox has been examined by Silvestris et al. (2003) and Hao et al. (2006), but it is still unresolved. The situation is even more complex since autoantibodies to FasL have been detected in sera of SLE patients which contribute to inhibit apoptotic cell death of lymphocytes (Suzuki et al., 1998). In our study (Turi et al, 2009) we confirmed that though slightly increased values of both sFas and sFasL are found in SLE patients compared to normal subjects, a very scattered distribution is observed. No definitive answer to the importance of these differences may derive from examining one factor when many contribute to the final effect, so we decided to derive and index from the ratio of the values of sFas to sFasL, which is about 50 in normal controls. This ratio has been found to be lower in younger subjects, being related to age, both in SLE patients and healthy controls. Apoptosis resistance is modulated during aging, and the changes in the sFas/sFasL ratio may be involved in this phenomenon. As clarified by the study by O'Reilly (2009), sFasL does not efficiently mediate Fas-induced apoptosis, therefore its increase in serum equals to an additive anti-apoptotic mechanism in conjunction with elevated sFas circulating levels and autoantibodies to FasL.

6. Conclusion

Systemic lupus erythematosus (SLE) is a chronic autoimmune disease characterized by the production of high-titer IgG autoantibodies directed against nuclear autoantigens. Type I interferon (IFN-I) has been shown to play an important pathogenic role in this disease. Common hypotheses about SLE pathogenesis suggest that environmental triggers, such as infectious agents, operate in the context of both susceptibility genes and epigenetic modifications, resulting in alterations in antigen presentation, lymphoid signaling, apoptosis, and antigen/IC clearance. Decreased numbers of neutrophils, dendritic cells, and lymphocytes are common features of SLE. pDCs accumulate at sites of inflammation such as the skin and the kidney, where they secrete type I interferon (IFN). Upon exposure to SLE serum, healthy monocytes differentiate into mature DCs in an IFN-I–dependent fashion. SLE display a type I IFN signature as measured by peripheral blood mononuclear cell (PBMC) gene expression profiling. The second most prevalent PBMC transcriptional signature corresponds to neutrophil-specific genes, and differential expression of these genes correlates with disease activity. Indeed, polymorphisms in genes expressed by neutrophils, such as ITGAM/CD11b, rank among the highest in the scale of SLE susceptibility. Polymorphisms in genes along the IFN and TLR signaling pathways (that is, IRF5, TLR7, IRAK1, STAT4, etc.) could amplify the response of SLE neutrophils to TLR7 triggering. Polymorphisms affecting thresholds of B cell activation and/or deficient removal of ICs might contribute to prolonged neutrophil exposure to activating ICs. Polymorphisms in FcgRIIa could affect the internalization and/or endosomal trafficking of SLE-specific ICs in neutrophils and pDCs.

Our review has highlighted some recent aspects of the main points relating to these issues, both at the cellular and molecular level, with discussion of the role of NETs formation, TLR 7/9 signaling, apoptosis increased proneness, and the induction both of autoantibodies and IFN-I overproduction. The consequences of these pathogenetic changes are then defined in terms of autoantigens presentation, B lymphocyte dysregulation and IC formation with organ damage. We mainly studied the alterations occurring at quantitative and functional level in the Fas/FasL apoptotic pathway, but also touched upon several other issues such as the relationship of newly identified B cell subsets to autoimmunity, and the role of nuclear cytokines in autoantibody stimulation. We believe that the key aspects of SLE pathogenesis have now been uncovered, and await the composition of their temporal sequence in a unified view of this multifaceted systemic autoimmune disorder.

7. Acknowledgments

Studies reported here have been supported by grants of the Faculty of Medicine of Chieti (60%) for 2009-11 and PRIN 2009 from the Italian Ministry of University (MIUR) to R.P. Studies on B reg have been carried out by M.C.T. as part of a PhD Fellowship at the University of Chieti.

8. Note added in proof

Since completion of this chapter, a review was published in the section of Clinical implications of Basic research of the N Engl J Med (Bosch X (2011). Systemic lupus erythematosus and the neutrophil. N Engl J Med 365;8 (Aug.25) 758-60) discussing the work of Lande and Garcia-Romo reviewed here. No mention of HMGB1 is to be found in the review, however much emphasis was put on antimicrobial peptides (LL-37, which is also implicated in psoriasis) and antagonistic molecules for TLR signalling; the main message was on the new therapeutic aspects and the generalization of these findings (of neutrophil NETosis as pathogenetic mechanism) to vasculitis with ANCA antibodies.

9. References

Arbuckle MR, Mc Clain MT, Rubertone MV, Scofield RH, Dennis GJ, James JA, Harley JB (2003). Development of autoantibodies before the clinical onset of systemic lupus erythematosus. N Engl J Med 349:1526-33.

Asadullah, K., Sterry, W., and Volk, H.D. (2003). Interleukin-10 therapy-review of a new approach. Pharmacol. Rev. 55, 241–269.

Badr G, Saad H, Waly H, Hassan K, Abdel-Tawab H, Alhazza IM, Ahmed EA. (2010). Type I interferon (IFN-alpha/beta) rescues B-lymphocytes from apoptosis via PI3Kdelta/Akt, Rho-A, NFkappaB and Bcl-2/Bcl(XL). Cell Immunol. 263:31-40.

Baekkevold, E.S. et al. (2003) Molecular characterization of NF-HEV, a nuclear factor preferentially expressed in human high endothelial venules. Am. J. Pathol. 163, 69–79

Banchereau J., V. Pascual (2006). Type I interferon in systemic lupus erythematosus and other autoimmune diseases. Immunity 25, 383–392

Baugh C. W., P. M. Kirol, M. V. Sachs, (1960). Demonstration and titration of anti-nuclear antibodies in systemic lupus erythematosus. Can. Med. Assoc. J. 83, 571–580.

Bengtsson AA, Gullstrand B, Truedsson L, Sturfelt G. (2008). SLE serum induces classical caspase-dependent apoptosis independent of death receptors. Clin Immunol. 126:57-66.

Bennett L., A. K. Palucka, E. Arce, V. Cantrell, J. Borvak, J. Banchereau, V. Pascual, (2003). Interferon and granulopoiesis signatures in systemic lupus erythematosus blood. J. Exp. Med. 197, 711–723

Berg, D.J., Leach, M.W., Kuhn, R., Rajewsky, K., Muller, W., Davidson, N.J., and Rennick, D. (1995). Interleukin 10 but not interleukin 4 is a natural suppressant of cutaneous inflammatory responses. J. Exp. Med. 182, 99–108.

Bijl M, van Lopik T, Limburg PC, Spronk PE, Jaegers SM, Aarden LA, Smeenk RJ, Kallenberg GG. (1998). Do elevated levels of serum-soluble fas contribute to the persistence of activated lymphocytes in systemic lupus erythematosus? J Autoimmun. 11:457-63.

Blair PA, Noreña LY, Flores-Borja F, Rawlings DJ, Isenberg DA, Ehrenstein MR, Mauri C. (2010). CD19(+) CD24(hi)CD38(hi) B cells exhibit regulatory capacity in healthy individuals but are functionally impaired in systemic Lupus Erythematosus patients. Immunity. 32:129-40.

Blanco P., A. K. Palucka, M. Gill, V. Pascual, J. Banchereau, (2001). Induction of dendritic cell differentiation by IFN-a in systemic lupus erythematosus. Science 294, 1540–1543

Bouaziz JD, Yanaba K, Tedder TF. (2008) Regulatory B cells as inhibitors of immune responses and inflammation. Immunol Rev. 224:201-14.

Brinkmann, V., U. Reichard, C. Goosmann, B. Fauler, Y. Uhlemann, D.S. Weiss, Y. Weinrauch, and A. Zychlinsky. (2004). Neutrophil extracellular traps kill bacteria. Science. 303:1532-1535.

Cancro MP, Y Hao, JL. Scholz, RL. Riley, D Frasca, DK. Dunn-Walters, BB. Blomberg (2009) B cells and aging: molecules and mechanisms. *Trends Immunol*. 30: 313–318.

Cantaert T, Baeten D, Tak PP and van Baarsen LGM. (2010). Type I IFN and TNFα cross-regulation in immune-mediated infl ammatory disease: basic concepts and clinical relevance. Arthr Res Ther 12:219.

Cariappa A, Pillai S. (2002). Antigen dependent B-cell development. *Curr Opin Immunol* 14:241–9.

Carriere, V. et al. (2007) IL-33, the IL-1-like cytokine ligand for ST2 receptor, is a chromatin-associated nuclear factor in vivo. Proc. Natl. Acad. Sci. U. S. A. 104, 282–287.

Carsetti R. (2004a) Characterization of B-cell maturation in the peripheral immune system. Methods Mol Biol. 271:25-35.

Carsetti R, Rosado MM, Wardmann H. (2004b) Peripheral development of B cells in mouse and man. Immunol Rev. 197:179-91.

Casciola-Rosen, L. A., G. Anhalt, and A. Rosen. (1994). Autoantigens targeted in systemic lupus erythematosus are clustered in two populations of surface structures on apoptotic keratinocytes. *J. Exp. Med.* 179: 1317–1330.

Colonna-Romano G, M Bulati, A Aquino, M Pellicanò, S Vitello, D Lio, G Candore and C Caruso (2009). A double-negative (IgD−CD27−) B cell population is increased in the peripheral blood of elderly people. Mech Ageing Dev 130: 681-90.

Craft J (2011). Dissecting the immune cell mayhem that drives lupus pathogenesis. Sci Transl Med 3, 73ps9.

Crow M.K. (2008). Collaboration, Genetic Associations, and Lupus Erythematosus. N Engl J Med 358: 956-61.

Ding C, Cai Y, Marroquin J, Ildstad ST, Yan J. (2009). Plasmacytoid dendritic cells regulate autoreactive B cell activation via soluble factors and in a cell-to-cell contact manner. J Immunol. 183:7140-9.

Duffau P., J. Seneschal, C. Nicco, C. Richez, E. Lazaro, I. Douchet, C. Bordes, J.-F. Viallard, C. Goulvestre, J.-L. Pellegrin, B. Weil, J.-F. Moreau, F. Batteux, P. Blanco (2010). Platelet CD154 potentiates interferon-a secretion by plasmacytoid dendritic cells in systemic lupus erythematosus. Sci. Transl. Med. 2, 47ra63.

Dumitriu, I. E., P. Baruah, A. A. Manfredi, M. E. Bianchi, and P. Rovere-Querini. (2005). HMGB1: guiding immunity from within. *Trends Immunol*. 26: 381–387.

Erlandsson Harris, H., and U. Andersson. (2004). Mini-review: the nuclear protein HMGB1 as a proinflammatory mediator. *Eur. J. Immunol.* 34: 1503–1512.

Fadok, V.A., Bratton, D.L., Guthrie, L., and Henson, P.M. (2001). Differential effects of apoptotic versus lysed cells on macrophage production of cytokines: role of proteases. J. Immunol. *166*, 6847-6854.

Ferguson, T.A., Dube, P., and Griffith, T.S. (1994). Regulation of contact hypersensitivity by interleukin 10. J. Exp. Med. 179, 1597-1604.

Fillatreau, S., Sweenie, C.H., McGeachy, M.J., Gray, D., and Anderton, S.M. (2002). B cells regulate autoimmunity by provision of IL-10. Nat. Immunol. 3, 944-950.

Fuchs TA,U Abed, C Goosmann, R Hurwitz, I Schulze, V Wahn, Y Weinrauch, V Brinkmann, A Zychlinsky (2007) Novel cell death program leads to neutrophil extracellular traps. J Cell Biol 176, 231–241.

Fujimoto M, Sato S. (2007). B cell signaling and autoimmune diseases: CD19/CD22 loop as a B cell signalling device to regulate the balance of autoimmunity. J Dermatol Sci. 46:1-9.

Gaipl, U.S., Kuhn, A., Sheriff, A., Munoz, L.E., Franz, S., Voll, R.E., Kalden, J.R., and Herrmann, M. (2006). Clearance of apoptotic cells in human SLE. Curr. Dir. Autoimmun. 9, 173–187.

Garcia-Romo G.S., S. Caielli, B. Vega, J. Connolly, F. Allantaz, Z. Xu, M. Punaro, J. Baisch, C.Guiducci, R. L.Coffman, F. J.Barrat, J. Banchereau,V. Pascual, (2011). Netting neutrophils are major inducers of type I IFN production in pediatric systemic lupus erythematosus. Sci. Transl. Med. 3, 73ra20

Goeken JA, T Layer, S Fleenor, M Laccheo and P Lenert (2010) B-cell receptor for antigen modulates B-cell responses to complex TLR9 agonists and antagonists: implications for systemic lupus erythematosus. Lupus 19, 1290–1301.

Gray M, Miles K, Salter D, Gray D, Savill J. (2007). Apoptotic cells protect mice from autoimmune inflammation by the induction of regulatory B cells. Proc Natl Acad Sci USA 104:14080–5

Groux, H., A. O'Garra, M. Bigler, M. Rouleau, S. Antonenko, J. E. de Vries, and M. G. Roncarolo. (1997). A CD4+ T cell subset inhibits antigen-specific T cell responses and prevents colitis. Nature 389: 737–742.

Habib HM, Taher TE, Isenberg DA, Mageed RA. (2009). Enhanced propensity of T lymphocytes in patients with systemic lupus erythematosus to apoptosis in the presence of tumour necrosis factor alpha. Scand J Rheumatol. 38:112-20.

Hadj-Slimane R, Chelbi-Alix MK, Tovey MG, Bobé P. (2004). An essential role for IFN-alpha in the overexpression of Fas ligand on MRL/lpr lymphocytes and on their spontaneous Fas-mediated cytotoxic potential. J Interferon Cytokine Res. 24:717-28.

Hahn BH (1998). Antibodies to DNA. N Engl J Med 338:1359-68.

Hanayama, R., Tanaka, M., Miyasaka, K., Aozasa, K., Koike, M., Uchiyama, Y., and Nagata, S. (2004). Autoimmune disease and impaired uptake of apoptotic cells in MFG-E8-deficient mice. Science 304, 1147–1150.

Hao, J.H., Ye, D.Q., Zhang, G.Q., Liu, H.H., Dai, H., Huang, F., Pan, F.M., Su, H., Dong, M.X., Chen, H., Wang, Q., Zhang, X.J. (2006): Elevated levels of serum soluble Fas are associated with organ and tissue damage in systemic lupus erythematosus among Chinese. Arch. Dermatol. Res. 297, 329-332.

Hao Y, O'Neill PJ, Naradikian MS, Scholz JL, Cancro MP. (2011). A B-cell subset uniquely responsive to innate stimuli accumulates in aged mice. Blood. 118:1294-304

Hardy RR, Hayakawa K. (2001). B cell development pathways. Annu. Rev. Immunol. 19:595–621

Hargraves M.M., H. Richmond, R. Morton, (1948). Presentation of two bone marrow elements; the tart cell and the L.E. cell. Mayo Clin. Proc. 23, 25–28

Harris, D.P., L. Haynes, P.C. Sayles, D.K. Duso, S.M. Eaton, N.M. Lepak, L.L. Johnson, S.L. Swain, and F.E. Lund. (2000). Reciprocal regulation of polarized cytokine production by effector B and T cells. Nat. Immunol. 1:475–482.

Haserick J.R., D. W. Bortz (1949a). A new diagnostic test for acute disseminated lupus erythematosus. Cleve. Clin. Q. 16, 158–161

Haserick J.R., D. W. Bortz, (1949b). Normal bone marrow inclusion phenomena induced by lupus erythematosus plasma. J. Invest. Dermatol. 13, 47–49.

Heyworth, P.G., A.R. Cross, and J.T. Curnutte. (2003). Chronic granulomatous disease. *Curr. Opin. Immunol.* 15:578–584.

Hom G, Graham RR, Modrek B, et al. (2008) Association of systemic lupus erythematosus with *C8orf13–BLK* and *ITGAM–ITGAX*. N Engl J Med 358: 900–909.

Huggins, M. L., I. Todd, M. A. Cavers, S. R. Pavuluri, P. J. Tighe, and R. J. Powell. (1999). Antibodies from systemic lupus erythematosus (SLE) sera define differential release of autoantigens from cell lines undergoing apoptosis. *Clin. Exp. Immunol.* 118: 322–328.

International Consortium for Systemic Lupus Erythematosus Genetics, Harley JB, Alarcon-Riquelme ME, et al. (2008). A genomewide association scan in women with systemic lupus erythematosus identifies risk variants in ITGAM, PXK, KIAA1542 and other loci and confirms multiple loci contributing to disease susceptibility. Nat Genet 40, 204–210

Ippolito A., DJ Wallace, D Gladman, PR Fortin, M Urowitz, V Werth, M Costner, C Gordon, GS Alarcón, R et al. (2011) Autoantibodies in systemic lupus erythematosus: comparison of historical and current assessment of seropositivity. Lupus 20, 250–255.

Kawane, K., Fukuyama, H., Kondoh, G., Takeda, J., Ohsawa, Y., Uchiyama, Y., and Nagata, S. (2001). Requirement of DNase II for definitive erythropoiesis in the mouse fetal liver. Science *292*, 1546–1549.

Kawane, K., Ohtani, M., Miwa, K., Kizawa, T., Kanbara, Y., Yoshioka, Y., Yoshikawa, H., and Nagata, S. (2006). Chronic polyarthritis caused by mammalian DNA that escapes from degradation in macrophages. Nature *443*,998–1002.

Kerr, J.F., Wyllie, A.H., and Currie, A.R. (1972). Apoptosis: a basic biological phenomenon with wide-ranging implications in tissue kinetics. Br. J. Cancer *26*, 239–257.

Klebanoff, S.J. (1999). Oxygen metabolites from phagocytes. *In* J.I. Gallin and R. Snyderman, editors. Infl ammation: Basic Principles and Clinical Correlates. Lippincott Williams & Wilkins, Philadelphia. 721–768

Kokkola R, Li J, Sundberg E, Aveberger AC, Palmblad K, Yang H, et al. (2003) Successful treatment of collagen-induced arthritis in mice and rats by targeting extracellular high mobility group box chromosomal protein 1 activity. Arthritis Rheum 48:2052–8.

Kozyrev SV, Abelson A-K, Wojcik J, et al. (2008) Functional variants in the B cell gene BANK1 are associated with systemic lupus erythematosus. Nat Genet 40: 211–216..

Krammer, P.H. (2000). CD95's deadly mission in the immune system. Nature *407*, 789–795.

Kraus M, Alimzhanov MB, Rajewsky N, Rajewsky K. (2004). Survival of resting mature B lymphocytes depends on BCR signaling via the Igα/β heterodimer. *Cell* 117:787–800

Kroemer, G., Galluzzi, L., Vandenabeele, P., Abrams, J., Alnemri, E.S., Baehrecke, E.H., Blagosklonny, M.V., El-Deiry, W.S., Golstein, P., Green, D.R., et al; Nomenclature Committee on Cell Death 2009. (2009). Classification of cell death: recommendations of the Nomenclature Committee on Cell Death 2009. Cell Death Differ. *16*, 3–11.

Kruse K, Janko C, Urbonaviciute V, Mierke CT, Winkler TH, Voll RE, Schett G, Muñoz LE, Herrmann M. (2010). Inefficient clearance of dying cells in patients with SLE: anti-dsDNA autoantibodies, MFG-E8, HMGB-1 and other players. Apoptosis. 15:1098-113.

Lande R, D. Ganguly, V. Facchinetti, L. Frasca, C. Conrad, J. Gregorio, S. Meller, G. Chamilos, R. Sebasigari, V. Riccieri, R. Bassett, H. Amuro, S. Fukuhara, T. Ito, Y.-J. Liu, M. Gilliet, (2011). Neutrophils activate plasmacytoid dendritic cells by releasing self-DNA–peptide complexes in systemic lupus erythematosus. Sci. Transl. Med. 3, 73ra19

Le Bon A., C. Thompson, E. Kamphuis, V. Durand, C. Rossmann, U. Kalinke, D. F. Tough (2006). Cutting edge: Enhancement of antibody responses through direct stimulation of B and T cells by type I IFN. J. Immunol. 176, 2074–2078.

Lenert, P., R. Brummel, E. H. Field, and R. F. Ashman. (2005). TLR-9 activation of marginal zone B cells in lupus mice regulates immunity through increased IL-10 production. J. Clin. Immunol. 25: 29–40.

Li LH, Li WX, Wu O, Zhang GQ, Pan HF, Li XP, Xu JH, Dai H, Ye DQ. (2009). Fas expression on peripheral blood lymphocytes in systemic lupus erythematosus: relation to the organ damage and lymphocytes apoptosis. Mol Biol Rep. 36:2047-52.

Loken MR, Shah VO, Hollander Z, Civin CI. (1988). Flow cytometric analysis of normal B lymphoid development. Pathol Immunopathol Res. 7:357-70.

Lüthi, A.U., and Martin, S.J. (2007). The CASBAH: a searchable database of caspase substrates. Cell Death Differ. 14, 641–650.

Martin F, Kearney JF. (2002). Marginal zone B cells. Nat. Rev. Immunol. 2:323– 35

Mauri, C., L.T. Mars, and M. Londei. (2000). Therapeutic activity of agonistic monoclonal antibodies against CD40 in a chronic autoimmune inflammatory process. Nat. Med. 6:673-679.

Mauri, C., Gray, D., Mushtaq, N., and Londei, M. (2003). Prevention of arthritis by interleukin 10-producing B cells. J. Exp. Med. 197, 489–501.

Mauri, C. and Ehrenstein, M.R. (2007) Cells of the synovium in rheumatoid arthritis. B cells. Arthritis Res. Ther. 9, 205-10.

Mauri C, Ehrenstein MR. (2008). The 'short' history of regulatory B cells. Trends Immunol 29:34–40.

Midgley A, McLaren Z, Moots RJ, Edwards SW, Beresford MW. (2009). The role of neutrophil apoptosis in juvenile-onset systemic lupus erythematosus. Arthritis Rheum. 60:2390-401.

Miret C, Font J, Molina R, Garcia-Carrasco M, Filella X, Ramos M, Cervera R, Ballesta A, Ingelmo M. (2001). Relationship of oncogenes (sFas, Bcl-2) and cytokines (IL-10, alfa-TNF) with the activity of systemic lupus erythematosus. Anticancer Res. 21(4B):3053-9.

Mizoguchi, A., Mizoguchi, E., Takedatsu, H., Blumberg, R.S., and Bhan, A.K. (2002). Chronic intestinal inflammatory condition generates IL-10-producing regulatory B cell subset characterized by CD1d upregulation. Immunity 16,219–230.

Mizoguchi A, Bhan AK. (2006). A case for regulatory B cells. J Immunol. 176:705-10.

Moschese V, Orlandi P, Di Matteo G, Chini L, Carsetti R, Di Cesare S, Rossi P. (2004). Insight into B cell development and differentiation. Acta Paediatr Suppl. 93(445):48-51.

Nagata, S. (1997). Apoptosis by death factor. Cell 88, 355–365.

Nagata S, Hanayama R, Kawane K (2010). Autoimmunity and the clearance of dead cells. Cell 140: 619-630.

Nicholas MW, Dooley MA, Hogan SL, Anolik J, Looney J, Sanz I, Clarke SH. (2008). A novel subset of memory B cells is enriched in autoreactivity and correlates with adverse outcomes in SLE. Clin Immunol. 126:189-201.

Niewold TB, Hua J, Lehman TJ, Harley JB, Crow MK. (2007). High serum IFN-alpha activity is a heritable risk factor for systemic lupus erythematosus. Genes Immun 8:492-502.

Nozawa, K., Kayagaki, N., Tokano, Y., Yagita, H., Okumura, K., Hasimoto, H. (1997): Soluble Fas (APO-1, CD95) and soluble Fas ligand in rheumatic diseases. Arthritis Rheum. 40, 1126-1129.

Obermoser G, Pascual V. (2010). The interferon-alpha signature of systemic lupus erythematosus. Lupus. 19:1012-9.

Oliver AM, Martin F, Gartland GL, Carter RH, Kearney JF. (1997). Marginal zone B cells exhibit unique activation, proliferative and immunoglobulin secretory responses. *Eur. J. Immunol.* 27:2366–74

Oliver AM, Martin F, Kearney JF. (1999). IgMhighCD21high lymphocytes enriched in the splenic marginal zone generate effector cells more rapidly than the bulk of follicular B cells. *J. Immunol.* 162:7198–207

O' Reilly LA, Tai L, Lee L, Kruse EA, Grabow S, Fairlie WD, Haynes NM, Tarlinton DM, Zhang JG, Belz GT, Smyth MJ, Bouillet P, Robb L, Strasser A. (2009). Membrane-bound Fas ligand only is essential for Fas-induced apoptosis. Nature. 461(7264):659-63.

Ow, Y.P., Green, D.R., Hao, Z., and Mak, T.W. (2008). Cytochrome c: functions beyond respiration. Nat. Rev. Mol. Cell Biol. 9, 532–542.

Pillai, S., A. Cariappa, and S. T. Moran. (2005). Marginal zone B cells. *Annu. Rev.Immunol.* 23: 161–196.

Ravichandran, K.S., and Lorenz, U. (2007). Engulfment of apoptotic cells: signals for a good meal. Nat. Rev. Immunol. 7, 964–974.

Remmers EF, Plenge RM, Lee AT, et al. (2007). *STAT4* and the risk of rheumatoid arthritis and systemic lupus erythematosus. N Engl J Med 357:977-86.

Rieck M, Arechiga A, Onengut-Gumuscu S, Greenbaum C, Concannon P, Buckner JH. (2007). Genetic variation in PTPN22 corresponds to altered function of T and B lymphocytes. J Immunol 179:4704-10.

Rönnblom L, Eloranta ML, Alm GV. (2006). The type I interferon system in systemic lupus erythematosus. Arthritis Rheum 54:408-20.

Rothman A, Isenberg DA (2008). Systemic lupus erythematosus. N Engl J Med 358:929-39.

Rubtsov A.V. , K Rubtsova, A Fischer, R T. Meehan, J Z. Gillis, JW. Kappler, and P Marrack (2011) TLR7-driven accumulation of a novel CD11c+ B-cell population is important for the development of autoimmunity. Blood. 118(5):1305-15

Rumore, P.M., and Steinman, C.R. (1990). Endogenous circulating DNA in systemic lupus erythematosus. Occurrence as multimeric complexes bound to histone. J. Clin. Invest. 86, 69–74.

Sahebari M, Rezaieyazdi Z, Nakhjavani MJ, Hatef M, Mahmoudi M, Akhlaghi S. (2010). Correlation between serum concentrations of soluble Fas (CD95/Apo-1) and IL-18 in patients with systemic lupus erythematosus. Rheumatol Int. DOI: 10.1007/s00296-010-1633-9

Sakaguchi, S. (2004). Naturally arising CD4_ regulatory T cells for immunologic self tolerance and negative control of immune responses. *Ann. Rev. Immunol.* 22:531–562.

Salmon JE, Millard S, Schacter LA, et al. (1996). Fc gamma RIIA alleles are heritable risk factors for lupus nephritis in African Americans. J Clin Invest 97:1348-54.

Santiago-Raber M-L, L Baudino and S Izui (2009). Emerging roles of TLR7 and TLR9 in murine SLE. J Autoimmunity 33:231-8.

Sato S, Hasegawa M, Fujimoto M, Tedder TF, Takehara K. (2000). Quantitative genetic variation in CD19 expression correlates with autoimmunity. J Immunol. 165:6635-43.

Savill, J., V. Fadok, P. Henson, and C. Haslett. (1993). Phagocyte recognition of cells undergoing apoptosis. *Immunol. Today* 14: 131–136.

Schmitz J, Owyang A, Oldham E, Song Y, Murphy E, McClanahan TK, Zurawski G, Moshrefi M, Qin J, Li X, Gorman DM, Bazan JF, Kastelein RA. (2005) IL-33, an interleukin-1-like cytokine that signals via the IL-1 receptor-related protein ST2 and induces T helper type 2-associated cytokines. Immunity 23, 479–490

Schneider P, Takatsuka H, Wilson A, Mackay F, Tardivel A, et al. (2001). Maturation of marginal zone and follicular B cells requires B cell activating factor of the tumor necrosis factor family and is independent of B cell maturation antigen. *J.Exp. Med.* 194:1691–97

Sheriff, A.,´Gaipl, U.S., Voll, R.E., Kalden, J.R., Herrmann, M. (2004): Apoptosis and systemic lupus erythematosus. Rheum. Dis. Clin. North Am. 30, 505-527.

Shevach, E. M. (2000). Regulatory T cells in autoimmunity. *Ann. Rev. Immunol.* 18:423–449.

Sigurdsson S, Göring HH, Kristjansdottir G, et al. (2008). Comprehensive evaluation of the genetic variants of interferon regulatory factor 5 reveals a novel 5bp length polymorphism as strong risk factor for systemic lupus erythematosus. Hum Mol Genet 17:872-81.

Silvestris, F., Grinello, D., Tucci, M., Cafforio, P., Dammacco, F. (2003): Enhancement of T cell apoptosis correlates with increased serum levels of soluble Fas (CD95/Apo-1)in active lupus. Lupus 12, 8-14.

Singh AK. (1995). Lupus in the Fas lane? J R Coll Physicians Lond. 29:475-8.

Singh R, Pradhan V, Patwardhan M, Ghosh K. (2009). APO-1/Fas gene: Structural and functional characteristics in systemic lupus erythematosus and other autoimmune diseases. Indian J Hum Genet. 15:98-102.

Sozzani S, Bosisio D, Scarsi M, Tincani A. (2010). Type I interferons in systemic autoimmunity. Autoimmunity. 43:196-203.

Strasser, A., Jost, P.J., and Nagata, S. (2009). The many roles of FAS receptor signaling in the immune system. Immunity 30, 180–192.

Su TT, Guo B, Wei B, Braun J, Rawlings DJ. (2004). Signaling in transitional type 2 B cells is critical for peripheral B-cell development. Immunol Rev. 197:161-78.

Suzuki, N., Ichino, M., Mihara, S., Kaneko, S., Sakane, T. (1998): Inhibition of Fas/Fas ligand-mediated apoptotic cell death of lymphocytes in vitro by circulating anti-Fas ligand autoantibodies in patients with systemic lupus erythematosus. Arthritis Rheum. 41, 344-353.

Tan EM, Cohen AS, Fries JF, et al. (1982). The 1982 revised criteria for the classification of systemic lupus erythematosus. Arthritis Rheum 25:1271-7

Telegina E, Reshetnyak T, Moshnikova A, Proussakova O, Zhukova A, Kuznetsova A, Ivanov A, Paltsev M, Beletsky I. (2009). A possible role of Fas-ligand-mediated "reverse signaling" in pathogenesis of rheumatoid arthritis and systemic lupus erythematosus. Immunol Lett. 122:12-7.

Theofilopoulos A,N., R. Baccala, B. Beutler, D. H. Kono (2005). Type I interferons (a/b) in immunity and autoimmunity. Annu. Rev. Immunol. 23, 307–336

Thibault DL, Graham KL, Lee LY, Balboni I, Hertzog PJ, Utz PJ. (2009). Type I interferon receptor controls B-cell expression of nucleic acid-sensing Toll-like receptors and autoantibody production in a murine model of lupus. Arthritis Res Ther. 11:R112.

Timmer, J.C., and Salvesen, G.S. (2007). Caspase substrates. Cell Death Differ. 14, 66–72.

Tinazzi, E., Puccetti, A., Gerli, R., Rigo, A., Migliorini, P., Simeoni, S., Beri, R., Dolcino, M., Martinelli, N., Corrocher, R., Lunardi, C. (2009): Serum DNase I, soluble Fas/FasL levels and cell surface Fas expression in patients with SLE: a possibile explanation for the lack of efficacy of hrDNase I treatment. Int. Immunol. 21, 237-243.

Tokano, Y., Miyake, S., Kayagaki, N., Nozawa, K., Morimoto, S., Azuma, M., Yagita, H., Takasaki, Y., Okumura, K., Hashimoto, H. (1996): Soluble Fas molecule in the serum of patients with systemic lupus erythematosus. J. Clin. Immunol. 16, 261-265.

Treml LS, Carlesso G, Hoek KL, Stadanlick JE, Kambayashi T, Bram RJ, Cancro MP, Khan WN. (2007). TLR stimulation modifies BLyS receptor expression in follicular and marginal zone B cells. J Immunol. 178:7531-9.

Turi MC, D'Urbano M, Celletti E, Alessandri C, Valesini G, Paganelli R. (2009). Serum Fas/FasL ratio in sistemi lupus erythematosus (SLE) is a function of age. Arch Gerontol Geriatr S1:221-6.

Ulloa L, D Messmer (2006). High-mobility group box 1 (HMGB1) protein: Friend and foe. Cytokine & Growth Factor Reviews 17:189–201

Urbonaviciute V, et al. (2008) Induction of infl amatory and immune responses by HMGB1 nucleosome complexes: implications for the pathogenesis of SLE. J. Exp. Med. 205:3007-3018

Voll , R.E. , M. Herrmann , E.A. Roth , C. Stach , J.R. Kalden , and I. Girkontaite . (1997). Immunosuppressive eff ects of apoptotic cells. Nature . 390 : 350 – 351 .

Wang, H., Bloom, O., Zhang, M., Vishnubhakat, J.M.,Ombrellino, M.,Che, J., Frazier, A., Yang, H., Ivanova, S., Borovikova, L., Abraham E, Andersson J, Andersson U, Molina PE, Abumrad NN, Sama A, Tracey KJ (1999). HMG-1 as a late mediator of endotoxin lethality in mice. Science 285:248 –251.

Wang H., H. Yang & K Tracey (2004). Extracellular role of HMGB1 in inflammation and sepsis. Journal of Internal Medicine 255: 320–331

Warnatz K, Wehr C, Dräger R, Schmidt S, Eibel H, Schlesier M, Peter HH. (2002). Expansion of CD19(hi)CD21(lo/neg) B cells in common variable immunodeficiency (CVID) patients with autoimmune cytopenia. Immunobiology. 206:502-13.

Yamada S, Maruyama I (2007). HMGB1, a novel inflammatory cytokine. Clin Chim Acta 375:36–42

Yanaba K, Bouaziz JD, Haas KM, Poe JC, Fujimoto M, Tedder TF. (2008). A regulatory B cell subset with a unique CD1dhiCD5+ phenotype controls T cell-dependent inflammatory responses. Immunity. 28:639-50.

Yang H, Ochani M, Li J, Qiang X, Tanovic M, Harris HE, et al. (2004). Reversing established sepsis with antagonists of endogenous high-mobility group box 1. Proc Natl Acad Sci USA 101:296–301.

6

Atherogenesis and Vascular Disease in SLE

Isabel Ferreira[1] and José Delgado Alves[1,2]
[1]*Systemic Immunomediated Diseases Unit*
Department of Medicine IV, Hospital Prof. Doutor Fernando Fonseca, Amadora
[2]*CEDOC-Centro de Estudos de Doenças Crónicas*
Faculdade de Ciências Médicas, Universidade Nova de Lisboa
Portugal

1. Introduction

SLE is the classical model of a chronic multi-systemic immune-mediated inflammatory disease. It affects mainly young women, a subgroup of the general population usually free of cardiovascular risk. Although survival rates have improved dramatically, mainly due to early diagnosis, improved treatment, and better management of complications, death rates for patients with SLE remain 3 to 5 times higher than in the general population (Haque & Bruce, 2009). Nevertheless, whilst the 5-year survival of SLE was below 50% in the 1950s, it is nowadays above 90% (Nikpour et al., 2005).

Atherosclerosis in SLE is a highly complex process with autoimmunity, local and systemic inflammation, and endothelial dysfunction playing critical roles in its initiation and propagation. In the particular case of SLE, the extremely intricate immune system deregulation involving all types of immune cells up to an increased autoantibody production seems to play a major role for the accelerated atheroma formation found in these patients.

Cardiovascular events are now the major cause of morbidity and mortality in SLE. The acceptance of the importance of vascular risk in this context came from the description of a bimodal mortality pattern (Urowitz et al., 1976), with the early peak (within 1 year of diagnosis) as a consequence of active lupus and its complications, and the later peak (more than 5 years after diagnosis) mainly attributable to atherosclerosis. SLE is now considered to be a coronary heart disease-risk equivalent, mainly due to accelerated atherosclerosis (Aranow & Ginzler, 2000; Bjornadal et al., 2004; Manzi et al., 1997; Esdaile et al., 2001; Fischer et al. 2004; Roman et al., 2003; Ward, 1999). This can be especially relevant in young women, where up to a 50-fold increase in cardiovascular risk over age and gender-matched controls has been reported (Manzi et al., 1997). In fact, the majority of those women were aged less than 55 years at the time of their first cardiac event.

Framingham risk factors do not explain entirely the atherosclerotic burden found in patients with SLE. Furthermore, traditional cardiovascular risk factors seem to be less important predictors of cardiovascular events than the activity of lupus (Esdaile et al., 2001). (see table 1).

The direct relation between conventional and SLE-related risk factors and the actual incidence of events has not been easy to establish for different reasons: most patients with

SLE are young or middle-age women, for whom the background rate of cardiovascular disease is low, SLE cohorts are small, the number of observed coronary heart disease events is also reduced, and may not provide statistical power for testing their associations with hypothetical SLE-specific risk factors (Karp et al., 2008). This is the main reason why recent studies are considering surrogate markers of cardiovascular risk, such as the presence of carotid plaques, coronary artery calcification and vascular stiffness.

TRADITIONAL RISK FACTORS	INFLAMMATION-RELATED RISK FACTORS	SLE-RELATED RISK FACTORS
Genetics	Vascular endothelial growth factor	Duration of disease
Gender		Disease activity
Post-menopausal status	Monocyte chemoattractant protein-1	Disease damage
Hypertension		Corticosteroids
Dyslipidemia	TNF-α, IL-1, IL-6	Auto-antibodies
Diabetes mellitus	VCAM-1, ICAM-1	Complement activation
Smoking	Matrix –degrading proteases	Lupus nephritis
Obesity	Acute phase reactants	Increased oxidative stress
Homocysteine	Vascular endothelial growth factor	
Sedentary life-style	Monocyte chemoattractant protein-1	
	TNF-α, IL-1, IL-6	
	VCAM-1, ICAM-1	
	Matrix –degrading proteases	

Table 1. Proposed cardiovascular risk factors in SLE

Both SLE-specific and non-specific mechanisms have been proposed to play a prominent role in the induction of premature vascular damage, but the exact etiology remains unclear. Chronic inflammation is a very appellative contributor for atherosclerosis, since the pathogenesis of the latter is, in part, mediated by inflammation (Ross, 1999).
A potential confounding factor is that clinically active lupus may also manifest itself with vascular inflammation and thrombosis in any vascular territory. However, when a significant large population is considered, premature vascular disease in SLE is not, as previously thought, just attributable to vasculitis. Actually, it presents mostly as premature atherosclerosis (Bacon et al., 2002; Ward, 1999), both clinically and histologically. Many authors believe that the rapid and progressive nature of vascular injury in patients with SLE makes this population ideal for the identification of mechanisms involved in general atherosclerosis and vascular damage.
This chapter aims at elucidating why patients with SLE are at high risk for cardiovascular events, what different types of vascular conditions may be more commonly found, and what treatments are more likely to help overcome such burden.

2. Burden of disease

Despite the fact that the overall survival of patients with SLE has reached over 90% in recent decades, the long term survival rate has not changed since the 1980s (Petri, 2002). SLE patients have mortality rates of 5-10% at 5 years and 15-30% at 10 years (Abu-Shakra et al., 1995; Jacobsen et al., 1998; Ståhl-Hallengren et al., 2000; Uramoto et al., 1999). This is particularly overwhelming in patients aged less than 55 years (Abu-Shakra et al., 1995). After the identification of the bimodal pattern of mortality in SLE, a more recent uptade from the Toronto group (Nikpour, 2005) showed that sudden death, congestive heart failure and vascular events are responsible for nearly 30% of late deaths in their SLE cohort. Currently, cardiovascular disease alone accounts for 20 to 30 % of deaths in patients with SLE (Rubin et al., 1985). Even with all-cause mortality declining during the last 20 years the risk of cardiovascular death remains unchanged. With the advent of more potent immunosuppressive and anti-inflammatory treatments, it is likely that the contribution of cardiovascular disease to morbidity and mortality in these patients will increase even further.

Using myocardial perfusion scintigraphy, subclinical coronary atherosclerosis can be present in 28-38% of patients with SLE (Manger et al., 2003; Sella et al., 2003) and the prevalence of symptomatic coronary heart disease (as defined by angina and myocardial infarction) ranges from 6,6% to 20% (Gladman & Urowitz, 1987; Jonsson et al., 1989; Manzi et al., 1997) . Women with SLE in the 35-44 year age group are over 50 times more likely to have a myocardial infarction than women of similar age in the Framingham Offspring Study (Manzi et al., 1997). The mean age at a first coronary event is 49 years in patients with SLE compared with 65-74 years in the general population, as the risk of development of coronary heart disease in the first decade after diagnosis is approximately 12% (Bruce et al., 1999).

There are significant racial disparities regarding age at the time of first hospital admission for a cardiovascular event and cardiovascular-related hospitalization resulting in death in patients with SLE (Scalzi et al., 2010). African-origin, in particular, is associated in an independent fashion with a worsened probability of survival.

The outcomes of hospitalization for acute myocardial infarction were thought to be identical between patients with and without SLE, despite women with SLE being less likely to undergo coronary artery bypass grafting (Ward, 2004). Whether this is due to a decreased need for the procedure or whether reflects a decreased referral or reduced access to the surgery, is not established. More recently it has been recognized that, like diabetes mellitus, SLE increases the risk of poor outcomes after acute myocardial infarction, and these patients should be considered for aggressive treatment. In fact, the risk for prolonged hospitalization is even higher for patients with SLE (OR 1.48, 95% CI 1.32-1.79) compared to those with diabetes mellitus (OR 1.30, 95% CI 1.28-1.32) (Shah et al., 2009).

Cerebrovascular disease has been identified in 2-15% of patients with SLE (Hermosillo-Romo & Brey, 2002; Manzi et al., 1999; Mok et al., 2001; Sanna et al., 2003), with a reported 2-10 times higher risk for stroke SLE (Jonsson et al., 1989; Manzi et al., 1997; Ward, 1999). A recent prospective study showed that the cumulative incidence of arterial thromboembolism in new-onset Caucasian SLE patients is 5,1%, with ischemic stroke and transient ischemic attack comprising 65% of them (Mok et al., 2005) . Cardiovascular risk is even higher in lupus patients who also have secondary antiphospholipid syndrome (APS), due to the additive effects of SLE- and APS-related risk factors. In fact, as APS is also related to accelerated atherosclerosis, it may be difficult to differentiate between SLE- and APS-associated risk factors in these patients.

3. Vascular disease in systemic lupus erythematosus

3.1 Atherosclerosis
3.1.1 Epidemiology
In cross-sectional studies, approximately one-third of patients with SLE has evidence of subclinical atheroma plaques in the carotid or coronary arteries (Asunuma et al., 2003) and

autopsy findings have showed an even higher prevalence of subclinical atherosclerosis (Bulkley & Roberts, 1975). More than 20% of SLE patients who had been on steroids for more than one year before death had a 50% occlusion of at least one major coronary artery. In a cohort of women with SLE, in whom 15% had already a cardiovascular event, 40% had at least one focal carotid artery plaque, a higher frequency than would be expected among healthy women (Manzi et al., 1999). Not surprisingly, the common carotid intima-media thickness (IMT) of patients with a history of cardiovascular disease is greater than that of SLE patients who had no such history and of healthy volunteers controls (Svenungsson et al., 2001). Using photon emission computed tomography (SPECT) and dual isotope myocardial perfusion imaging (DIMPI), 40% of all women with SLE and 35% of women with SLE and no history of coronary artery disease had abnormalities in myocardial perfusion, reinforcing the idea of a high prevalence of early coronary artery disease (Bruce et al., 2000). Also, coronary-artery calcification, as detected by electron-beam computed tomography (Roman et al., 2003), occurs more frequently and at a younger age in patients with SLE than in healthy controls. Aortic stiffness overall and at any level of the aortic artery was higher in patients with SLE than in controls, even after adjusting for age (Roldan et al., 2010). Furthermore, increased aortic stiffness seems to be an early manifestation of lupus vasculopathy that seems to precede the development of hypertension and atherosclerosis. Whether we consider the SLE context or not, better biomarkers for measuring disease burden are needed. They should be non-invasive, have a good sensitivity and specificity, predict disease in asymptomatic individuals and be available for widespread application.

In clinical practice, diagnosis of atherosclerosis is usually made after the presence of symptoms. Pre-symptomatic screening could identify subclinical disease, allowing for a more aggressive treatment of the different atherothrombotic risk factors.

3.1.2 Atheroma formation

Atherosclerosis is not an age-related process with passive accumulation of lipids in the vessel wall. It must be understood as a dynamic and complex biochemical and anatomical process. It is characterized by changes in lipoprotein metabolism, activation of the immune system and consequent proliferation of smooth-muscle cells, atheroma formation and arterial narrowing. In atheroma formation, inflammation and autoimmunity are at the forefront of the initiation, progression, and rupture of the plaque (Libby et al., 2010; van Leuven et al., 2008). Patients suffering from chronic inflammatory diseases have accelerated atherosclerosis, and the high level of inflammation to which patients with auto-immune diseases are exposed may induce and accelerate endothelial cell injury. Furthermore, biomechanic shear forces enhanced by classic cardiovascular risk factors, such as hypertension, hypercholesterolemia, diabetes and smoking are known to contribute to endothelium dysfunction (Ando & Yamamoto, 2011). In fact, the earliest manifestation of atherothrombosis can be the result of a single disturbance on the physiologic pattern of blood flow at an arterial bending on bifurcation site.

Endothelium regulates anti-inflammatory, mitogenic and contractility activities of the vessel wall; also, it has a role in the the hemostatic process within the vessel lumen. A dysfunctional endothelium is characterized by an increase in oxidative stress. It facilitates oxidation, the uptake of circulating lipoproteins by monocytes, and the migration of these cells to the vessel wall, resulting in the proliferation of smooth muscle cells. The expression of adhesion molecules (such as ICAM and VCAM) induces the binding of monocytes to the endothelial wall (Lusis, 2000). This, when submitted to shear stress forces is also susceptible to permeation and subendothelial accumulation of apolipoprotein-B-containing lipoproteins, such as low density lipoproteins (LDL) and remnant lipoproteins, that become targets for oxidative and enzymatic attack. After monocyte-endothelial binding takes place, the blood cells are internalized and differentiated into macrophages. Retained pro-atherogenic LDL leads to an enhanced selective leukocyte recruitment and attachment to the endothelial layer, further contributing to their transmigration across the endothelium into the intima. Lipoprotein uptake promotes the accumulation of lipid droplets in the cytoplasm of the macrophages, transforming them into foam cells. The consequent inflammatory response leads to the recruitment of more monocytes, T cells, mast cells and neutrophiles. A fibrous cap is produced by collagen secreting myofibroblasts that populate the intima, and the developing lesion is contained, most of the times, by a fibrous cap. At the beginning, the atherosclerotic lesions are asymptomatic and not at risk for rupture and induction of thrombosis. Atheroma lesions submitted to a chronic inflammatory state will become unstable and may result in an acute vascular event (Virmani et al., 2002). Within those plaques, apoptotic macrophages will suffer necrosis and perpetuate inflammation, with the formation of necrotic cores. These vulnerable or unstable plaques may rupture, exposing pro-coagulant and pro-thrombogenic molecules into the intima and initiating platelet activation and aggregation. This, in turn, will lead to thrombosis and to the clinical manifestation of atherothrombotic disease.

Inflammation plays a major role during all stages of atherosclerosis: endothelial dysfunction, endothelial and cytokine activation, recruitment of inflammatory cells, macrophage uptake of oxidized low-density lipoprotein (oxLDL), development of fatty streaks and fibrous plaque, and finally plaque rupture. Being so, it becomes obvious why SLE and atherosclerosis are so closely related.

3.1.3 Lipids and humoral response towards lipoproteins

Lipid abnormalities are one of the major contributors for atherosclerosis in SLE and different patterns of dyslipoproteinemia have been reported in this disease (Ilowite et al., 1988; Svenungsson et al., 2003). Dyslipoproteinemia in active lupus is characterized by depressed high density lipoprotein cholesterol and apolipoprotein A1 (ApoA1) with elevated very low density lipoprotein cholesterol (VLDL) and triglyceride; on the other hand, the dyslipoproteinemia associated with corticosteroid treatment is characterized by increased total cholesterol, VLDL, and triglycerides. The pattern of dyslipoproteinemia typical of SLE is closely related to disease activity. An enhanced activity in the TNFalpha/soluble TNF-receptor system seems to be an important underlying factor (Svenungsson et al., 2003).

Oxidative stress is also a key factor in atherogenesis, and it is increased in patients with SLE. Interactions between anticardiolipin (aCL) antibodies and anti-oxidant endothelial cells antibodies with the production of pro-oxidant substances suggestes that the interactive mechanisms linking plasma lipoproteins, the immune system, and the endothelium are one of the missing links that can unveil atheroma plaque formation in SLE. Oxidation profile in SLE is reflection of a pro-oxidant status and the presence of aCL antibodies is just one of the potential contributors. A direct effect of aCL antibodies with endothelial cells (inducing inducible nitric oxide synthase expression) leads to an enhanced peroxynitrite synthesis, a pro-oxidant substance, associated with vascular dysfunction and atherogenesis (Delgado Alves et al., 2005).

The primary lipid components involved in atherosclerosis are lipoproteins. Among these, low-density lipoprotein (LDL) and high-density lipoprotein (HDL) assume a central role. HDL are thought to have an anti-atherothrombogenic effect by stimulating endothelial nitric oxide and inhibiting oxidative stress and inflammation (Yuhanna et al., 2001), thus preventing LDL oxidation. LDL is the most pro-atherogenic lipoprotein, due to its ability to capture free radicals becoming itself a powerful pro-oxidant. HDL-associated ApoA1 has known anti-inflammatory properties (Ashby et al., 1998; Hyka et al., 2001) by promoting reverse cholesterol transport from macrophages *in vivo* as well as by blocking contact mediated activation of monocytes by T lymphocytes. Its anti-atherosclerotic actions is also associated with the stabilization of paraoxonase (James & Deakin, 2000). Paraoxonase is an anti-oxidant enzyme that prevents the formation of lipid peroxidation products, such as oxLDL. Higher paraoxonase activity is associated with a lower incidence of cardiovascular events (Soran et al., 2009).

HDL has several other antiatherogenic properties, including the transport of cholesterol from peripheral tissues to the liver. The concept that macrophage-cholesterol efflux has a significant role in cardiovascular disease prevention was recently suggested by the finding of a strong inverse association between HDL-mediated cholesterol efflux from macrophages, carotid intima media thickness (IMT) and the likelihood of coronary heart disease (Khera et al., 2011). These effects were shown to be independent of HDL-cholesterol level. Nevertheless, low levels of HDL increase the cholesterol burden and macrophage-driven inflammation, being strongly associated with the risk of coronary artery disease. Another condition that increases that risk involves the conversion of HDL to a dysfunctional form that is no longer cardioprotective (Barter et al., 2004), but instead acquire a pro-inflammatory and pro-oxidant phenotype promoting atherosclerosis (Delgado Alves et al., 2002, 2009). Regardless of all these data, the underlying mechanisms are still unclear, and no widely accepted methods for determining HDL function have been recognized. Other possible mechanisms for HDL dysfunction may be the increased glycation with the consequent ApoA1 multimerization and decreased phospholipid content (Parker & Cho, 2011). This proinflammatory form of HDL (piHDL) has been described in SLE (Navab et al., 2001) High levels of piHDL increases the risk of developing subclinical atherosclerosis in SLE (MacMahon et al., 2009).

A new concept has merged recently that might account for the higher risk of atherosclerosis in SLE: the humoral response towards HDL. It has been confirmed the presence of IgG antibodies towards HDL and its main protein component ApoA1 in patients with SLE. By interfering with the anti-atherogenic properties of HDL, anti-HDL and ApoA1 antibodies enhance oxidative stress and the consequent SLE-related atherosclerotic lesions. Anti-HDL antibodies are associated with decreased paraoxonase activity, increased biomarkers of endothelial dysfunction (nitric oxide, adhesion molecules VCAM-1 and ICAM-1), reduced total antioxidant capacity, and also increased disease-related damage and activity (Batuca et al., 2009). Both anti-HDL and anti-apolipoprotein A1 antibodies cross react with aCL. Theoretically, anti-HDL and anti-ApoA1 antibodies that cross react with aCL antibodies may contribute to endothelial dysfunction by favouring the oxidation of LDL.

Anti-ApoA1 antibodies have also been described in acute coronary syndromes (Vuilleumier et al., 2008), and they be potential markers of plaque instability (Montecucco et al., 2011).

LDL is the major cholesterol carrying lipoprotein in plasma and may exist in different forms. OxLDL injures cells in artery walls, and promotes atheroma formation (Colles et al., 2001; Hessler et al., 1979). Small dense LDL, when compared with its larger, normal-size counterpart, is more easily oxidized, has a higher affinity for extracellular matrix, and is subject to a higher degree of retention in the arterial wall (Berneis & Krauss, 2002; Hurt-Camejo et al., 2001; Packard & Sheperd, 1997). Also, smaller LDL has reduced binding to LDL receptors (Chapman et al., 1998) and a longer "half-life". These facts may lead to a greater degree of structural modification, which further increases its atherogenic profile.

In SLE, antibodies to oxidized LDL (anti-oxLDL) have been demonstrated in up to one half of patients with SLE (Romero et al., 1998). Also, anti-oxLDL antibody levels correlate with complement activation, disease activity scores, anti-double-stranded DNA antibody titres (Gómez-Zumaquero et al., 2004) and were found to facilitate the formation of foam cells(Matsuura et al., 2006)

3.1.4 Inflammation and acute response

It is already established that inflammation plays a pivotal role in the pathogenesis of atherosclerosis. It mediates several of the stages of atheroma development from initial leukocyte recruitment to eventual rupture of the unstable atherosclerotic plaque. SLE is characterized by a low-grade persistent pro-inflammatory state, present not only during flares but also during stable disease. The chronic burden of activated inflammatory mediators may have a considerable impact on endothelial cell function and blood coagulation. Several inflammatory circulating intermediates in SLE have been identified as highly atherogenic, such as IL-1, IL-6, IL-18, monocyte chemotatic protein 1, interferon γ and TNFα, among others (Asanuma et al., 2006; Blake &Ridker, 2001; Aringer & Smolen, 2004).

C-Reactive protein (CRP) is an acute phase protein that plays a major role in the regulation of the inflammatory response. It has been implicated in the promotion of both leukocyte adhesion and migration and also in vascular endothelial dysfunction by inducing adhesion molecules, chemokines and cytokines(Pasceri et al., 2000, 2001). Levels of C-reactive protein (CRP) have been shown to be predictive of cardiovascular disease in the general population (Ridker et al., 2002). High-sensitivity CRP and ICAM-1 have been associated with increased coronary artery calcification in SLE patients (Kao et al., 2008). The interaction of anti-monomeric CRP with monomeric CRP in blood vessel walls may also contribute to development of cardiovascular disease in SLE (O'Neill et al., 2007).

As compared with other auto-immune diseases, such as rheumatoid arthritis, the magnitude of CRP elevation is less important. It has been proposed that the relatively low CRP levels in SLE patients can be explained by increased clearance or decreased production of this protein. Autoantibodies to CRP in SLE patients support its increased clearance (Bell et al, 1998; Sjowall et al, 2004); however, the plasma clearance rate of CRP is the same in patients with active lupus and normal individuals, which makes this hypothesis less likely (Vigushin et al, 1993).

3.1.5 Insulin resistance and the metabolic syndrome

The metabolic syndrome is a new defined cluster of risk factors associated with increased insulin resistance, higher risk of developing type II diabetes mellitus and cardio and cerebrovascular events. It is an independent predictor of cardiovascular morbidity and mortality. These risk factors include abdominal obesity, pro-atherogenic dyslipidemia and elevated blood pressure. Even though individually these abnormalities may contribute little, as a risk-factor cluster it is very important and aggressive treatment should be considered in these patients. It is estimated that this syndrome may affect 20-25% of the overall population in the United States and the prevalence increases with age (Ford et al., 2002).

Insulin resistance is characterized by an impaired response to insulin in several insulin-sensitive tissue, such as muscle, liver, fat and endothelium (Simonson et al., 2005). Insulin has anti-inflammatory properties, mainly due to its ability to suppress several proinflammatory transcription factors, such as nuclear factor kappa-light-chain-enhancer of activated B cells (NF-κB) , early growth response protein 1 (Egr-1) and activator protein 1 (AP-1) (Aliada et al., 2002). Insulin resistance is a main contributor to the increased cardiovascular risk attributed to the metabolic syndrome (Hanley et al., 2002). There is a link between high levels of proinflammatory cytokines and cardiovascular disease through metabolic pathways. The exact mechanisms linking insulin resistance and inflammation are not fully established. A possible candidate is TNF- α. It is over-expressed in the adipose tissues of animal models of obesity (Hotamisligi et al., 1993). Adipose tissue act as an endocrine secretory gland, producing several inflammatory mediators, responsible for a pro-inflammatory state and thus to an increased cardiovascular risk (Després & Lemieux, 2006).

Tumor necrosis factor-α (TNF-α), IL-1β, IL-4, IL-6, IL-11, Interferon-γ (INF-γ), acting on sensitive adipocytes, can lead to the activation of inflammatory signaling cascades (Rajala & Sherer, 2003). As a response to fat activation, there is enhanced expression and secretion of several acute phase reactants and also mediators of inflammation, such as TNF-α, IL-1β, IL-6, IL-8, IL- 10, prostaglandin E2 (PGE2). Leptin, adiponectin, and resistin (Fain et al., 2004) can perpetuate in the highly pro-inflammatory state.

SLE is associated with an increased prevalence of the metabolic syndrome (El-Magdami et al., 2006). The frequency of metabolic syndrome amongst patients with SLE varies from 16,7% in Mexico(Zonana-Nacah e tal., 2008), 28,6 % in Argentina to 29,4 % in USA (Chung et al., 2007) and 32,1 % in Brazil (Telles et al., 2010), with other cohorts showing similar results. Other metabolic-associated changes such as insulin resistance, premature menopause, renal impairment and high triglyceridemia also occur more frequently in SLE. Controversy still remains regarding the exact role of metabolic syndrome in predicting long-term risk for coronary heart disease in SLE. The major benefit in recognising this syndrome in the context of SLE is related to the identification of patients more in need for lifestyle interventions and specific therapeutic approach.

There is no clear association between treatment with steroids and the development of metabolic syndrome (Telles et al., 2007. However, prednisone in dosages higher than 10 mg/ day and high dosages of intravenous methylprednisone has been previously associated with this condition (Négron et al., 2008). These findings are still not definitive as they can be a reflection of lupus activity and severity. In fact, low-dose steroids may still be of value, due to its anti-inflammatory effects.

3.1.6 Traditional risk factors for cardiovascular disease in SLE

A patient with SLE and cardiovascular disease has on average one less traditional risk factor than people in the general population with a similar cardiovascular condition (Bruce, 2005; Urowitz et al., 2007) and the baseline 10-year coronary heart disease and stroke risk (after adjusting for Framingham score) for all patients with SLE is 7.5–17-fold higher (Esdaile et al., 2001). This is one of the reasons why the relative importance of the individual traditional risk factors differs between patients with SLE and the general population.

Hypertension

Hypertension is a predictor of mortality and vascular events in SLE (Petri et al., 1992; Rahman et al., 2000). It is more common than in the general population with a relative risk of 2.59 (95% CI 1.79–3.75) (Bruce et al., 2003), independently of whatever treatment for SLE is being administred.

Smoking

Smoking, a well known risk factor for atherosclerosis, is not more frequent in patients with SLE than in the general population (RR 0.86, 95% CI 0.59–1.24) (Boyer et al., 2011), but in the Systemic Lupus International Collaborating Clinics registry (SLICC) (Urowitz et al., 2008) the prevalence of smokers increased from 13.7% at baseline to 18.7%.

Dyslipidemia

Hpercholesterolemia in lupus patients is associated with an 18-fold increased risk of myocardial infarction as compared with the general population (Fischer et al., 2004).

Body composition and low physical exercise

Patients with lupus are more likely to have a sedentary lifestyle, with consequent obesity and hypercholesterolemia (Petri et al., 1992). Low physical activity is associated with increased subclinical atherosclerosis and proinflammatory HDL levels in patients with SLE. Despite the common presence of fatigue as a symptom of the disease, there is reason to believe that exercise should be included in the rehabilitation of patients with mild to moderate SLE (Yuen et al., 2011). Exercise, if well tolerated, may reduce the risk of atherosclerosis in SLE (Volkmann et al., 2010).

3.1.7 Other risk factors

Treatment of SLE and its most common co-morbidities has become more and more complex with drug interactions and side effects becoming a very important issue. Apart from the classical complications of steroid and immunosuppressive treatment, new associations between drugs and clinical adverse effects have been identified. Azathioprine, as an example, was associated with arterial events (hazard ratio of 1.45 (95% CI 1.21–10.4) (Toloza et al., 2004) and with the presence of carotid plaques (Ahmad et al., 2004). Although we should keep these results in mind, the fact is that azathioprine is used in more active disease and it may be just a surrogate for more severe inflammation.

Hyperhomocysteinemia is a well known risk factor for cardiovascular disease and it is a possible marker of atherosclerosis progression and more-active lupus (Bultink et al., 2005; Kianai et al., 2007; Roman et al., 2007). It decreases the availability of endothelial cell-derived nitric oxide, impairs endothelial-dependent vasodilatation, induces oxidative stress, and increases the risk of thrombosis (Maron & Loscalzo, 2009). Homocystein actions on endothelial cells are partly mediated by asymmetric dimethylarginine (ADMA), an intrinsic inhibitor of nitric oxide synthase (Stuhlinger et al., 2003). High levels of ADMA have been described in patients with renal and heart failure, diabetes mellitus, hypertension, and acute coronary events and may predict stroke, coronary artery disease, and also cardiovascular-related death (Laier et al. 2008; Wilson et al., 2008). Among patients with SLE, higher ADMA levels are linked to a higher prevalence of cardiovascular disease.

Hyperuricemia correlates with arterial stiffness and inflammation markers in patients with SLE without symptomatic atherosclerotic disease. It has been showed that women with SLE and hyperuricemia have a high risk cardiovascular profile with metabolic syndrome and renal failure.

3.2 Vasculitis

In the absence of clinically significant coronary atherosclerosis, two other major mechanisms of vascular damage may occur: vasculitis and thrombosis.

The prevalence of vasculitis in SLE patients ranges from 11% to 20% (Cardinali et al., 2000; Wisnieki, 2000). Small vessels (both arteries and venules) of the skin are the most commoly involved (Gonzalez-Gay et al., 2005); medium-sized vessel involvement is less frequent (D'Cruz et al., 1993), and large vessel involvement is rare (Goldberger et al., 1992). Although vasculitis presents mainly as cutaneous lesions, the clinical spectrum is wide, and lifethreatening ischemic injury may result from vasculitis of medium-sized vessels in the gastrointestinal, cardiac, pulmonary, or cerebrovascular regions (D'Cruz, 1998).

Coronary vascular damage may be related to coronary arteritis, affecting preferentially small-size coronary arteries (Bulkley & Roberts, 1975) or, rarely, the medium-size coronary arteries (Bonfiglio et al., 1992); and/ or coronary artery thrombosis. Acute myocardial infarction due to coronary arteritis is reported in SLE, although the incidence is very low.

Immune complex deposition and complement activation play important roles in the pathogenesis of vasculitis in general and coronary arteritis in particular. In patients with both SLE and antiphospholipid syndrome, microvascular thrombi of the coronary circulation, with discrete atherosclerosis and vasculitis, have been observed (Brown et al., 1988).

The distinction between atherosclerosis and arteritis is a difficult task, because coronary vasculitis often occurs in the absence of a clinical SLE flare and also with minimal serologic evidence of disease activity (Wilson et al., 1992).

Central nervous system (CNS) vasculitis in the context of SLE is rare, although it has been found in autopsies in SLE in 7-12% of cases (Johnson & Richardson, 1968; Ellis & Verity, 1979).

Stroke (both ischaemic and haemorrhagic) and SLE cerebral vasculopathy are far more frequent. While ischaemic stroke in SLE is strongly associated to antiphospholipid syndrome, atherosclerosis (Bruce, 2005) and Libman-Sacks endocarditis (Moyassaki et al., 2007), factors that contribute to hemorrhagic stroke are less clear.

The predominant pathology finding in CNS vessels in SLE patients is a noninflammatory small vessel vasculopathy involving small arterioles and capillaries. At autopsy, 50% of the patients have cerebral vasculopathy, characterized by hyaline thickening and eosinophilia of the vessel wall, fibrinoid degeneration without vasculitis, and endothelial proliferation, sometimes accompanied by microhemorrhages (Devinsky et al., 1988; Ellison et al. 1993; Hanly et al., 1992).

3.3 Thrombosis

Thrombotic events are reported in 7-12% of patients with SLE (Somers et al., 1999). During the first year of disease, the incidence of both arterial and venous thrombotic events increases. Several reasons have been pointed out, and include aPL antibodies, circulating immune complexes, high levels of disease activity, and chronic inflammation (Manger et al., 2002). When associated with SLE, antiphospholipid syndrome is a relevant predictor of organ damage and death in patients (Ruiz-Irastorza et al., 2004). Anti-cardiolipin (aCL) antibodies, lupus anticoagulant (LAC) and anti-beta2-glycoprotein 1 antibodies (anti-B2GPI) are detected in approximately one-third of patients with SLE (Love & Santoro, 1990), especially in the context of the antiphospholipid syndrome. The best predictors for thrombotic events in SLE are persistent aPL antibodies, the presence of LAC (Somers et al., 2002), and high titers of aCL antibodies (Ginsburg et al., 1992).

Not all thrombotic phenomena are associated with the presence of aPL antibodies and some patients may develop venous and arterial thrombosis without aCL positivity. The relevance of traditional and SLE-related thrombotic risk factors in aPL positive patients is still under investigation. Most of the patients with SLE and aPL antibodies who developed thrombosis had other thrombotic risk factors (Erkan et al., 2007). Interestingly, after adjusting for other risk factors, SLE itself remains independently associated with thrombotic events (Bruce, 2005). Thrombosis is frequent in early SLE and is associated with a significant mortality; therefore, the identification of possible modifiable risk factors and the establishment of efficacious strategies of prevention and treatment are vital.

4. Treatment

The impact of cardiovascular disease has been under-recognized in the context of SLE, with limited attention on aggressive management of possible modifiable risk factors. Despite a general awareness of coronary vascular disease in SLE patients, physicians do not address risk factors in a comprehensive fashion. Also, the management of conventional cardiovascular risk factors such as diabetes mellitus, smoking, hypercholesterolemia and hypertension is not at the same level of non-SLE patients. This is reinforced by the fact that recruiting and retaining patients with SLE for clinical trials regarding preventive measures has been proven to be extremely difficult.

It is therefore of great importance to identify in each patient the modifiable risk factors and introduce in clinical practice guidelines to help clinicians reducing long-term cardiovascular morbidity and mortality. In this chapter, we analyze the potential impact of some of the most commonly used drugs in SLE and their effects in the cardiovascular system.

The general approach suggested in the overall population for primary and secondary prophylaxis of vascular disease should be proposed to every patient and should include (table 2):

4.1 Corticosteroids: Are they good or bad for lupus?

Corticosteroids still remain a first line treatment for lupus, despite having numerous detrimental side effects on blood pressure, blood glucose and lipid profile (Manzi et al., 2000). Corticosteroids have a particular deleterious effect on the heart (Bulkley et al., 1975). Prednisone dosage superior to 7,5 mg/d increases insulin levels, a risk factor for cardiovascular disease (Karp et al., 2008) and total cholesterol, triglycerides and apolipoprotein B levels increase significantly with a daily prednisone dose higher than 10 mg (Petri et al., 1992). The estimated 2-year coronary risk for a patient treated with anved an average dosage of 30 mg/day of prednisone for 1 year, is approximately 60% higher than it would be for a patient with the same levels of SLE activity and similar risk factors who received no corticosteroids (Karp et al., 2008).

When compared to a baseline chronic inflammatory status, low dose corticosteroids may exert an anti-inflammatory action which might be beneficial. In fact, such exposure may improve the lipid profile and increase insulin levels, whithout having a negative effect on blood pressure and atherosclerosis. A weak association between low-dose corticosteroids and cardiovascular risk factors has been established, and identified a dose-related trend for increasing major cardiovascular events (Ruyssen-Witrand et al., 2010). Furthermore, subclinical atherosclerosis is correlated with lower mean dose of corticosteroids and lesser immunossupressants (Roman et al., 2003).

Cholesterol	1. 2. 3. 4.	Screening: fasting lipid profile every year; For LDL cholesterol <2.6 mmol/l: no treatment; For LDL cholesterol 2.6–3.4 mmol/l: therapeutic lifestyle changes. Consider statins when LDL is >3.4 mmol/l with or without other risk factors; or when LDL is persistently >2.6 mmol/l despite therapeutic lifestyle changes.
Hypertension	1. 2. 3. 4.	Blood pressure assessments at every visit to the outpatients clinic; Ideal target is defined as blood pressure at <130 mmHg systolic and <80 mmHg diastolic. If elevated blood pressure (>140 mmHg systolic or >90 mmHg diastolic): lifestyle modification.; If, despite previous measures, the blood pressure is persistently found to be elevated: start antihypertensive medication.
Diabetes mellitus	1. 2. 3.	Regular testing for diabetes (1-2 /year); In patients with a fasting glucose ≥6.1 mmol/l: glucose tolerance test and lifestyle changes; Referral to a specialist in diabetes.
Weight control	1. 2. 3.	Screening for obesity; Lifestyle changes, exercise programmes and behavioral support; If, despite efforts, obesity remains, refer to drug/ bariatric surgery by a multidisciplinary team.

Table 2. Summary of some therapeutic interventions.

There are some important limitations in addressing the role of steroids in cardiovascular risk. Corticosteroid use is more common in patients with moderate to severe disease (Bruce, 2006) and the duration of exposure to this drug may function as a surrogate for disease duration. Further work is needed to assess if there are doses or regimes of corticosteroid therapy that can optimise their anti-inflammatory effects whilst minimizing their multiple adverse effects.

4.2 Statins

Pleotropic actions of hydroxyl-3-methylglutaryl coenzyme A (HMG-CoA) inhibitors (statins) have been thourougly reported and is now accepted that their benefits go beyond cholesterol lowering and include immunomodulatory and immunossupressive properties. Statins inhibit HMG-CoA reductase, an enzyme that converts HMG-CoA to mevalonate, a fundamental step in cholesterol synthesis. The mevalonate pathway is involved in posttranslational modification of cell-signaling proteins during cell division and maturation, with inhibition of proinflammatory effects. It then promotes anti-inflammatory activities through the direct inhibition/activation of chemokyne, cytokine-, and acute-phase reactant-driven intracellular pathways in several cell types involved in inflammation. Statins modulate the activity of cells involved in both innate and adaptive immune responses, affecting the production of cytokines and cellular adhesion molecules (e.g. ICAM-a, IL-6, TNF-α, IL-1 and selectin levels (Mira & Mañes, 2009) and have an antithrombotic effect by inhibiting platelet activation (Ferroni et al., 2006). In the general population, statins have shown efficacy in primary and secondary prevention of acute myocardial infarction and stroke (Amarenco et al., 2006; Ridker et al., 2008).

Following the identification of their mechanisms of action, statins became a potential drug for treating SLE patients despite cardiovascular involvement. Low dose rosuvastatin induced a significant reduction in LDL and CRP after 12 months treatment (Mok et al., 2011). In patients with low disease activity, rosuvastatin decreased plasma levels of endothelial activation markers such as P-selectin and VCAM-1. Unexpectedly, in 2011, the results from the Lupus Atherosclerosis Prevention Study (Petri et al., 2011) offered no evidence that atorvastatin could reduce markers of subclinical atherosclerosis or disease activity over 2 years and the anti-inflammatory effects of statins observed in the general population were not replicated in this SLE clinical trial. However, comments were raised regarding the homogeneity of both treatment arms which may limit the final interpretation. Importantly, there was no information about the treatments received by patients during the 2 years follow-up, regarding the use of prednisone, immunosupresive agents and hydroxychloroquine, all of them having a direct effect on inflammation and disease activity and potentially on subclinical atherosclerosis. Hence, the negative results in this clinical trial could be caused by an imbalance in the use of these drugs in both arms, rather than by the lack of efficacy of atorvastatin.

4.3 Low dose salicylic acid

Most of SLE patients with aPL, but without a history of thrombosis, do not receive any preventive therapeutic, while some receive low dose salicylic acid (ASA) (Kamashta, 2000). Prophylactic treatment with ASA in SLE patients may prevent both arterial and venous thrombotic manifestations, especially in patients with positive aPL (Wahl et al., 2000). In fact, ASA decreases the probability of thrombosis in asymptomatic individuals with aPL (Erkan et al., 2002). The use of low-dose ASA has been recommended by the expert committee in the recent European League Against Rheumatism guidelines for the management of SLE (Bertsias et al., 2008).

4.4 Hydroxychloroquine

Hydroxychloroquine is an anti-malarial drug also used to treat SLE, Sjögren's syndrome and other immune mediate diseases. Several mechanisms have been proposed to explain its beneficial effect, which is not fully established. Hydroxychloroquine can inhibit the binding of antiphospholipid antibody–β2-glycoprotein I complexes to phospholipid bilayers (Rand et al., 2008), reverse platelet activation induced by human IgG aPL antibodies (Espinola et al., 2002), and reduce of aPL antibody–induced thrombosis (Edwards et al., 1996). There is no consistent data regarding whether this antithrombotic effect is present both for arterial and venous events.

A beneficial effect on serum lipid levels, including patients taking corticosteroid therapy (Borba et al., 2001; Hodis et al., 1993; Sachet et al., 2007; Tam et al., 2000), was shown by a few observational studies. However, the strenght of evidence supporting a clinically meaningful beneficial effect was rated as low. Also, there is no data supporting any protective effect of this drug on the development of metabolic syndrome (Ruiz-Irastorza et al., 2010).

Regarding the effect of hydroxychloroquine on atherosclerosis, most studies are limited by the low consistency and lack of specific design (Ahmad et al., 2007; Maksimowicz-McKinnon et al, 2006). The effect was not quantified in most cases and the exposure to hydroxychloroquine has been heterogeneously defined, without taking into account the time of exposure or a possible dose effect.

Because of its beneficial effects on reducing SLE activity and mortality, most of the authors recommend hydroxychloroquine for most patients with SLE, starting as soon as the diagnosis is made. Its application for the specific prevention of thrombosis and treatment of atherosclerosis requires validation in future clinical trials.

4.5 B-cell depletion therapy

Rituximab, a drug that had no previously documented lipid-lowering effect, was recently investigated in patients with SLE who had failed standard immunosuppressive therapy (Pego-Reigosa et al., 2010). An increase in HDL cholesterol and a fall in the total cholesterol/HDL ratio and triglyceride levels was documented in a significant proportion of the 12 patients studied. Furthermore, this improvement in lipid profile mirrored a decrease in disease activity; this suggests a positive effect of rituximab related to a reduction in the overall high inflammatory status. Still, larger prospective studies should aim to evaluate if this observed favorable effect contributes to a lower incidence of cardiovascular events.

5. Conclusion

Patients with SLE are at increased risk for cardiovascular complications. Atherosclerosis occurs prematurely in patients with systemic lupus erythematosus and is independent of the traditional risk factors for cardiovascular disease. Premature atherosclerosis has emerged as a leading cause of morbidity and mortality in SLE. Traditional risk factors, such as hypertension, smoking, diabetes, obesity and dyslipidemia are common in SLE but they fail to explain entirely the atherosclerotic burden found in these patients. Increased understanding of the mechanisms underlying vascular damage, plaque formation and stability, and thrombosis, will greatly facilitate the long-term care of patients with lupus. The clinical profile of patients with lupus and atherosclerosis suggests a role for disease-related factors in atherogenesis and underscores the need better trials targeting atherosclerosis in a specific fashion.

An early identification of subclinical atherosclerosis in SLE is warranted to help to identify patients with higher risk to undergo major vascular complications, who might benefit from more aggressive treatment and lifestyle modifications.

6. References

Abu-Shakra, M, Urowitz, MB, Gladman, DD, et al. (1995). Mortality studies in systemic lupus erythematosus. Results from a single center. II. Predictor variables for mortality. *J Rheumatol*, Vol.22, No.7, (July 1995), pp. 1265-70, ISSN 1499-2752.

Aranow, C, Ginzler, EM. (2000). Epidemiology of cardiovascular disease in systemic lupus erythematosus. *Lupus*. Vol.9, No.3, (April 2000). pp.166–169, ISSN 1477-0962.

Asanuma, Y, Oeser, A, Shintani, AK, et al. (2003). Premature coronary-artery atherosclerosis in systemic lupus erythematosus. *N Engl J Med*. Vol.349, No.25, (December 2003), pp. 2407-2415, ISSN 1533-4406.

Ahmad, Y, Shelmerdine, J, Bodill, H, et al. (2007). Subclinical atherosclerosis in systemic lupus erythematosus (SLE): the relative contribution of classic risk factors and the lupus phenotype. *Rheumatology* (Oxford), Vol. 46, No.6, (June 2007), pp. 983–988, ISSN 1499-2752.

Amarenco, P, Bogousslavsky, J, Callahan, A 3rd, et al. (2006). Stroke Prevention by Aggressive Reduction in Cholesterol Levels (SPARCL) Investigators High-dose atorvastatin after stroke or transient ischemic attack. *N Engl J Med*, (August 2006), Vol.355, No.6, pp. 549-559, ISSN 1533-4406.

Ahmad ,Y, Bodill ,H, Shelmerdine ,J, et al. (2004). Antiphospholipid antibodies (APLA) contribute to atherogenesis in SLE. *Arthritis Rheum*, (2004), Vol. 50, Suppl. 1, pp. S191, ISSN 1529-013.

Aljada, A, Ghanim, H, Mohanty, P, et al. (2002). Insulin inhibits the pro-inflammatory transcription factor early growth response gene-1 (Egr-1) expression in mononuclear cells and reduces plasma tissue factor (TF) and plasminogen activator inhibitor-1 (PAI-1) concentrations. *J Clin Endocrinol Metab*, (March 2002), Vol.87, No.3, pp. 1419–1422, ISSN 1945-7197.

Asanuma,Y, Chung, CP, Oeser, A, et al. (2006). Increased concentration of proatherogenic inflammatory cytokines in systemic lupus erythematosus: relationship to cardiovascular risk factors. *J Rheumatol*. (March 2006), Vol.33, No.3, pp. 539-545, ISSN 1499-2752.

Aringer, M, Smolen, JS. (2004). Tumour necrosis factor and other proinflammatory cytokines in systemic lupus erythematosus: a rationale for therapeutic intervention. *Lupus*, (2004), Vol.13, Vol.5, pp. 344-347, ISSN 1477-0962.

Ashby, DT, Rye, KA, Clay, MA, et al. (1998). Factors influencing the ability of HDL to inhibit expression of vascular cell adhesion molecule-1 in endothelial cells. *Arterioscler Thromb Vasc Biol*, Vol.18, No.9, (September 1998), pp. 1450–1455, ISSN 0276-5047.

Ando, J, Yamamoto, K (2001). Effects of shear stress and stretch on endothelial function. *Antioxid Redox Signal*, (February 2011), ISSN 1523-0864.

Bacon, PA, Stevens, RJ, Carruthers, DM, et al. (2002). Accelerated atherogenesis in autoimmune rheumatic diseases. *Autoimmun Rev*, Vol.1, No.6, (December 2002), pp.338–347, ISSN 1568-9972.

Barter, PJ, Nicholls, S, Rye, KA, et al. (2004). Antiinflammatory properties of HDL. *Circ Res*, Vol.95, No.8, (October 2004), pp.764-772, ISSN 0009-7300.

Batuca, JR, Ames, PR, Amaral, M, et al. (2009). Anti-atherogenic and anti-inflammatory properties of high-density lipoprotein are affected by specific antibodies in systemic lupus erythematosus. *Rheumatology* (Oxford), (January 2009), Vol.48, No.1, pp. 26-31, ISSN 1499-2752.

Bell, SA, Faust, H, Schmid, A, et al. (1998). Autoantibodies to C-reactive protein (CRP) and other acute-phase proteins in systemic autoimmune diseases. *Clin Exp Immunol*, (September 1998), Vol.113, No.3, pp. 327–332, ISSN 1365-2249.

Berneis, KK, Krauss, RM. (2001). Metabolic origins and clinical significance of LDL heterogeneity. *J Lipid Res*, (September 2001), Vol.43, No.9, pp.1363–1379, ISSN 1539-7262.

Bertsias, G, Ioannidis, JP, Boletis, J, et al. (2008). Task Force of the EULAR Standing Committee for International Clinical Studies Including Therapeutics. EULAR recommendations for the management of systemic lupus erythematosus. Report of a Task Force of the EULAR Standing Committee for International Clinical Studies Including Therapeutics. *Ann Rheum Dis*, / February 2008), Vol. 67, No.2, pp. 195-205, ISSN 1468-2060.

Bjornadal, L, Yin, L, Granath, F, et al. (2004). Cardiovascular disease a hazard despite improved prognosis in patients with systemic lupus erythematosus: results from a Swedish population based study 1964–1995. *J Rheumatol.* Vol.31, No.4, (April 2004), pp. 713–719, ISSN 0263-7103

Blake, GJ, Ridker, PM. (2001). Novel clinical markers of vascular wall inflammation. *Circ Res*, (October 2001), Vol.89, No.9, pp. 763-771, ISSN 0009-7300.

Bonfiglio, TA, Botti, RE, Hagstrom, JWC. (1992). Coronary arteritis, occlusion and myocardial infarction due to lupus erythematosus. *Am Heart J*, (February 1992), Vol.183, No.2, pp.153-158, ISSN 0002-8703.

Boyer, JF., Gourraud, PA., Cantagrel, A, et al. (2011). Traditional cardiovascular risk factors in rheumatoid arthritis: A meta-analysis. *Joint Bone Spine*, (March 2011), Vol. 78, No.12, pp.179–183 (2011), ISSN 1297-319X.

Brown, JH, Doherty ,CC, Allen ,DC, et al. (1988). Fatal cardiac failure due to myocardial microthrombi in systemic lupus erythematosus. *Br Med J (Clin Res)*, (May 1988), Vol.296, No.6635, pp.1505-1510, ISSN 0267-0623.

Bruce, IN, Urowitz, MB, Gladman, DD, et al. (1999). Natural history of hypercholesterolemia in systemic lupus erythematosus. *J Rheumatol*, Vol.26, No.10, (October 1999), pp. 2137-2143, ISSN 1499-2752.

Bruce, IN, Burns, RJ, Gladman, DD, et al. (2000). Single photon emission computed tomography dual isotope myocardial perfusion imaging in women with systemic lupus erythematosus. I. Prevalence and distribution of abnormalities. *J Rheumatol*, Vol. 27, No.10, (October 2010), pp. 2372-2377. ISSN 1499-2752.

Bruce, IN, Urowitz, MB, Gladman, DD, et al. (2003). Risk factors for coronary heart disease in women with systemic lupus erythematosus: the Toronto Risk Factor Study. *Arthritis Rheum*, (November 2003), Vol.48, No.11, pp. 3159–3167, ISSN 1529-013.

Bruce IN. (2005). Atherogenesis and autoimmune disease: the model of lupus. *Lupus*, (2005), Vol.14, No.9, pp. 687–690, ISSN 1477-0962

Bruce IN. (2006). The influence of other drugs on coronary heart disease (CHD) risk in systemic lupus erythematosus. *Lupus*, (November 2006), Vol. 15, No.11, pp. suppl. 23-26, ISSN 1477-0962.

Bulkley, BH, Roberts, WC. (1975). The heart in systemic lupus erythematosus and the changes induced in it by corticosteroid therapy. A study of 36 necropsy patients. *Am J Med*, (February 1975), Vol.58, No.2, pp. 243-264, ISSN 0002-9343.

Bultink, EM, Teerlink, T, Heijst, JA, et al. (2005). Raised plasma levels of asymmetric dimethylarginine are associated with cardiovascular events, disease activity, and organ damage in patients with systemic lupus erythematosus. *Ann Rheum Dis*, (September 2005), Vol.64, No.9, pp. 1362–1365, ISSN 1468-2060.

Bultink, IE, Turkstra, F, Diamant, M, et al. (2008). Prevalence of and risk factors for the metabolic syndrome in women with systemic lupus erythematosus. *Clin Exp Rheumatol*, (January-February, 2008); Vol.26, No.1, pp. 32-38, ISSN 1593-098

Cardinali C, Caproni M, Bernacchi E, et al. (2000). The spectrum of cutaneous manifestations in lupus erythematosus—the Italian experience. *Lupus*, (2000), Vol.9, No.6, pp. 417-423, ISSN 1477-0962.

D'Cruz D. (1998). Vasculitis in systemic lupus erythematosus. *Lupus,* (1998), Vol.7, No.4, pp. 270–274, ISSN 1477-0962.

Chapman, MJ, Guerin, M, Bruckert, E. et al. (1998). Atherogenic, dense low-density lipoproteins: pathophysiology and new therapeutic approaches. *Eur Heart J,* (February 1998), Vol.19, Suppl.A, pp. A24–A30, ISSN 1522-9645.

Chung, CP, Avalos, I, Oeser, A, et al. (2007). High prevalence of the metabolic syndrome in patients with systemic lupus erythematosus: association with disease characteristics and cardiovascular risk factors. Ann Rheum Dis, (February 2007), Vol.66, No.2, pp. 208-214, ISSN 1468-2060.

Colles, SM, Maxson, JM, Carlson, SG,et al. (2001). Oxidized LDL-induced injury and apoptosis in atherosclerosis. Potential roles for oxysterols. *Trends Cardiovasc Med.* (April-May 2001), Vol.11, No.3-4, pp. 131-138, ISSN 1050-1738.

Costenbader, KH, Karlson, EW, Gall, V, et al. (2005). Barriers to a trial of atherosclerosis prevention in systemic lupus erythematosus. *Arthritis Rheum,* (October 2005), Vol.53, No.5, pp. 718-723, ISSN 1529-013.

D'Cruz, D, Cervera, R, Olcay Aydintug, A, et al. (1993). Systemic lupus erythematosus evolving into systemic vasculitis: a report of five cases. Br J Rheumatol, (February 1993), Vol.32, No.2, pp. 154–157, ISSN 1460-2172.

Delgado Alves, J, Ames, PR, Donohue, S, et al. (2002). Antibodies to high-density lipoprotein and beta2-glycoprotein I are inversely correlated with paraoxonase activity in systemic lupus erythematosus and primary antiphospholipid syndrome. *Arthritis Rheum,* Vol.46, No.10, (October 2002), pp. 2686-2694, ISSN 1529-013.

Delgado Alves, J, Kumar, S, Isenberg, DA. (2003). Cross-reactivity between anti-cardiolipin, anti-high-density lipoprotein and anti-apolipoprotein A-I IgG antibodies in patients with systemic lupus erythematosus and primary antiphospholipid syndrome. *Rheumatology* (Oxford), (July 2003), Vol. 42, No.7, pp. 893-899, ISSN 1499-2752.

Delgado Alves, J, Mason, LJ, Ames, PR, et al. (2005). Antiphospholipid antibodies are associated with enhanced oxidative stress, decreased plasma nitric oxide and paraoxonase activity in an experimental mouse model. *Rheumatology* (Oxford), Vol.44, No.10, (October 2005), pp.1238-44; ISSN 1462-0332.

Després, JP, Lemieux, I. (2006). Abdominal obesity and metabolic syndrome. *Nature,* (December 2006), Vol.14, No.444(7121), pp. 881-887, ISSN 0028-0836.

Devinsky, O, Petito, CK, Alonso, DR. (1088). Clinical and neuropathological findings in systemic lupus erythematosus: the role of vasculitis, heart emboli, and thrombotic thrombocytopenic purpura. *Ann Neurol,* (April 1988),Vol.23, No.4, pp.380–384, ISSN 0364-5134.

Edwards, MH, Pierangeli, S, Liu, X, et al. (1996), Hydroxychloroquine reverses thrombogenic properties of antiphospholipid antibodies in mice. *Circulation,* (December 1996), Vol.96, No.12, pp. 4380–4384, ISSN 0009-7322.

Ellis, SG, Verity, MA (1979) Central nervous system involvement in systemic lupus erythematosus: a review of neuropathologic findings is 57 cases, 1955-1977. *Semin Arthritis Rheum,* (February 1979), Vol.8, No.3, pp. 212-221, ISSN 0049-0172.

Ellison, D, Gatter, K, Heryet, A, et al. (1993). Intramural platelet deposition in cerebral vasculopathy of systemic lupus erythematosus. *J Clin . Pathol,* (January 1993), Vol.46, No.1, pp. 37–40, ISSN 0021-9738.

El Magadmi, M, Ahmad, Y, Turkie, W, et al. (2006). Hyperinsulinemia, insulin resistance, and circulating oxidized low density lipoprotein in women with systemic lupus erythematosus. *J Rheumatol*, (January 2006), Vol.33, No.1, pp.50-56, ISSN 1499-2752.

Erkan, D, Yazici, MG, Peterson, L, et al. (2002). A cross-sectional study of clinical thrombotic risk factors and preventive treatments in antiphospholipid syndrome. *Rheumatology* , (August 2002), Vol.41, No.8, pp. 924–929, ISSN 1462-0332.

Esdaile, JM, Abrahamowicz M, Grodzicky T, et al. (2001). Traditional Framingham risk factors fail to fully account for accelerated atherosclerosis in systemic lupus erythematosus. *Arthritis Rheum*, Vol.44, No.10, (October 2001), pp. 2331–2337, ISSN 1529-013.

Espinola, RG, Pierangeli, SS, Ghara, AE, et al. (2002). Hydroxychloroquine reverses platelet activation induced by human IgG antiphospholipid antibodies. *Thromb Haemost*, Vol.83, No. 3, pp. 518–522, ISSN 0340-6245.

Fain, JN, Madan, AK, Hiler, ML, et al. (2004). Comparison of the release of adipokynes by adipose tissue, adipose tissue matrix, and adipocytes form visceral and subcutaneous abdominal adipose tissue of obese humans. *Endocrinology*, (May 2004), Vol.145, No.5, 2273–2782, ISSN 1945-7170.

Ferroni, P, Basili, S, Santilli, F, et al. (2006). Low-density lipoprotein-lowering medication and platelet function. *Pathophysiol Haemost Thromb*, (2006), Vol. 35, No.3-4, pp. 346-354, ISSN 1424-8840.

Fischer, L. M., Schlienger, R. G., Matter, C.,et al. (2004). Effect of rheumatoid arthritis or systemic lupus erythematosus on the risk of first-time acute myocardial infarction. Am J Cardiol (January 2004), Vol.93, No.2, pp. 198–200, ISSN 0735-1097.

Ford, ES, Giles, WH, Dietz, WH. (2002). Prevalence of metabolic syndrome among US adults: findings from the third National Health and Nutrition Examination Survey. *JAMA*, (January 2002), Vol.287, No.3, pp. 356–359, ISSN 1538-3598.

Ginsburg, KS, Liang, MH, Newcomer, L, et al. (1992). Anticardiolipin antibodies and the risk for ischemic stroke and venous thrombosis. *Ann Intern Med*, (December 1992), Vol.117, No.12, pp. 997-1002, ISSN 1539-3704.

Gladman, DD, Urowitz, MB. (1987). Morbidity in systemic lupus erythematosus. *J Rheumatol Suppl*, Vol.14, (June 1987), pp. 223-226, ISSN 0380-0903.

Goldberger, E, Elder, RC, Schwartz, RA, (1992). Vasculitis in the antiphospholipid syndrome. A cause of ischemia responding to corticosteroids. *Arthritis Rheum*, (May 1992), Vol.35, No.5, pp. 569–572, ISSN 1529-013.

Gómez-Zumaquero, JM, Tinahones, FJ, De Ramón, E. (2004). Association of biological markers of activity of systemic lupus erythematosus with levels of anti-oxidized low-density lipoprotein antibodies. *Rheumatology* (Oxford), (April 2004), Vol.43, No.4, pp. 510-513, ISSN 1499-2752.

Gonzalez-Gay, MA, Garcia-Porrua, C, Pujol, RM. (2005). Clinical approach to cutaneous vasculitis. *Curr Opin Rheumatol*, (January 2005), Vol.17, No.1, pp. 56–61, ISSN 1531-6963.

Hanley, AJ, Williams, K, Stern, MP, et al. (2002). Homeostasis model assessment of insulin resistance in relation to the incidence of cardiovascular disease: the San Antonio Heart Study. *Diabetes Care*, (July 2002), Vol.25, No.7, pp.1177-1184, ISSN 1935-5548.

Hanly, JG, Walsh, NM, Sangalang, V. (1992). Brain pathology in systemic lupus erythematosus. *J Rheumatol*, (May 1992), Vol.19, No. 5, pp. 732–741, ISSN 1499-2752.

Harrison, MJ, Levy, R, Peterson, M, et al. (2007). Aspirin for primary thrombosis prevention in the antiphospholipid syndrome: a randomized, double-blind, placebo-controlled trial in asymptomatic antiphospholipid antibody-positive individuals. *Arthritis Rheum*, (July 2007), Vol.56, No.7, pp. 2382-2391, ISSN 1529-013.

Haque, S, Bruce, IN. (2009). Cardiovascular outcomes in systemic lupus erythematosus: big studies for big questions. *J. Rheumatol*. Vol.36, No.3, (March 2009), pp. 467–469, ISSN 1499-2752.

Harrison, MJ, Levy, R, Peterson, M, et al. (2007). Aspirin for primary thrombosis prevention in the antiphospholipid syndrome: a randomized, double-blind, placebo-controlled trial in asymptomatic antiphospholipid antibody-positive individuals. *Arthritis Rheum*, (July 2007), Vol.56, No.7, pp. 2382-2391, ISSN 1529-013.

Hermosillo-Romo, D, Brey, RL. (2002). Neuropsychiatric involvement in systemic lupus erythematosus. *Curr Rheumatol Rep*, Vol.4, No.4. (August 2002), pp. 337-344, ISSN 1534-6307.

Hessler, JR, Robertson, AL Jr, Chisolm, GM 3rd. (1979). LDL induced cytotoxicity and its inhibition by HDL in human vascular smooth muscle and endothelial cells in culture. *Atherosclerosis*. (March 1979), Vol.32, No.3, pp. 213- 229, ISSN 0021-9150.

Hotamisligil, GS, Shargill, NS, Spiegelman BM. et al. (1993). Adipose expression of tumor necrosis factor alpha: a direct role in obesity-linked insulin resistance. *Science*, (January 1993), Vol.259, No.5091, pp. 87–91, ISSN 1095-9203.

Hyka, N, Dayer, JM, Modoux, C et al. (2001). Apolipoprotein A-I inhibits the production of interleukin-1β and tumor necrosis factor-α by blocking contact-mediated activation of monocytes by T lymphocytes. *Blood*. Vol.97, No.8, (April, 2001), pp. 2381–2389, ISSN 1528-0020.

Hurt-Camejo, E, Camejo, G, Sartipy, P. (2001). Phospholipase: A2 and small, dense low-density lipoprotein. *Curr Opin Lipidol*. (October 2001), Vol.11, No.5, pp.465–471, ISSN 1473-6535.

Ilowite NT, Samuel P, Ginzler E, et a. (1988). Dyslipoproteinemia in pediatric systemic lupus erythematosus. *Arthritis Rheum*. Vol.31, No.7, (July 1988), pp. 859-863, ISSN 1529-013.

Jacobsen S, Petersen J, Ullman S, et al. (1998). A multicentre study of 513 Danish patients with systemic lupus erythematosus. II. Disease mortality and clinical factors of prognostic value. *Clin Rheumatol*, Vol.17, No.6, (June 1998), pp. 478-484, ISSN 1434-9949.

James, RW, Deakin, SP. (2004). The importance of high-density lipoproteins for paraoxonase-1 secretion, stability, and activity. *Free Radical Biol. Med*, Vol. 37, No. 12, (December 2004), pp.1986–1994, ISSN 0891-5849.

Johnson, RT, Richardson, EP. (1968). Theneurological manifestations of systemic lupus erythematosus: a clinical-pathological study of 24 cases and review of the literature. *Medicine* (Baltimore), Vol.47, No.4, pp. 337-369, ISSN 1536-5964.

Jonsson, H, Nived, O, Sturfelt, G. (1989). Outcome in systemic lupus erythematosus: a prospective study of patients from a defined population. *Medicine* (Baltimore), Vol.68, No.3, (May 1989), pp. 141-150, ISSN 1536-5964.

Khamashta, MA. (2000). Primary prevention of thrombosis in subjects with positive antiphospholipid antibodies. *J Autoimmun*, (September 2000), Vol.15, No.2, pp. 249-253, ISSN 1095-9157.

Karp, I, Abrahamowicz, M, Fortin, PR, et al. (2008). Recent corticosteroid use and recent disease activity: independent determinants of coronary heart disease risk factors in systemic lupus erythematosus? *Arthritis Rheum*, (February 2008), Vol.59, No.2, pp. 169-175, ISSN 1529-013.

Kao, AH, Wasko MC, Krishnaswami, S, et al. (2008). C-reactive protein and coronary artery calcium in asymptomatic women with systemic lupus erythematosus or rheumatoid arthritis. *Am J Cardiol*, (September 2008), Vol.102, No.6, pp. 755–760, ISSN 0002-9149.

Khera, A, Cuchel M, de la Llera-Moya M et al. (2011). Cholesterol efflux capacity, high-density lipoprotein function, and atherosclerosis. *N Engl J Med*, Vol.364, No.2, (January 2011), pp.127-135, ISSN 1533-4406.

Kianai, AN, Mahoney, JA, Petri, M. (2007). Asymmetric dimethylarginine isa marker of poor prognosis and coronary calcium in systemic lúpus erythematosus. *J Rheumatol*, (July 2007), Vol.34, No.7, pp. 1502–1505, ISSN 1499-2752

Lajer, M, Tarnow, L, Jorsal, A, et al. (2008). Plasma concentration of asymmetric dimethylarginine (ADMA) predicts cardiovascular morbidity and mortality in type 1 diabetic patients with diabetic nephropathy. *Diabetes Care*, (April 2008), Vol.31, No.4, pp. 747–752, ISSN 1935-5548.

Libby, P, Okamoto, Y, Rocha, VZ, et al. (2010). Inflammation in atherosclerosis: transition from theory to practice. *Circ J. Vol*, Vol.74, No.2, (February 2010), pp. 213-220, ISSN 1346-9843.

Love, PE, Santoro, SA. (1990). Antiphospholipid antibodies: anticardiolipin and the lupus anticoagulant in systemic lupus erythematosus (SLE) and in non-SLE disorders. Prevalence and clinical significance. *Ann Intern Med*, (May 1990), Vol.112, No.9, pp. 682-698, ISSN 1539-3704.

Lusis, AJ. (2000). Atherosclerosis. *Nature*. Vol. 407, No. 6801, (September 2000), pp. 233-241, ISSN 0028-0836.

Mackness, MI, Durrington, PN, Mackness, B. (2000). How high-density lipoprotein protects against the effects of lipid peroxidation. *Curr Opin Lipidol*. Vol.11, No. 4, (August 2000), pp. 383–388, ISSN 1473-6535.

Maksimowicz-McKinnon, K, Magder, L, Petri, M. (2006). Predictors of carotid atherosclerosis in systemic lupus erythematosus. *J Rheumatol*, Vol.33, No.12, (December, 2006), pp. 2458–2463, ISSN 1499-2752.

Manger, K, Kusus, M, Forster, C, et al. (2003). Factors associated with coronary artery calcification in young female patients with SLE. *Ann Rheum Dis*, Vol.62, No.9, (September 2003), pp. 846-850, ISSN 1468-2060.

Manger, K, Manger, B, Repp, R, et al. (2002). Definition of risk factors for death, end stage renal disease, and thromboembolic events in a monocentric cohort of 338 patients with systemic lupus erythematosus. *Ann Rheum Dis*, (December), Vol. 61, No.12, pp. 1065-70, ISSN 1468-2060.

Manzi, S, Meilahn, EN, Rairie, JE, et al. (1997). Age-specific incidence rates of myocardial infarction and angina in women with systemic lupus erythematosus: comparison with the Framingham Study. *Am J Epidemiol*, Vol.145, No.5, (March 1997), pp. 408-415, ISSN 1476-6256.

Manzi, S, Selzer F, Sutton-Tyrrell, K, et al. (1999). Prevalence and risk factors of carotid plaque in women with systemic lupus erythematosus. *Arthritis Rheum*, Vol. 42, No.1, (January 1999), pp. 51-60, ISSN 1529-013.

Manzi, S, Kuller, LH, Edmundowicz, D, et al. (2000). Vascular imaging: changing the face of cardiovascular research. *Lupus*, (2000), Vol.9, No.3, pp. 176-178, ISSN 1477-0962.

Maron, BA, Loscalzo, J. (2009). The treatment of hyperhomocysteinemia. *Annu Rev Med.* (July 2009), Vol.60, pp.39–54, ISSN 0785-3890.

Matsuura, E, Kobayashi, K, Tabuchi, M. (2006). Oxidative modification of low-density lipoprotein and immune regulation of atherosclerosis. *Prog Lipid Res*, (November 2006), Vol.45, No.6, pp. 466-486, ISSN 1873-2194.

McMahon, M, Grossman, J, Skaggs, B, et al. (2009). Dysfunctional proinflammatory high-density lipoproteins confer increased risk of atherosclerosis in women with systemic lupus erythematosus. *Arthritis Rheum*, (August 2009), Vol.60, No. 8, pp. 2428-2437, ISSN 1529-013.

Mira, E, Mañes, S. (2009). Immunomodulatory and anti-inflammatory activities of statins. *Endocr Metab Immune Disord Drug Targets*, (September 2009), Vol.9, No.3, pp. 237-247, ISSN 1871-5303.

Mok, CC, Lau, CS, Wong, RW. (2001). Neuropsychiatric manifestations and their clinical associations in southern Chinese patients with systemic lupus erythematosus. *J Rheumatol*, Vol.28, No.4, (April 2001), pp.766-771, ISSN 1499-2752.

Mok, CC, Tang, SS, To, CH, et al. (2005). Incidence and risk factors of thromboembolism in systemic lupus erythematosus: a comparison of three ethnic groups. *Arthritis Rheum*, Vol.52, No.9, (September 2005), pp. 2774-2782, ISSN 1529-013.

Mok, CC, Wong, CK, To, CH, et al. (2011). Effects of rosuvastatin on vascular biomarkers and carotid atherosclerosis in lupus: A randomized, double-blind, placebo-controlled trial. *Arthritis Care Res*, (June 2022), Vol.63, No.6, pp. 875-883, ISSN 0893-7524.

Montecucco, F, Vuilleumier, N, Pagano, S, et al. (2011). Anti-Apolipoprotein A-1 auto-antibodies are active mediators of atherosclerotic plaque vulnerability. *Eur Heart J*, (February 2011), Vol. 32, No.4, pp. 412-421, ISSN 1522-9645.

Moyssakis, I, Tektonidou, MG, Vasilliou, VA, et al.(2007). Libman-Sacks endocarditis in systemic lupus erythematosus: prevalence, associations, and evolution. *Am J Med*, (July 2007), Vol.120, No.7, pp. 636–642, ISSN 0002-9343.

Navab, M, Hama, SY, Hough, GP, (2001). A cell-free assay for detecting HDL that is dysfunctional in preventing the formation of or inactivating oxidized phospholipids. J *Lipid Res*, (August 2001), Vol.42, No. 8, pp. 1308-1317, ISSN 1539-7262.

Negrón, AM, Molina, MJ, Mayor, AM, (2008). Factors associated with metabolic syndrome in patients with systemic lupus erythematosus from Puerto Rico. *Lupus*, (April 2008), Vol.17, No.4, pp. 348-54, ISSN 1477-0962.

Nikpour, M, Urowitz, MB, Gladman, DD. (2005). Premature atherosclerosis in systemic lupus erythematosus. *Rheum Dis Clin North Am*, Vol.31, No.2, (May 2005), pp.329-354, ISSN 1558-3163.

O'Neill, SG, Isenberg, DA, Rahman, A. (2007). Could antibodies to Creactive protein link inflammation and cardiovascular disease in patients with systemic lupus erythematosus? Ann Rheum Dis, (August 2007), Vol.66, No.8, pp. 989–991, ISSN 1468-2060.

Packard, CJ, Shepherd, J. (1997). Lipoprotein heterogeneity and apolipoprotein B metabolism. *Arterioscler Thromb Vasc Biol,* (December 1997), Vol.17, No.12, pp. 3542–3556, ISSN 0276-5047

Pasceri, V, Willerson, JT, Yeh ET. (2000). Direct proinflammatory effect of C-reactive protein on human endothelial cells. *Circulation,* (October 2000), Vol.102, No.18, pp. 2165–2168, ISSN 0009-7322.

Pasceri, V, Cheng, JS, Willerson, JT, (2001). Modulation of C-reactive protein-mediated monocyte chemoattractant protein-1 induction in human endothelial cells by anti-atherosclerosis drugs. *Circulation,* (May 2001), Vol.103, No.21, pp. 2531–2534, ISSN 0009-7322.

Park, KH, Cho, KH. (2011). High-density lipoprotein (HDL) from elderly and reconstituted HDL containing glycated apolipoproteins A-I share proatherosclerotic and prosenescent properties with increased cholesterol influx. *J Gerontol A Biol Sci Med Sci.* (May 2011), Vol. 66, No.5, pp. 511-520, ISSN 1079-5006.

Petri ,M, Spence ,D, Bone, LR, et al. (1992). Coronary artery disease risk factors in the Johns Hopkins Lupus Cohort: prevalence, recognition by patients, and preventive practices. *Medicine* (Baltimore), (September 1992), Vol.71, No.5, pp. 291-302. ISSN 1536-5964.

Petri, M. (2002). Epidemiology of systemic lupus erythematosus. *Best Pract Res Clin Rheumatol,* Vol.16, No.5, (December 2002), pp.847-858, ISSN 1521-6942.

Petri, MA, Kiani, AN, Post, W, et al (2011). Lupus Atherosclerosis Prevention Study (LAPS). *Ann Rheum Dis,* (May 2011), Vol.70, No.5, pp. 760-765, ISSN ISSN 1468-2060.

Pego-Reigosa, JM, Lu, TY, Fontanillo, MF, et al. (2010). Long-term improvement of lipid profile in patients with refractory systemic lupus erythematosus treated with B-cell depletion therapy: a retrospective observational study. *Rheumatology* (Oxford), Vol. 49, No.4, (October 2010), pp. 691-696; SSN 1499-2752.

Rahman, P., Aguero, S., Gladman, D. D., et al. (2000). Vascular events in hypertensive patients with systemic lupus erythematosus. *Lupus,* (2000), Vol.9, No.9, pp. 672–675, ISSN 1477-0962.

Rajala, MW, Sherer, PE. (2003). Minireview: the adipocyte at the crossroads of energy homeostasis, inflammation, and atherosclerosis. *Endocrinology,* (September 2003), Vol.144, No.9, 3765–3773, ISSN 1945-7170.

Rand, JH, Wu, XX, Quinn, AS, et al. Hydroxychloroquine directly reduces the binding of antiphospholipid antibody–β2-glycoprotein I complexes to phospholipid bilayers. *Blood,* Vol.112, No.5, pp. 1687–1695, ISSN 1528-0020.

Ridker, PM, Rifai, N, Rose L, et al. (2002). Comparison of C-reactive protein and low-density lipoprotein cholesterol levels in the prediction of first cardiovascular events. *N Engl J Med,* (November 2002), Vol.347, No.20, pp.1557–1565, ISSN 1533-4406.

Ridker, PM, Danielson, E, Fonseca FA, et al. (2008). JUPITER Study Group Rosuvastatin to prevent vascular events in men and women with elevated C-reactive protein. *N Engl J Med,* (November 2008), Vol.329, No.20, pp. 2195-2207, ISSN 1533-4406.

Roldan, CA, Joson, J, Qualls, CR, et al. (2010). Premature aortic stiffness in systemic lupus erythematosus by transesophageal echocardiography. *Lupus.* Vol.19, No.14, (December 2010), pp.1599-1605, ISSN 1477-0962.

Roman, MJ, Shanker, BA, Davis, A, et al. (2003). Prevalence and correlates of accelerated atherosclerosis in systemic lupus erythematosus. *N Engl J Med,* (December 2003), Vol.349, No.25, pp. 2399-2406, ISSN ISSN 1533-4406.

Roman, MJ, Crow, MK, Lockshin, MD, et al. (2007). Rate and determinants of progression of atherosclerosis in systemic lupus erythematosus. *Arthritis Rheum,* (October 2007), Vol.56, No.10, pp.3412-3419, ISSN 1529-013.

Romero, FI, Amengual, O, Atsumi, T. et al. (1998). Arterial disease in lupus and secondary antiphospholipid syndrome: association with anti-beta2-glycoprotein I antibodies but not with antibodies against oxidized low-density lipoprotein. *Br J Rheumatol,* (August 1998), Vol.37, No.8, pp. 883-888, ISSN 1460-2172.

Ross R. (1999). Atherosclerosis--an inflammatory disease. *N Engl J Med,* Vol.340, No.2, (January 1999), pp. 115-26, ISSN 1533-4406.

Rubin, LA, Urowitz, MB, Gladman DD. (1985). Mortality in systemic lupus erythematosus: the bimodal pattern revisited. *Q J Med,* Vol.55, (April 1985), pp. 87-98, ISSN 1460-2393.

Ruiz-Irastorza, G, Egurbide, MV, Ugalde, J, et al. (2004). (High impact of antiphospholipid syndrome on irreversible organ damage and survival of patients with systemic lupus erythematosus. *Arch Intern Med,* (January 2004), Vol.164, No.1, pp. 77-82, ISSN 1538-3679.

Ruiz-Irastorza G, Ramos-Casals, M, Brito-Zeron, P, et al. (2010). Clinical efficacy and side effects of antimalarials in systemic lupus erythematosus: a systematic review. *Ann Rheum Dis,* Vol.69, No.1, (January 2010), pp. 20-28, ISSN 1468-2060.

Ruyssen-Witrand, A, Fautrel, B, Sarauxc, A, et al. (2010).Cardiovascular risk induced by low-dose corticosteroids in rheumatoid arthritis: a systematic literature review. *Joint Bone Spine,* (January 2010), pp. 23-30, ISSN 1297-319X.

Sabio, JM, Vargas-Hitos, JA, Mediavilla, JD, et al. (2010). Correlation of asymptomatic hyperuricaemia and serum uric acid levels with arterial stiffness in women with systemic lupus erythematosus without clinically evident atherosclerotic cardiovascular disease. *Lupus,* (April 2010), Vol.19, No.5, pp. 591-598, ISSN 1477-0962.

Sachet, J, Borba, E, Bonfa, E, et al. Chloroquine increases low-density lipoprotein removal from plasma in systemic lupus patients. *Lupus,* Vol.16, No.4, (2007), pp. 273-278, ISSN 1477-0962.

Sanna, G, Bertolaccini, ML, Cuadrado, MJ, et al. (2003). Neuropsychiatric manifestations in systemic lupus erythematosus: prevalence and association with antiphospholipid antibodies. *J Rheumatol,* Vol.30, No.5, (May 2003), pp. 985-992, ISSN 1499-2752.

Scalzi, LV, Hollenbeak, CS, Wang, L. (2010). Racial disparities in age at time of cardiovascular events and cardiovascular-related death in patients with systemic lupus erythematosus. *Arthritis Rheum,* Vol.62, No.9, (September 2010), pp. 2767-2775, ISSN 1529-013.

Sella, EM, Sato, EI, Leite, WA, et al. (2003). Myocardial perfusion scintigraphy and coronary disease risk factors in systemic lupus erythematosus. *Ann Rheum Dis,* Vol.62, No.11, (November 2003), pp.1066-1070, ISSN 1468-2060.

Shah, MA, Shah, AM, Krishnan, E. (2009). Poor outcomes after acute myocardial infarction in systemic lupus erythematosus. *J Rheumatol,* Vol.36, No.3, (March 2009), pp. 570-575, ISSN 1499-2752.

Simonson, GD, Kendall, DM. (2005). Diagnosis of insulin resistance and associated syndromes: the spectrum from the metabolic syndrome to type 2 diabetes mellitus. *Coron Artery Dis*, (December 2005), Vol.16, No.8, pp. 465–472, ISSN 1473-5830.

Sjowall, C, Bengtsson, AA, Sturfelt, G, et al. (2004). Serum levels of autoantibodies against monomeric C-reactive protein are correlated with disease activity in systemic lupus erythematosus. *Arthritis Res Ther*, (December 2004), Vol. 6, No.2, pp. R87–R94, ISSN 1478-6362

Ståhl-Hallengren, C, Jönsen, A, Nived, O, et al. (2000). Incidence studies of systemic lupus erythematosus in Southern Sweden: increasing age, decreasing frequency of renal manifestations and good prognosis. *J Rheumatol*. Vol.27, No.3, (March 2000), pp. 685-691, ISSN 1499-2752.

Somers, E, Magder, LS, Petri, M, et al. (1999). Morbidity and mortality in systemic lupus erythematosus during a 5-year period. A multicenter prospective study of 1,000 patients. European Working Party on Systemic Lupus Erythematosus. *Medicine* (Baltimore), (May 1999), Vol.78, No.3, pp.167-175, ISSN 1536-5964.

Somers, E, Magder, LS, Petri, M. (2002). Antiphospholipid antibodies and incidence of venous thrombosis in a cohort of patients with systemic lupus erythematosus. *J Rheumatol*, (December 2002), Vol.29, No.12, pp. 2531-2536, ISSN 1499-2752

Soran, H, Younis, NN, Charlton-Menys, V, et al. (2009). Variation in paraoxonase-1 activity and atherosclerosis. *Curr Opin Lipidol*, Vol. 20, No.4, (August 2009), pp.265–274, ISSN 1473-6535.

Stuhlinger, MC, Oka, RK, Graf, EE, et al. (2003). Endothelial dysfunction induced by hyperhomocysteinemia: role of asymmetric dimethylarginine. *Circulation*, (August 2003), Vol.108, No.8, pp. 933–938, ISSN 0009-7322.

Svenungsson, E, Jensen-Urstad, K, Heimburger, M, et al. (2001). Risk factors for cardiovascular disease in systemic lupus erythematosus. *Circulation*, Vol. 104, No.16, (October 2001), pp. 1887-1893, ISSN 0009-7322.

Svenungsson, E, Gunnarsson, I, Fei, GZ, et al. (2003). Elevated triglycerides and low levels of high-density lipoprotein as markers of disease activity in association with up-regulation of the tumor necrosis factor alpha/tumor necrosis factor receptor system in systemic lupus erythematosus. *Arthritis Rheum*, Vol. 48, No. 9, (September 2003), pp. 2533-2540, ISSN 1529-013.

Telles, R, Lanna C, Ferreira, G, et al. (2010). Metabolic syndrome in patients with systemic lupus erythematosus: association with traditional risk factors for coronary heart disease and lupus characteristics. Lupus, (June 2010), Vol.19, No.7, pp.803-809, ISSN 1477-0962.

Toloza, SM, Uribe, AG, McGWin, G Jr, et al. (2004). Systemic lupus erythematosus in a multiethnic US cohort (LUMINA). XXIII. Baseline predictors of vascular events. *Arthritis Rheum*, (October 2004), Vol.50, No.10, pp. 3947–3957, ISSN 1529-013.

Tuhrim S. (2004). Antiphospholipid antibodies and stroke. *Curr Cardiol Rep*, (March 2004), Vol.6, No.2, pp.130–134, ISSN 1534-3170.

Uramoto KM, Michet CJ Jr, Thumboo J, et al. (1999). Trends in the incidence and mortality of systemic lupus erythematosus, 1950-1992. *Arthritis Rheum*, Vol.42, No.1, (January 1999), pp. 46-5, ISSN 1529-013.

Urowitz, MB, Bookman, AA, Koehler, BE, et al. (1976). The bimodal mortality pattern of systemic lupus erythematosus. *Am J Med*, Vol.60, No.2, (February 1976), pp.221-225, ISSN 0002-9343.

Urowitz, MB., Ibanez, D, Gladman, DD. (2007). Atherosclerotic vascular events in a single large lupus cohort: prevalence and risk factors. *J. Rheumatol*, (January 2007), Vol.34, No.1, pp. 70–75, ISSN 1499-2752.

Urowitz, MB, Gladman, D, Ibañez, D, et al. (2008). Systemic Lupus International Collaborating Clinics. Accumulation of coronary artery disease risk factors over three years: data from an international inception cohort. *Arthritis Rheum*, (February 2008), Vol.59, No.2, pp. 176–180, ISSN 1529-013.

van Leuven, SI, Franssen, R, Kastelein, JJ, et al. (2008). Systemic inflammation as a risk factor for atherothrombosis. *Rheumatology* (Oxford), Vol.47, No.1, (January 2008), pp. 3-7, ISSN 1499-2752.

Virmani, R, Burke, AP, Kolodgie, FD, et al. (2002). Vulnerable plaque: the pathology of unstable coronary lesions. *J Interv Cardiol*. Vol.15, No.6, (December 2002), pp. 439–446, ISSN 1540-8183.

Vlachoyiannopoulos, PG, Karassa, FB, Karakostas, KX, et al. (1993). Systemic lupus erythematosus in Greece. Clinical features, evolution and outcome: a descriptive analysis of 292 patients. *Lupus*, (1993), Vol.2, No.5 , pp. 303–312, ISSN 1477-0962.

Volkmann, ER, Grossman JM, Sahakian, LJ, et al. (2010). Low physical activity is associated with proinflammatory high-density lipoprotein and increased subclinical atherosclerosis in women with systemic lupus erythematosus. *Arthritis Care Res*, (February 2010), Vol.62, No.2, pp. 258-265, ISSN 2151-4658.

Vuilleumier N, Charbonney, E, Fontao, L, et al (2008). Anti-(apoA-1) IgG are associated with high levels of oxidized low-density lipoprotein in acute coronary syndrome. *Clin Sci*. (July 2008), Vol.115 ,No.1 ,pp. 25-33, ISSN 1470-8736.

Vigushin, DM, Pepys, MB, Hawkins, PN. (1993). Metabolic and scintigraphic studies of radioiodinated human C-reactive protein in health and disease. *J Clin Invest*, (April 1993), Vol.91, No.4, pp. 1351–1357, ISSN 1558-8238.

Wahl, DG, Bounameaux, H, de Moerloose, P, et al. (2000). Prophylactic antithrombotic therapy for patients with systemic lupus erythematosus with or without antiphospholipid antibodies: do the benefits outweigh the risks? A decision analysis. *Arch Intern Med*, (July 2000), Vol.160, No. 3, pp. 2042–2048, ISSN 1538-3679.

Ward, MM. (1999). Premature morbidity from cardiovascular and cerebrovascular diseases in women with systemic lupus erythematosus. *Arthritis Rheum*, Vol.42, No.2, (February 1999), pp. 338–346, ISSN 1529-013.

Ward, MM. (2004). Outcomes of hospitalizations for myocardial infarctions and cerebrovascular accidents in patients with systemic lupus erythematosus. *Arthritis Rheum*, Vol.50, No.10, (October 2004), pp. 3170-3176, ISSN 1529-013.

Wilson ,VE, Eck ,SL, Bates ,ER. (1992). Evaluation and treatment of acute myocardial infarction complicating systemic lupus erythematosus. *Chest*, (February 1992), Vol.101, No.2, pp. 420–424, ISSN 1931-3543.

Wilson Tang ,WH, Tong ,W, Shrestha ,K, et al. (2008). Differential effects of arginine methylation on diastolic dysfunction and disease progression in patients with chronic systolic heart failure. *Eur Heart J*, (October 2008), Vol.29, No.20, pp. 2506–2513, ISSN 1554-2815

Wisnieski ,JJ. (2000). Urticarial vasculitis. *Curr Opin Rheumatol*, (January 2000), Vol.12, No.1, pp.24–31, ISSN 1531-6963

Yuen, H, Holthaus, K, Kamen ,DL, (2011). Using Wii Fit to reduce fatigue among African American women with systemic lupus erythematosus: A pilot study. *Lupus*, (June 2011), ISSN 1477-0962.

Yuhanna ,IS, Zhu, Y, Cox ,BE, et al. (2001). High density lipoprotein binding to scavenger receptor-BI activates endothelial nitric oxide synthase. *Nat Med*, Vol.7, No.7, (July 2001), pp. 853-857, ISSN 1078-895.

Zonana-Nacach, A, Santana-Sahagún, E, Jiménez-Balderas, FJ, et al. (2008). Prevalence and factors associated with metabolic syndrome in patients with rheumatoid arthritis and systemic lupus erythematosus. *J Clin Rheumatol*, (April 2008), Vol.14, No.2, 74-77, ISSN 1536-7355

7

Tyrosine-Based Monitoring of Glucocorticoid Therapy of Systemic Lupus Erythematosus

I. T. Rass

Center of Theoretical Pharmacology, Russian Academy of Sciences, Moscow
Russia

1. Introduction

The present chapter considers only one aspect of glucocorticoid therapy of patients with systemic lupus erythematosus (SLE): a possibility of using blood level of tyrosine for monitoring glucocorticoid therapy. Thus, problems of SLE etiology and pathogenesis, as well as numerous schemes of SLE therapy are beyond the limits of this chapter. In the chapter normal catabolism of tyrosine and some congenital disturbances in catabolism of this amino acid are considered. But in the great majority of cases, specific features of tyrosine catabolism allow us to admit that tyrosine content in blood should be determined by the liver functional competence, in particular, its ability to synthesize an adaptive enzyme tyrosine aminotransferase and by entrance into the liver of glucocorticoids, natural hormones or glucocorticoid preparations. This chapter also presents experimental data obtained on adrenalectomized rats and observations on children with adrenogenital syndrome which clearly demonstrate blood tyrosine dependence on glucocorticoids and support the idea of using blood tyrosine content as a promising laboratory parameter for monitoring glucocorticoid therapy, similar to blood glucose for insulin. Some observations on glucocorticoid therapy in patients with SLE compared with changes in their blood tyrosine level which were earlier published only in Russian are presented, as well as the imaginary tyrosine-based monitoring of these cases.

2. Approaches to treatment of systemic lupus erythematosus

Systemic lupus erythematosus (SLE) seems to be the most striking example of using corticosteroid, or glucocorticoid, preparations in non-endocrine diseases as the most powerful anti-inflammatory, immunosuppressive, anti-allergic, antitoxic, etc. agents. Sixty years ago glucocorticoids allowed clinicians to radically change the fate of patients with SLE – this collagen disease stopped to be virtually lethal (Dubois, 1974; Schroeder & Euler, 1997; Ioannou & Isenberg, 2002; Goldblatt & Isenberg, 2005; Nived et al., 2008). In modern schemes of SLE treatment glucocorticoids are usually combined with various other preparations: cyclophosphamide, mycophenolate mofettil, rituximab, cyclosporine, azathioprine, etc. (Ntali et al., 2009; Ponticelli et al., 2010). In addition to their specific effects, all these preparations are given, in particular, in order to lower the dose of steroids, however, up to now glucocorticoids remain the cornerstone in the schemes of SLE treatment. Therefore, in SLE all problems associated with using glucocorticoid preparations in non-endocrine diseases are clearly pronounced and still urgent: the unpredictability of efficiency of glucocorticoids and nearly inevitable serious side effects, difficulties and sometimes even the impossibility to abolish glucocorticoids, and glucocorticoid resistance of some patients – such was the situation at the beginning of the "steroid era" and it is nearly the same nowadays, and the same problems are still urgent.

Since 1966, life-threatening exacerbations of SLE are sometimes treated by pulse-therapy – intravenous injection of very high doses of glucocorticoid preparations – up to 1 mg methylprednisolone daily for three days. However, the rapid immunosuppressive effect is often accompanied by various infections. But this regimen of pulse-therapy has been formed historically, although it is not excluded that lower doses of glucocorticoids would be similarly effective (Badscha & Edwards, 2003; Franchin & Diamond, 2006).

It is obvious that the existent schemes of using glucocorticoids in SLE are far from optimal, and to specify and refine therapeutical approaches there are some attempts to compare the glucocorticoid efficiency in SLE with different individual characteristics of the patients, such as the number and type of glucocorticoid receptors (Li et al., 2010; Deng & Tsao, 2010; Oakley & Cidlowski, 2011), titers of antibodies to double-stranded DNA (Rahman & Isenberg, 2008), specific features of T- and B-cells, etc. It seems clear that responsiveness to glucocorticoids should be associated with some individual specific features of the patients. Moreover, glucocorticoid sensitivity is not steady in the same patient, but can vary from time to time and can be much more changeable than it has been believed earlier (De Rijk & Sternberg, 1997).

It is rather strange but a very essential aspect of action of glucocorticoid preparations has been neglected during the whole period of using glucocorticoids in clinical medicine. It is extremely important that glucocorticoid preparations, as discriminated from all other pharmaceuticals used in the treatment of SLE, are synthetic copies of *natural products* of the organism – of glucocorticoid hormones synthesized in the adrenal cortex. Glucocorticoid preparations possessing the unique combination of therapeutic properties also inevitably retain the features of their natural prototypes, i.e. they are directly or indirectly involved in regulation of many if not all physiological processes and metabolic reactions and their using interferes the negative feedback regulation in the hypothalamus–pituitary–adrenocortical system. Therefore, it should be noted and emphasized that the inevitable complications of glucocorticoid therapy really are not "side effects", on the contrary, they are natural manifestations of just hormonal properties of glucocorticoid preparations, either of their excess or of induced disorders in the feedback regulation of the hypothalamus–pituitary–adrenocortical system. Possibly, this neglecting was reasoned by a surprising and somewhat discouraging discovery in the beginning of "the glucocorticoid era" that the therapeutical effect of glucocorticoid preparations did not depend on the level of a patient's own hormones?

However, not the level of glucocorticoid hormones should be important, but the tissue provision with these hormones, especially on taking into account that glucocorticoids are hormones of virtually total action. Nevertheless, for glucocorticoids there is no parameter to characterize the tissue provision with these hormones (or with glucocorticoid preparations) and to determine the real need in them of a subject under various circumstances, in particular, under stress situations or in disease. This is especially important because glucocorticoids play a determinative role in stress situations. For glucocorticoids an indirect parameter is required *which would be similar to blood glucose for insulin.*

Naturally, this parameter must be easily determinable in blood, have rather narrow normal limits in healthy persons, and clearly depend on glucocorticoids, natural hormones or preparations. In particular, the glucocorticoid-dependent hepatic enzyme tyrosine aminotransferase and the resulting tyrosine level in blood which is directly determined by the activity of this enzyme deserve a special attention.

3. Blood tyrosine levels in some non-endocrine diseases

In the late 1950s Japanese researchers of the Nishimura group found increased levels of tyrosine in blood and urine of patients with collagen diseases (Nishimura et al., 1958; Nishimura et al., 1961) and supposed that disorders in tyrosine catabolism could be a biochemical basis of these diseases. These reports stimulated intensive studies on tyrosine catabolism in collagenoses and some other diseases, especially in Russia. As it was reasonably to expect, tyrosine catabolism was disturbed in patients with liver disorders, such as infectious hepatitis, chronic hepatitis, and liver cirrhosis, and blood tyrosine level was two-threefold increased in them (Levine & Kohn, 1967; Powell & Axelsen, 1972; Nordlinger et al., 1979).

The hypothesis about the role of tyrosine catabolism disorders in pathogenesis of collagen diseases was not confirmed, but very interesting observations were described, in particular, by A.S. Kainova (Kainova, 1974): tyrosine levels in blood of patients with rheumatism decreased to normal values on successful hormonal and/or medicamentous therapy, and abolishment of glucocorticoid preparations in some cases was accompanied by an increase in the blood tyrosine level.

4. Observations on blood tyrosine levels and glucocorticoid treatment in patients with SLE

Systemic Lupus Erythematosus (SLE) was a problem for the Clinics of Therapy and Occupational Diseases, I Moscow Medical Institute, where I entered as a biochemist in 1968 and had been working until 1978. Naturally, the disorders in tyrosine metabolism observed by Nishimura et al. in patients with collagen diseases and observations by Kainova on blood tyrosine changes in patients with rheumatism seemed to me a possible biochemical approach to start my study on SLE.

Sixteen healthy donors (14 women and 2 men in the age from 20 to 40 years old) were used for determination the normal level of blood tyrosine, and it was found to be 16.2 ± 0.9 $\mu g/ml$. Note, that the repeated measurements of blood tyrosine levels in the same donors gave virtually the same values, i.e. it occurred to be rather a stable parameter.

Altogether 80 patients with SLE, 70 women and 10 men in the age range from 16 to 53 years old, were observed at 134 hospitalizations over the period of 1973–1976. Some patients were under observation repeatedly. The patients were not selected previously basing on their case history and severity and character of the disease. Tyrosine was determined in the serum from blood samples taken from patients with SLE at 8.00–8.30 a.m. on the empty stomach, usually once during 7-14 days over the period of hospitalization. The work was not a part of a previously approved plan of investigations, therefore, no blood samples were taken specially to determine the tyrosine content. Initially, levels of tyrosine and of its transamination product p-oxyphenylpyruvic acid were determined in parallel samples of blood and 24-h urine. The determination of tyrosine was performed spectrophotometrically by the method of Udenfriend & Cooper (1952), p-oxyphenylpyruvic acid was determined as described in the work (Knox & Pitt , 1957). It was shown that the increase in blood tyrosine level was caused by disturbance in transamination (Rass, 1976), whereas the further stages of tyrosine oxidation in the patients under study were virtually unaffected.

Changes in blood tyrosine in every patient were compared with the clinical and laboratory data recorded in their case histories after the patients' discharge from the hospital, with a special attention to using glucocorticoid preparations, i.e. a kind of the retrospective experiment was performed. The results were published in Russian in the work (Rass et al., 1977). Thirty-six patients were observed in the state of clinical remission; blood tyrosine was in normal limits in 23 of them and was steadily elevated in three patients (two of them had the affected liver); 28 patients obtained a supporting dose of glucocorticoids (not more than 15 mg prednisolone per day).

In 44 patients with SLE short-term "splashes" in blood tyrosine level were observed, and the retrospective analysis revealed that these "splashes" occurred simultaneously with some extraordinary events, such as a concurrent infection, aggravation of symptoms, or on the other day of a severe diagnostic procedure (e.g. the kidney biopsy), during the reaction to a new preparation, etc. Thus, these "splashes" were associated with a "stress-situation" when the need in glucocorticoid hormones was increased and in healthy subjects the synthesis of glucocorticoid hormones should increase. Thus, in a patient with chronic SLE who obtained 5 mg/day prednisolone as a supporting dose over the period of 50 days of hospitalization blood tyrosine values were 25, 20, 22 μg/ml, and a "splash" to 53 μg/ml was recorded on the day after the diagnostic intravenous urography. At the other hospitalization two years later this patient obtained the daily dose of 10 mg prednisolone and had blood tyrosine level of 8 μg/ml (possibly, the supporting dose of 10 mg prednisolone/day was too high – the previous supporting dose of 5 mg/day seemed sufficient to maintain the level of blood tyrosine in normal limits of 20-25 μg/ml). Similar "splashes" in blood tyrosine level were also observed in patients with glomerulonephritis under similar situations.

A very demonstrative was an attempt to even slightly lower the dose of glucocorticoid preparations in a clinically steroid-dependent patient with subacute SLE (Fig. 1). This "splash" in blood tyrosine was observed concurrently with the aggravation of her condition. In this patient the high background content of tyrosine was thought to be associated with the liver affection.

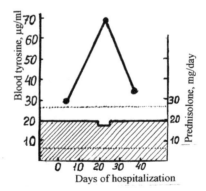

Fig. 1. Changes in the blood tyrosine content in a clinically steroid-dependent 40-year-old patient with subacute SLE. The attempt to decrease the dose of prednisolone was associated with an aggravation of the patient's condition. Dotted lines here and in the further Figures show normal limits of blood tyrosine contents.

"Splashes" in blood tyrosine were also observed in some patients with SLE at the alternate-day scheme of hormonal treatment on the next morning after glucocorticoid-free day.

But comparing results of glucocorticoid therapy with the initial level and behavior of blood tyrosine in patients with SLE seems to be the most interesting and informative. Changes in blood tyrosine upon prescribing or increasing the dose of glucocorticoids (40-60 mg/day calculated per prednisolone) because of SLE exacerbation were followed in 32 patients. Glucocorticoid preparations were prescribed according to the conventional schemes. The post-discharge analysis of the case histories revealed that to 20 patients glucocorticoids were prescribed at the significantly increased level of blood tyrosine (49.1 ± 0.8 µg/ml as compared to 16.2 ± 0.9 µg/ml in 16 healthy donors) and an essential improvement of clinical and laboratory parameters was recorded in 17 of them. In 13 patients this improvement was accompanied by a decrease in blood tyrosine, and this decrease was recorded before appearance of signs of Cushing's syndrome; in four patients with markedly affected liver functions the level of blood tyrosine remained elevated although their general condition became somewhat better. It should be noted that the "improvement" in all cases concerned only parameters of SLE activity, and side effects were considered as inevitable.

Twelve patients were given glucocorticoids on the background of normal blood tyrosine (≤ 26.5 µg/ml); glucocorticoids were inefficient in nine of them, and in four patients signs of Cushing's syndrome appeared very rapidly. Some improvement was recorded in three patients but this improvement could be due to other preparations given to them concurrently with glucocorticoids: azathioprine, heparin, cyclophosphamide, etc.

Let us consider some real cases.

Patient M., 27 years old, suffering from SLE for nine years was hospitalized because of aggravation of chronic SLE. Blood tyrosine at the first determination was 47.5 µg/ml. She was given prednisolone (30 mg/day) and antibiotics because of catarrhal state, however, 20 days later the immunologic activity was still present, as well as arthralgia and myalgia, blood tyrosine remains increased - 40 µg/ml; because of a continued aggravation of her condition 15 days later the prednisolone dose was increased to 40 mg/day, and *in a week a pronounced clinical improvement was recorded, together with a decrease in the blood tyrosine level to normal (25 µg/ml).* She received 40 mg/day prednisolone for 20 days, and then the lowering prednisolone dose was started – and blood tyrosine slightly increased. The patient was discharged with the improved clinical and laboratory data (Fig. 2).

The following case (Fig. 3) presents a 21-year-old patient Zh., suffering of SLE during five years. She received long-term courses of prednisolone earlier in the maximal dose of 30 mg/day. A progressing osteonecrosis was observed. This time she was hospitalized because of an acute flare. At the first determination blood tyrosine level was somewhat increased (34.0 µg/ml), on the next day she was prescribed with prednisolone – 45 mg/day, and this dose was maintained *during 20 days. Five days* after the beginning of glucocorticoid therapy blood tyrosine decreased to 20.0 µg/ml, and *two days later a moon-like face appeared and elevations of arterial pressure up to 170/100 mm Hg* were recorded. GG therapy for 1.5 months was considered to be unfavorable; moreover, pains in femoral joints increased. Clinical improvement in this patient was obtained on prescribing heparin.

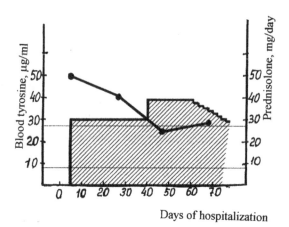

Fig. 2. Changes in the blood tyrosine content and regimen of glucocorticoid therapy (hatched) in a 27-year-old patient with chronic SLE.

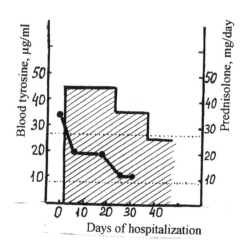

Fig. 3. Changes in the blood tyrosine content and regimen of glucocorticoid therapy (hatched) in a 21-year-old patient with chronic SLE.

Figure 4 shows changes in blood tyrosine level observed at withdrawal syndrome in a 22-year-old patient P. with subacute SLE (Fig. 4). The patient was in the state of a relative clinical and laboratory remission at the supporting dose of prednisolone (15 mg/day) for rather a long time. Such a rapid abolishment of prednisolone at the hospitalization in 1974 was forced by development of a pronounced aseptic osteonecrosis of femoral heads, and this abolishment was associated with a sharp aggravation of SLE symptoms associated with a sharp increase in blood tyrosine level.

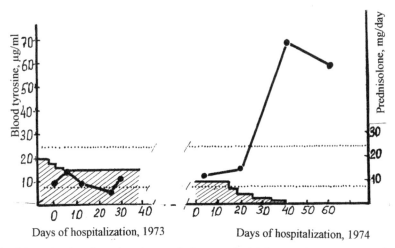

Fig. 4. Blood tyrosine levels and regimen of glucocorticoid therapy in a patient with subacute SLE during two hospitalizations, at the state of relative remission in 1973, and at withdrawal syndrome in 1974.

Thus, a certain association obviously occurred between the therapeutic effect of glucocorticoid preparations and their regulatory effect manifested by changes in the blood level of tyrosine. Moreover, such association cannot be occasional, exclusive, or SLE-specific, because the dependence of tyrosine catabolism on glucocorticoids is fundamentally the same in humans and in other mammals. Such an association must be significantly most common. In particular, blood tyrosine level was also increased in patients with bronchial asthma (not receiving glucocorticoids) during the period of attacks and was normal during the state of remission (Rass et al., 1978).

If so, may be blood tyrosine content can be used as a representative index of action of glucocorticoid hormones on metabolism, as an index of tissue provision with these hormones, and of real need of a subject in these hormones? May be blood tyrosine level can be used as a parameter (index) of glucocorticoid action, similarly to blood glucose which is a parameter of insulin action?

5. Tyrosine catabolism and blood tyrosine level as an index of glucocorticoid hormone action

This idea induced by observations on changes in blood tyrosine levels and regimens of glucocorticoid therapy in patients with SLE was for the first time published in the above-mentioned work (Rass et al., 1977) and was theoretically considered in the paper (Rass, 1978); then this idea was confirmed by experimental studies on adrenalectomized rats (Rass, 1980; Rass, 1983) and by observations on children with adrenogenital syndrome receiving long-life substitutive glucocorticoid therapy (Rass et al., 1979). In 1991 the hazard of glucocorticoid hormone application in non-endocrine diseases was considered to be mainly due to the absence of a test for sufficiency and real need in these hormones, and introduction of blood tyrosine as such a test was proposed as a safety basis for the individualized strategy of glucocorticoid therapy (Piruzian & Rass, 1991). However, all these works were published only in Russian, and this apparently promising idea remained virtually not called for until the review (Rass, 2010) was published in English.

Let us consider some specific features of tyrosine catabolism, especially those which allow us to consider the blood level of this amino acid as a promising laboratory parameter for monitoring glucocorticoid therapy.

Tyrosine is produced in the organism as a result of hydrolysis of food protein immediately or after hydrolysis of phenylalanine. About 30% of produced tyrosine is used for synthesis of catecholamines, melanin, and thyroid hormones, a portion is used for renewal of tissue proteins, and more than 60% is oxidized in the liver (Knox, 1955). And the first reaction in the major oxidation pathway of tyrosine is its transamination with alpha-ketoglutaric acid under the influence of tyrosine aminotransferase with production of p-oxyphenylpyruvic acid. Then p-oxyphenylpyruvic acid is oxidized under the influence of the appropriate oxidase in the presence of ascorbic acid with production of 2,5-dioxyphenylpyruvic, or homogentisic acid. The terminal products of the major pathway of tyrosine oxidation are acetoacetic and fumaric acids (Fig. 5).

Most frequently, tyrosine content in blood is determined using its reaction with alpha-nitroso-beta-naphthol with a subsequent recording by spectrophotometry (Udenfriend & Cooper, 1952) or by fluorimetry (Grenier & Laberge, 1974; Gavrilov et al., 1998). In some works HPLC (Kand'ar & Zakova, 2009), ion-exchange chromatography (Allard et al., 2004), and gas chromatography – mass-spectrometry (Deng et al., 2002) are also used. In some of the above-listed works tyrosine was determined in blood samples dried on filter paper discs.

The interest for determination of tyrosine level in blood is caused by necessity of early diagnosis of congenital disturbances of phenylalanine–tyrosine catabolism which result in severe disorders in the mental and physical development of the affected children. Phenylketonuria is caused by deficiency of the enzyme phenylalanine hydroxylase and is characterized by an extremely low level of blood tyrosine (< 0.05 µg/ml), tyrosinosis which is caused by an insufficient elimination of p-oxyphenylpyruvate acid due to deficiency of the appropriate oxidase (Scriver, 1967; Cerone at al., 1997) is manifested by a stable hypertyrosinemia up to 100 µg/ml, and in Richner–Hanhart syndrome caused by an inborn insufficiency of tyrosine aminotransferase blood tyrosine level can reach 600 µg/ml (Goldsmith, 1978; Natt et al., 1992). Incidence of phenylketonuria throughout the world is, on average, 1 : 15'000, and of the two other disorders in tyrosine catabolism are, respectively, 1 : 100'000 and 1 : 250'000, but in Canada they are recorded more frequently.

Tyrosine aminotransferase is an adaptive enzyme synthesized by the liver cells in response to entrance of the substrate – tyrosine, but for the substrate induction of this enzyme the entrance of glucocorticoids in the liver is necessary (Rosen and Nichol, 1963; Gelehrter, 1973; Thompson, 1979). Synthesis of hepatic tyrosine aminotransferase is a well-known example of the so-called gene-mediated action of glucocorticoids, and this enzyme is the most demonstrative and beloved object for studies of such effects of glucocorticoids (Sun at al., 1998; Grange et al., 2001; Hazra et al., 2007). Tyrosine aminotransferase is also used for testing on cell cultures and on intact and adrenalectomized animals of newly synthesized preparations which are expected to have less adverse effects than "classic" glucocorticoid preparations (Schacke et al., 2004; Zimmermann et al., 2009). The synthesis of tyrosine aminotransferase quantitatively depends on glucocorticoids, but being a hepatic enzyme, it cannot be determined in blood. However, tyrosine aminotransferase is a key enzyme in the major pathway of tyrosine catabolism and its activity determines the level of free tyrosine in blood. As a result, blood tyrosine level also depends on glucocorticoids (and, naturally, also on the functional competence of the liver cells).

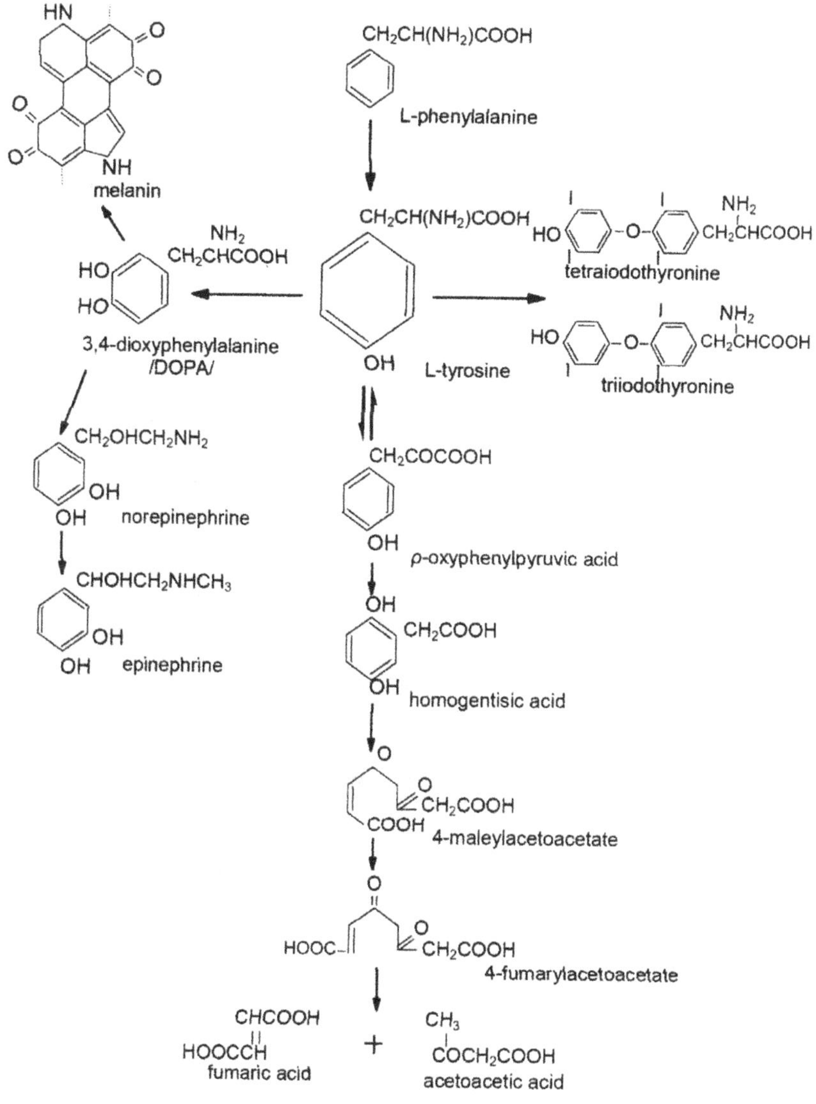

Fig. 5. Tyrosine catabolism (Scheme).

Due to substrate induction of tyrosine aminotransferase, even on tenfold increase in protein amount in the diet the blood content of tyrosine increases no more than by 50% above the basal level (Scriver et al., 1971), whereas circadian variations in blood tyrosine level mainly depending on circadian variations in production of natural glucocorticoids are in the limit of ± 25% (Wurtman et al., 1968).

But in the majority of cases and under real conditions an increase in blood tyrosine can be mainly determined by two factors: 1) a functional inferiority of the liver leading to a disturbed reception of glucocorticoids and inability of the liver cells to synthesize some enzymes including tyrosine aminotransferase, and 2) an insufficient entrance of glucocorticoids in the liver. As a result, under conditions of physiological rest, in the absence of extreme fluctuations in the diet, and on determination on the empty stomach in the morning the levels of free tyrosine in blood are similar in healthy animals and humans and do not depend on age and sex (Table 1).

Subjects under study	The number of subjects	μg/ml
Men	91	13.0 ± 2.7
Women	103	12.3 ± 2.4
Boys 6-18 yr	75	12.3 ± 1.8
Girls 6-18 yr	65	11.4 ± 2.0

Table 1. Blood tyrosine levels in humans, after (Armstrong & Stave, 1973a)

Moreover, it should be noted that blood samples taken from the same subjects (35 boys and 26 girls) four times over the period of 3–3½ years displayed characteristic individual patterns for the most of plasma amino acids, in particular, the content of blood tyrosine was virtually constant in the same subject (Armstrong & Stave, 1973b). We have also observed virtually the same values of blood tyrosine level in the samples taken repeatedly from the same healthy donors, as well as in blood samples from patients with SLE on supporting dose of glucocorticoids in the state of remission.

Injection of glucocorticoid preparations induced a 20–40% dose-dependent decrease in blood tyrosine in both animals and humans (Rivlin & Melmon, 1965; Betheil et al., 1965), and this decrease was the most pronounced 4-5 h after the injection, i.e. at the maximum of the glucocorticoid-induced synthesis of tyrosine aminotransferase. A decrease in the content of blood tyrosine was also recorded under stress conditions (Nemeth, 1978), obviously, due to a well-known increase in the glucocorticoid production by the adrenal cortex. Effects of hydrocortisone injection to healthy volunteers recorded by changes in the blood tyrosine levels and in the peripheral lymphocyte counts were considered as manifestations of genomic and nongenomic effects of glucocorticoids, respectively (Derks et al., 1999).

It is interesting to note that injections of hepatotoxins caused in rats an increase in the level of blood tyrosine, and the more pronounced was the liver necrosis the higher was this increase (Clayton et al., 2007).

6. Blood tyrosine content is an index of tissue provision with glucocorticoids: Confirmation on the experimental and clinical models

The dependence of blood tyrosine content on glucocorticoids was demonstrated experimentally on adrenalectomized rats (Rass, 1980; Rass, 2010). In intact rats blood tyrosine level was 15.0 ± 1.4 μg/ml. After bilateral adrenalectomy the blood level of tyrosine began to increase and reached, on average, 37.9 ± 6.4 μg/ml on the 5th day concurrently with the worst condition of the animals; then blood tyrosine level began to decrease most likely due to synthesis of corticosterone in the brown fat tissue in response to the increased synthesis of ACTH after adrenalectomy; on the 10th day blood tyrosine level was the same as initially (under conditions of physiological rest!). Thus, the tyrosine level in blood manifested a pronounced dependence on production of natural glucocorticoids.

Starting from the 7th day after the operation, adrenalectomized rats were injected daily intraperitoneally with hydrocortisone in the dose of 2 mg per kg body weight (this dose approximately corresponded to the supporting dose 15 mg/day of prednisolone). Daily injections of hydrocortisone during 20 days resulted in a decrease in the tyrosine level in blood to undeterminable level, the abolishment of the injections and their absence during 5 days caused an increase in blood tyrosine, and the recommencement of hydrocortisone injections (5 mg per kg body weight) was accompanied by a decrease in blood tyrosine (Fig. 6).

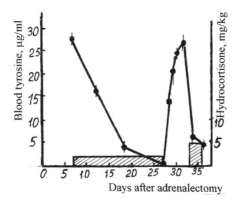

Fig. 6. Changes in tyrosine content in blood of adrenalectomized rats subjected to daily injections of hydrocortisone (hatched), upon abolishment of the injections, and on their recommencement.

And it seems that the only clinical situation exists (the model was recommended by Prof. M.A. Zhukovsky) which allows a physician (endocrinologist) to control the entrance of glucocorticoids in the organism and to some degree assess the adequacy of tissue provision with glucocorticoids to real needs of just this patient. This unique situation is presented by adrenogenital syndrome (synonyms: congenital adrenal hyperplasia, congenital virilizing adrenal cortex dysfunction) in children. The disease is caused by a genetically determined deficiency of glucocorticoid biosynthesis enzymes in the adrenal cortex, most frequently of 21-beta-hydroxylase, and a resulting shift to synthesis of androgens, mainly of dehydroepiandrosterone. The decreased production of glucocorticoids induces an increased synthesis of ACTH in the adenohypophysis that permanently stimulates the adrenal cortex with a resulting surplus synthesis of androgens (Brooks, 1979). The excess of androgens is displayed by a characteristic clinical picture: an abnormal structure of external sex organs, an accelerated body growth with an overdevelopment of masculine type muscles during the first years of life, the early arresting of growth because of premature ossification of tubular bones, etc. In the affected girls a picture of pseudohermaphroditism is developed.

The lifelong substitutive glucocorticoid therapy is the only pathogenetically reasonable treatment of this disease (Lo et al., 1999; Stikkelbroeck et al., 2003; Hughes, 2007). Glucocorticoid preparations break the vicious circle: recompensing the shortage of endogenous glucocorticoids they inhibit synthesis of ACTH responsible for overproduction of androgens. Glucocorticoid therapy started as early as possible after the birth and the appropriate dose can provide the normal physical and sexual maturation of the affected children according to their genetic sex, with a possibility of normal pregnancy and labor in females. The dose of glucocorticoids must be strictly individualized, and it can vary from 2.5 to 15 mg prednisolone per day.

On the other hand, changes in the clinical picture observed in children with adrenogenital syndrome – the rate of growth, ossification, and sexual maturation – allow a physician to relatively objectively and faultlessly estimate the correctness of the dose. In adult patients with this syndrome and in other conditions which obviously require the substitutive glucocorticoid therapy, after bilateral adrenalectomy or in chronic hypocorticism of various etiology, the dose of glucocorticoids can be prescribed only "according to the patient's self-feeling". According to B. Lukert (Lukert, 2006), "The problem for the clinician is the lack of objective criteria for determining adequate, but not excessive doses of glucocorticoids... In current practice, the clinician must rely on surrogate markers of glucocorticoid excess (early changes of Cushing's syndrome) rather than definitive end points".

Our study was performed with participation of 38 children with virilizing adrenogenital syndrome (33 girls and five boys of 3–18 years old hospitalized in the Pediatric Department of the Institute of Experimental Endocrinology and Chemistry of Hormones, the USSR Academy of Medical Sciences). Tyrosine levels were determined in blood samples taken in the morning on empty stomach and compared with clinical picture which characterized the degree of compensation of the genetic defect. The results were published in Russian (Rass et al., 1979) and republished in English in the review (Rass, 2010). The main results are presented in Fig. 7.

Figure 7 shows that in 17 children with adrenogenital syndrome at the complete clinical compensation blood contents of tyrosine were the same as in healthy donors (16 adults and seven children of 7–13 years old). In a girl with signs of Cushing's syndrome blood tyrosine was below the normal level. In untreated patients and in non-compensated patients because of irregular treatment blood tyrosine was significantly increased. In three non-compensated patients a pronounced melanodermia was observed along with the normal level of blood tyrosine, i.e. a part of excessive tyrosine was not oxidized through the major pathway but was converted into melanin (compare with the Scheme in Fig. 5!). Prescribing glucocorticoids resulted in "whitening" of such patients. Normalization of skin color in patients with hypocorticism upon taking glucocorticoids was also described in the literature (Snell, 1967).

In two compensated patients who initially displayed normal levels of blood tyrosine, transient increases to 29.0 and 45.0 μg/ml were recorded in association with a concurrent acute respiratory disease. Obviously, these increases are very alike "splashes" observed in patients with SLE, and can be explained by increased requirements for glucocorticoid hormones under conditions of stress or concurrent disease. Such observations justify the empirical recommendation to increase the dose of glucocorticoid preparations in the case of stress situations.

Two previously untreated girls were prescribed with glucocorticoids, and the determinations of blood tyrosine levels were helpful for choosing the optimal dose. Note that in patients with hypocorticism an acute withdrawal of the substitutive hydrocortisone injections resulted on the next day in a 25-30% increase in the level of blood tyrosine, whereas the levels of other amino acids remained virtually unchanged (Christiansen et al., 2007). The data presented in this section show that the normal level of blood tyrosine seems to indicate a sufficient provision of tissues and glucocorticoid-dependent reactions and processes with these hormones, whereas an increased level of blood tyrosine seems to be due to insufficient level of glucocorticoids. This seems rather clear for endocrine diseases.

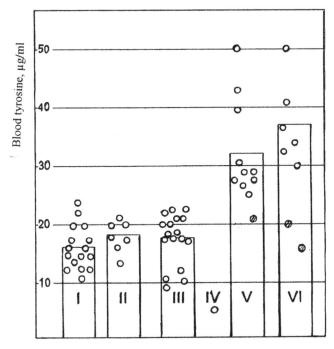

Fig. 7. Tyrosine contents in blood of healthy donors and children with adrenogenital syndrome. The columns present arithmetic means for the corresponding groups; the circles show individual values: I) healthy adults; II) healthy children; III) patients with the complete clinical compensation; IV) a girl patient with overdosed glucocorticoids; V) irregularly treated non-compensated patients; VI) untreated patients. Hatched circles in the columns V and VI show patients with a pronounced melanodermia.

However, it is also reasonable to expect that blood content of tyrosine could be a promising candidate for the role of an indirect marker for prescribing the correct dose in non-endocrine diseases. Unfortunately, for non-endocrine diseases there are no similar data, nevertheless, let us admit that blood tyrosine level could be used as an index of tissue provision and real need in glucocorticoid hormones (or glucocorticoid preparations) – in our patients with SLE described in the Section 4.

7. The imaginary tyrosine-based monitoring of glucocorticoid therapy in the above-presented cases of SLE (reconsideration of cases presented in Figs. 2–4)

Thus, keeping in mind the blood tyrosine as an index of the real need in glucocorticoids, let us look again at Figs. 2–4 and *imagine* the tyrosine-based monitoring of glucocorticoid treatment in these patients with SLE.

Fig. 2 – the imaginary monitoring. The patient M. was prescribed with 30 mg prednisolone daily on the background of a rather high initial level of blood tyrosine (47.5 µg/ml); she received this dose during 35 days without a pronounced clinical effect and on retention of the increased blood tyrosine (40.0 µg/ml). The improvement was achieved as soon as a week after increasing the prednisolone dose to 40 mg/day and this improvement was accompanied by normalization of blood tyrosine. The patient continued to receive 40 mg prednisolone for the following 15 days. Thus, in total, the patient M. received *30-40 mg prednisolone daily within two months.* But, taking into account the initial high level of blood tyrosine, as well as its retention at the second determination 20 days later, *it would have been reasonable to give her 40 mg prednisolone earlier and to start lowering the dose on normalization of blood tyrosine, i.e. the course of hormonal therapy could be much shorter.*

Fig. 3 – the imaginary monitoring. The increased level of blood tyrosine (34 µg/ml) at the first determination on the next day after the hospitalization could be a kind of "splash" – the reaction to hospitalization-associated procedure. The patient was prescribed 45 mg prednisolone per day and obtained this dose for 20 days. Blood tyrosine became normal very rapidly – on the 5th day after the hospitalization (even *earlier than the recorded in the case history appearance of the moon-like face and elevations in blood pressure!*) and continued to decrease to very low level during the treatment with glucocorticoids. After 1.5 months, glucocorticoid therapy was qualified as unfavorable. Was it a case of steroid-resistance or simply a manifestation of a sufficient provision with own hormones? In any case, *this patient did not need such a prolonged and rather intensive glucocorticoid therapy.*

Fig. 4 – the imaginary monitoring. Withdrawal syndrome in a 22-year-old patient with subacute SLE. The normal blood tyrosine level during the hospitalization the year before at the supporting dose of prednisolone 15 mg/day made it possible to think about at least *of decreasing the supporting dose of glucocorticoids, or even of trying to abolish hormonal preparations the year earlier!*

8. And the real successful course of glucocorticoid therapy *without side effects*

The next case (Fig. 8) exemplifies a successful course of glucocorticoid therapy performed by Dr. I.A. Borisov (described in detail in the work (Rass et al., 1977)) in a 48-year-old patient E. who had been suffering of SLE for 12 years. This hospitalization was because of a serious flare of SLE after an acute respiratory disease. *All previous courses of glucocorticoids in this patient resulted in a rapid development of Cushing's syndrome.* On the entrance blood tyrosine was 45–79 µg/ml. She was given prednisolone (40 mg/day) within a week and then transferred to alternate-day scheme of the dose lowering (the increase in blood tyrosine to 100 µg/ml was recorded in the morning two days after the abolishment of daily prednisolone). The alternate-day scheme was started from daily dose of 75 mg with a stepwise decreasing to 25 mg/day (combined with methindol on prednisolone-free days). Blood tyrosine decreased to the normal level (16 µg/ml) alongside with a general improvement of all clinical and laboratory data. The increase in the blood tyrosine level to 35 µg/ml concurrently with the SLE activation was recorded when prednisolone was replaced by decortilene; then a respiratory disease was associated with blood tyrosine increases to 30–45 µg/ml; and prednisolone was prescribed again in the daily dose of 30 mg during a week followed by the alternate-day lowering the prednisolone dose starting from 55 mg. The patient was discharged with an essential improvement *without any side effect of glucocorticoid therapy.*

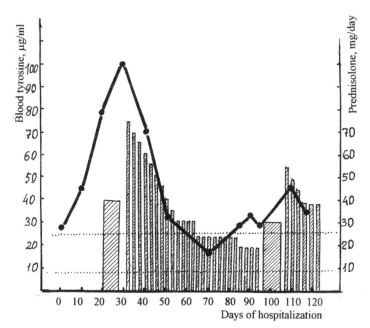

Fig. 8. Changes in the blood tyrosine content and regimen of glucocorticoid therapy (hatched) in a 48-year-old patient with SLE.

It should be underlined that in this case two specific hormonal features of the glucocorticoid preparations were taken into account: the organism's provision with glucocorticoids characterized by blood tyrosine level and using the alternate-day scheme for lowering the dose of hormonal preparation dose to promote the recovery of the negative feedback regulation in the hypothalamus-pituitary-adrenocortical system.

9. Conclusion

Preparations of glucocorticoid hormones for more than 60 years remain one of cornerstones of modern medicine as the most effective anti-inflammatory drugs also possessing anti-allergic, immunosuppressive, antitoxic, and anti-shock properties. Glucocorticoid preparations are widely used in all fields of clinical medicine and are virtually indispensable, although very serious complications are associated with their application. The number of works concerning glucocorticoid treatment of various diseases is innumerable. However, despite the extreme importance and indispensability of glucocorticoid preparations, up to now there is no objective laboratory parameter, similar to blood glucose for insulin, which would allow a clinician to foresee the effect of hormonal therapy in a given patient and realize a reasonable monitoring of the dose of glucocorticoid preparations.

The problem of safety of glucocorticoid therapy arose concurrently with the first usage of glucocorticoids by Dr. P. Hench and colleagues in 1948 (Hench et al, 1949) and difficulties which should be inevitable on using glucocorticoids were predicted and described in their large publication (Hench et al., 1950). Unfortunately, multiple refined studies on glucocorticoids by biochemists, geneticists, endocrinologists, physiologists, although very informative, are not frequently intersected with real need of clinical medicine.

Just the permanent critical state of glucocorticoid therapy made me reconsider my old works published in Russian in 1976–1983 which remained unnoticed and unknown. And only the publication in English (Rass, 2010) has attracted the attention to the still urgent problem of absence of a laboratory parameter extremely required for glucocorticoid therapy of both endocrine and non-endocrine diseases.

I hope that rather an easy determination of blood tyrosine level will be at last used as a suitable laboratory parameter for many situations in clinical medicine, endocrinology, and physiology of the hypothalamus–pituitary–adrenal cortex system. In physiology blood tyrosine determination can supplement measurements of levels of the hormonal participants of this system by data on adequacy of this system functioning to the organism's needs under different situations.

And finally some speculations.

The comparison of therapeutic effect of glucocorticoid preparations in SLE with their regulatory influence on the blood tyrosine level suggests that the therapeutic action of these preparations cannot be conditioned by an exclusive combination of pharmacological properties; on the contrary, the unique combination of therapeutic properties of these preparations is caused by retention of specific hormonal properties.

Glucocorticoid hormones are essentially responsible for supporting homeostasis – they directly or indirectly participate in regulation of the majority (if not all) biochemical reactions and physiological processes. They are hormones of total action and of vital importance. But in addition to supporting homeostasis under conditions of health and physiological rest, glucocorticoid hormones play a very important and sometimes a decisive role under conditions of stress or disease when, as a rule, their secretion increases. Under stress situations or in disease glucocorticoid hormones can realize their effects acting via the evolutionary selected best pathways, and, no doubt, a certain optimum of the adrenal cortex activity must exist for every subject (a human or animal) under extraordinary conditions. However, it seems that the optimum of this individual adrenocortical response can be revealed not by determination of functions of the hypothalamus-pituitary-adrenocortical system links, but only using a result of this system activity - an indirect glucocorticoid-dependent parameter, which can indicate whether this response is sufficient or not just for the concrete subject in a specific situation.

Glucocorticoid preparations retain the fundamental features of their natural prototypes, including their physiological and regulatory functions and can act via the same pathways. Therefore, it seems very likely that glucocorticoid therapy in non-endocrine diseases must imitate the optimal hormonal response of a given patient under conditions of disease – as if his adrenals could realize such a response. Glucocorticoid therapy must compensate an insufficient response of the patient's own adrenals, it can be life-saving within these limits and dangerous beyond them. The determination of blood tyrosine level which is a manifestation of the regulatory effect of glucocorticoid can allow a clinician to assess the correspondence of the hormonal provision to real needs of the patient.

10. References

Allard, P.; Cowell, L., Zytkovicz, T., Korson, M. & Ampola, M. (2004). Determination of Phenylalanine and Tyrosine in Dried Blood Specimens by Ion-Exchange Chromatography Using the Hitachi L-8800 Analyzer. *Clinical Biochemistry*, Vol.37, No.10, (October 2004), pp. 857-862, ISSN 0009-9120

Armstrong, M. & Stave, U. (1973). A Study of Plasma Free Amino Acid Levels. II. Normal Values for Children and Adults. *Metabolism.* Vol.22, No.4, (April 1973), pp. 561-569, ISSN 0026-0495

Armstrong, M. & Stave, U. (1973). A Study of Plasma Free Amino Acid Levels. IV. Characteristic Individual Levels of the Amino Acids. *Metabolism.* Vol. 22, No.6, (June 1973), pp. 821-825, ISSN 0026-0495

Badsha, H. & Edwards, C. (2003). Intravenous Pulses of Methylprednisolone for Systemic Lupus Erythematosus. *Seminars in Arthritis and Rheumatism.* Vol.32, No.6, (June 1973), pp. 1370-377, ISSN 0049-0172

Betheil, J.; Feigelson, M. & Feigelson, P. (1965). The Differential Effect of Glucocorticoids on Tissue and Plasma Amino Acid Levels. *Biochemica et Biophysica Acta.* Vol.104, No. 1, (January 1965), pp. 92-97, ISSN 0006-3002

Brooks, R. (1979). Biosynthesis and Metabolism of Adrenocortical Steroids. In: *The Human Adrenal Gland*, V.H.T. James, (Ed.), 67-92, ISBN 0861963628, Academic Press, London

Cerone, R; Holme, E., Schiaffino, M., Caruso, U., Maritano, L. & Romano, C. (1997). Tyrosinemia Type III: diagnosis and ten-year follow-up. *Acta Paediatrica.* Vol.86, No.9, (September 1997), pp. 1013-1015, ISSN 0340-6717

Christiansen, J.J.; Djurhuus, C., Gravholt, C., Iversen, P., Christiansen, J.S., Schmitz, O., Weeke, J., Lunde, J., Jergensen, J. & Meller, N. (2007). Effects of Cortisol on Carbohydrate, Lipid, and Protein Metabolism: Studies of Acute Cortisol Withdrawal in Adrenocortical Failure. *Journal of Clinical Endocrinology and Metabolism.* Vol.92, No.9, (September 2009), pp. 3553-3559, ISSN 0021-972X

Clayton, T.; Lindon, J., Everett, J., Charuel, C., Hanton, G., Le Net, L., Provost, J. & Nicholson, J. (2007). Hepatotoxin-Induced Hypertyrosinemia and Its Toxicological Significance. *Archive of Toxicolology.* Vol.81, No.3, (March 2007), pp. 201-210, ISSN 0340-5760 (doi)

Deng, Y. & Tsao, B. (2010). Genetic Susceptibility to Systemic Lupus Erythematosus in the Genomic Era. *National Reviews of Rheumatology.* Vol. 6, No.12, (December 2010), pp. 683-692, ISSN 1759-4790

De Rijk, R. & Sternberg, E. Corticosteroid Resistance and Disease. (1997) *Annals of Medicine.* Vol.29, No.1, (January 1997), pp. 79-82, ISSN 0785-3890

Derks, M; Dubois, E.F., Koomans, P. & Boxtel, C. (1999). Effect of Hydrocortisone on Plasma Tyrosine Concentration and Lymphocyte Counts in Healthy Volunteers. *Clinical Drug Investigations.* Vol.18, No.5, (November 1999), pp. 391-401. ISSN 1058-4838

Dubois, E.L. (1974). *Lupus Erythematosus.* 2nd Edition, ISBN 0781793947, University of Southern California Press, Los Angeles, USA

Franchin, G. & Diamond, B. (2006). Pulse Steroids: How Much is Enough? *Autoimmunity Reviews.* Vol. 5, no. 2, (February 2006), pp. 111-113, ISSN 0022-1767

Gavrilov, V.; Lychkovskii, E., Shostak, E. & Konev, S. (1998). Fluorescence Assay of Tyrosine in Blood Plasma. *Journal of Applied Spectroscopy.* Vol. 65, No. 3, (March 1998), pp. 379-384, ISSN 0021-9037

Gelehrter, T. (1973). Mechanisms of Hormonal Induction of Enzymes. *Metabolism.* Vol.22, No.1, (January 1973), pp. 85-100, ISSN 0026-0495

Godblatt, F. & Isenberg, D. (2005). New Therapies for Systemic Lupus Erythematosus. *Clinical and Experimental Immunology.* Vol.140, No.2 (May 140), pp. 205-212, ISSN 0268-3369

Goldsmith, L. (1978). Molecular Biology and Molecular Pathology of a Newly Described Molecular Disease – Tyrosinemia II (the Richner–Hanhart Syndrome). *Experimental Cell Biology.* Vol.46, No.1-2, (January-February 1978), pp. 96-113, ISSN 0304-3568

Grenier, A. & Laberge, C. (1974). A Modified Automated Fluorimetric Method for Tyrosine Determination in Blood Spotted on Paper: A Mass Screening Procedure for Tyrosinemia. *Clinica et Chimica Acta.* Vol.57, No.1, (January 1974), pp. 71-75, ISSN 0022-2275

Hazra, A.; Pyszeznsli, N., DuBois, D., Almon, R. & Jusko, W. (2007). Modeling Receptor/Gene-Mediated Effect of Corticosteroids on Hepatic Tyrosine Aminotransferase Dynamics in Rats: Dual Regulation by Endogenous and Exogenous Corticosteroids. *Journal of Pharmacokinetetics and Pharmacodynamics.* Vol.34, No.5, (May 2007), pp. 643-647, ISSN 0344-5704

Hench, P.; Kendall, E., Slocumb, C. & Polley, H. (1949). The Effect of a Hormone of the Adrenal Cortex (17-Hydroxy-11-dehydrocorticosterone, Compound E) and of Pituitary Adrenocorticotrophic Hormone on Rheumatoid Arthritis. Preliminary Report. *Proceedings of the Staff Meetings of Mayo Clinic.* Vol.24, No.1, (January 1949), pp. 181-197, ISSN 1462-0324

Hench, P.; Kendall, E., Slocumb, C. & Polley, H. (1950). Effect of Cortisone Acetate and Pituitary ACTH on Rheumatoid Arthritis, Rheumatic fever, and Certain Other conditions; Studies in Clinical Physiology. *Archives of Internal Medicine.* Vol.85, No.4, (April 1950), pp. 545-666, ISSN 1462-0324

Hughes, I. (2007). Congenital Adrenal Hyperplasia: a Lifelong Disorder. *Hormone Research.* Vol. 68, Supplement 5, pp. 84-89, DOI 000110585

Ioannou, Y, & Isenberg, D. (2002). Current Concepts for the Management of Systemic Lupus Erythematosus in Adults: a Therapeutic Challenge. *Postgraduated Medicne Journal.* Vol.78, No.924, (July 2002), pp. 599-606, ISSN 0032 - 5473

Kainova, A. (1974) Amino Acid Metabolism in Patients with Collagen Diseases. *Voprosy Revmatizma.* 1974; Vol.14, No.1, pp. 68-73, ISSN 0040-3660

Kand'ar, R. & Zakova, P. (2009). Determination of Phenylalanine and Tyrosine in Plasma and Dried Blood Samples Using HPLC with Fluorescence Detection. *Journal of Chromatography. B. Analytic Technology for Biomedical Life Sciences.* Vol.877, No.30, (November 2009), pp. 3926-3929, ISSN 1873-376X

Knox, W. (1955). Metabolism of Phenylalanine and Tyrosine. In: *Symposium on Amino Acid Metabolism.* pp. 836-866, ISSN 0022-3166, Baltimora, USA, April 1955.

Knox, W. & Pitt, B. (1957). Enzymic Catalysis of the Keto-enol-Tautomerization of Phenylpyruvic Acid. *Journal of Biological Chemistry.* Vol.225, No.2, (April 1957), pp. 675-688, ISSN 0021-9258

Levine, R. & Kohn, H. (1967). Tyrosine Metabolism in Patients with Liver Diseases. *Journal of Clinical Investigations.* Vol.46, No.12, (December 1967), pp. 2012-2030, ISSN 0021-9738

Li, X; Zhang, F., Zhang, J. & Wang, J. (2010). Negative Relationship between Expression of Glucocorticoid Receptor alpha and Disease Activity: Glucocorticoid Treatment of Patients with Systemic Lupus Erythematosus. *Journal of Rheumatolology.* Vol.37, No.2, (March 2010), pp. 316-321, ISSN 0315-162X

Lo, J.; Schwitzgebel, V., Tyrrell, V., Fitzgerald, P., Kaplan, S., Conte, F. & Grumbach, M. (1999). Normal Female Infants Born of Mothers with Classic Congenital Adrenal Hyperplasia due to 21-Hydroxylase Deficiency. *Journal of Clinical Endocrinology and Metabolism.* Vol.84, No.3, (March 1999), pp. 930-936, ISSN 0021-972X

Lukert, B. (2006) Glucocorticoid Replacement – How Much is Enough? *Journal of Clinical Endocrinology and Metabolism.* Vol.91, No.3, pp. 793-794, ISSN 0021-972X

Natt, E.; Kida, K., Odievre, M., Di Rocco, M. & Scherer G. (1992). Point Mutations in the Tyrosine Aminotransferase Gene in Tyrosinemia Type II. *Proceedings of the National Academy of Sciences of USA.* Vol.89, No.19, (October 1992), pp. 9297-9301, ISSN 0027-8424

Nemeth, S. (1978). The Effect of Stress or Glucose Feeding on Hepatic Tyrosine Aminotransferase Activity and Liver and Plasma Tyrosine Level of Intact and Adrenalectomized Rats. *Hormone and Metabolism Research.* Vol.10, No.2, (March 1978), pp. 144-147, ISSN 0018-5043

Nishimura, N.; Yasui, M., Okamoto, H., Kanazawa, M., Kotaka, Y. & Shibata, Y. (1958). Intermediary Metabolism of Phenylalanine and Tyrosine in Diffuse Collagen Diseases. *Archives of Dermatology.* 1958; Vol.77, No.2, (February 1958), pp. 255-262, ISSN 0003-4819

Nishimura, N.; Maeda, K., Yasui, M., Okamoto, H., Matsukawa, M. & Toshina, H. (1961). Phenylalanine and Tyrosine in Collagen Diseases. *Archives of Dermatology.* Vol.83, No.4, (April 1961), pp. 644-652, ISSN 0003-4819

Nived, O.; Sturfelt, G. & Bengtsson, A. Improved Lupus Outcome. We Are Doing a Good Job, But Could We Do Better? (2008). *Journal of Rheumatology.* Vol.59, No.2, (February 2008), pp. 176-180, ISSN 0315-162X

Nordlinger, B.; Fulenwider, J., Ivey, J., Faraj, B., Ali, F., Kutner, M., Henderson, J. & Rudman, D. (1979). Tyrosine Metabolism in Cirrhosis. *Journal of Laboratory and Clinical Medicine.* Vol.94, No.6, (December 1979), pp. 832-840, ISSN 0022-2143

Ntali, S.; Tzanakakis, M., Bertsias, G. & Boumpas, D. (2009). What's New in Clinical Trials in Lupus? *International Journal of Clinical Rheumatology.* Vol.4, No.4, (April 2009), pp. 473-485, ISSN 1462-0324

Oakley, R. & Cidlowski, J. (2011). Cellular Processing of the Glucocorticoid Receptor Gene and Protein: New Mechanisms for Generating Tissue Specific Action of Glucocorticoids. *Journal of Biological Chemistry.* Vol.286, No.5, (February 2011), pp. 3177-3184, ISSN 0270-7306.

Piruzian, L. & Rass, I. (1991). The Safety Problem and a Physiological Strategy for Using Glucocorticoid Hormones. *Izvestiya Akademii Nauk SSSR, Seriya Biologicheskaya.* No.5, (October 1991), pp. 735-743, ISSN 0002-3329

Ponticelli, C.; Glassock, R. & Moroni, G. (2010). Induction and Maintenance Therapy in Proliferative Lupus Nephritis. *Journal of Nephrology.* Vol.23, No.1, (January 2010), pp. 9-16, ISSN 0250-8095.

Powell, L. & Axelsen, E. (1972). Corticosteroids in Liver Diseases: Studies on the Biological Conversion of Prednisone to Prednisolone and Plasma Protein Binding. *Gut.* Vol.13, No.9, (September 1972), pp. 690-696, ISSN 0003-4819

Rahman, A. & Isenberg, D. (2008) Severe Lupus Erythematosus. *New England Journal of Medicine.* Vol.358, No. 9, (September 2009), pp. 929-939, ISSN 0961-2033.

Rass, I. (1976). Character of Tyrosine Metabolism Disorder in Systemic Lupus Erythematosus. *Voprosy Revmatizma.* Vol.16, No.4, (April 1976), pp. 21-23, ISSN 0040-3660

Rass, I. (1978). The Usage of Corticosteroid Hormones and Tyrosine Metabolism. *Patologicheskaya Fiziologiya.* No.2, pp. 87-91, ISSN 0040-3660

Rass, I. (1980). Changes in Blood Tyrosine Content in Rats upon Adrenalectomy and on Substitution Injection of Hydrocortisone. *Doklady Akademii Nauk SSSR.* Vol.250, No.6, (June 1983), pp. 1497-1499, ISSN 0869-5652

Rass, I. (1983). Changes in Blood Tyrosine Levels in Response to Stress in Intact and Adrenalectomized Rats. *Byulleten Eksperimental'noi Biologii i Meditsiny.* Vol.95, No.3, (March 1983), pp. 29-31, ISSN 0365-9615

Rass, I. (2010). Blood Content of Tyrosine is an Index of Glucocorticoid Action on Metabolism, *Biochemistry (Moscow).* Vol.75, No.3, (March 2010), pp. 353-366, ISSN 0006-2979

Rass, I.; Borisov, I., Nikishova, T. & Sura, V. (1977). Blood Tyrosine Dynamics and Treatment with Corticosteroids in Systemic Lupus Erythematosus. *Terapevticheskii Arkhiv.* Vol.59, No.8, (August 1977), pp. 110-115, ISSN 0040-3660

Rass, I.; Bunyatyan, A., Kornev, B. & Turusina, T. (1978). Tyrosine, 11-Oxycorticosteroids, and Cortisol in Blood of Patients with Bronchial Asthma. *Terapevticheskii Arkhiv.* Vol.60, No.11, (November 1978), pp. 98-101, ISSN 0040-3660

Rass, I.; Kuznetsova, E. & Zhukovskii, M. (1979). Blood Tyrosine as an Index of Adequacy of the Glucocorticoid Substitution Therapy in Congenital Adrenal Cortex Dysfunction in Children. *Pediatriya.* Vol.58, No.9, (September 1979), pp. 26-29, ISSN 0031-403X

Rivlin, R. & Melmon, K. (1965). Cortisone-Provoked Depression of Plasma Tyrosine Concentration: Relation to Enzyme Induction in Man. *Journal of Clinical Investions.* Vol.44, No.3, (March 1965), pp. 1690-1698, ISSN 0021-9738

Rosen, F. & Nichol, C. (1963). Corticosteroids and Enzyme Activity. *Vitamins and Hormones.* Vol.21, No.1, (January 1963), pp. 135-214, ISSN 0042-7543

Schacke, H.; Schottelius, A., Docke, W., Strehlke, P., Jaroch, S., Schmees, N., Rehwinkel, H., Hennekes, H. & Khusru, A. (2004). Dissociation of Transactivation from Transrepression by a Selective Glucocorticoid Agonist Leads to Separation of Therapeutic Effects from Side Effects. *Proceedings of National Academy of Sciences of USA.* Vol.101, No.1, (January 2004), pp. 227-232, ISSN 0027-8424

Schroeder, J. & Euler, H. (1997). Recognition and Management of Systemic Lupus Erythematosus. *Drugs.* Vol.54, No.3, (March 1997), pp. 422-434, ISSN 1525-6359

Scriver, C. (1967). The Phenotypic Manifestions of Hereditary Tyrosinemia and Tyrosyluria. A Hypothesis. *Canadian Medical Association Journal.* Vol.97, No.18, (October 1967), pp. 1045-1101, ISSN 0003-4819

Scriver, C.; Clow, C. & Lamm, P. (1971). Plasma Amino Acids. Screening, Quantitation, and Interpretation. *American Journal of Clinical Nutrition.* Vol.24, No.7, (July 1971), pp. 826-890, ISSN 0002-9165

Snell, R. (1967). Hormonal Control of Pigmentation in Man and Other Mammals. *Advances in Biology of Skin.* Vol. 8, No. 4, (April 1967), pp. 447-466, ISSN 0906-6705

Stikkelbroeck, N.; van't Hof Grootenboer, B., Hermus, A., Otten, B., & van't Hof, M. (2003). Growth Inhibition by Glucocorticoid Treatment in Salt Wasting 21-Hydroxylase Deficiency: in Early Infancy and (Pre)puberty. *Journal of Clinical Endocrinology and Metabolism.* Vol.88, No.7, (July 2003), pp. 3525-3530, ISSN 0021-972X

Sun, Y.; DuBois, D., Almon, R., Pyszeznsli, N. & Jusko, W. (1998). Dose-Dependence and Repeated-Dose Studies for Receptor/Gene-mediated Pharmacodynamics of Methylprednisolone on Glucocorticoid Receptor Down-regulation and Tyrosine Aminotransferase Induction in Rat Liver. *Journal of Pharmacokinetics and Biopharmacology.* Vol. 26, No.6, (June 1998), pp. 619-648, ISSN 0090-466X

Thompson, E. (1979). Glucocorticoid Induction of Tyrosine Aminotransferase in Cultured Cells. In: *Glucocorticoid Hormone Action,* J. D. Baxter & G. G. Rousseau, (Eds.), 203-213, Springer Verlag, ISBN 038708973X Berlin/Heidelberg/New York

Udenfriend, S. & Cooper J. (1952). The Chemical Estimation of Tyrosine and Tyramine. *Journal of Biological Chemistry.* Vol.196, No.1, (January 1952), pp. 227-233, ISSN 0022-1767

Wurtman, R.; Rose, C., Chou, C. & Larin, F. (1968). Daily Rhythms in the Concentration of Various Amino Acids in Human Plasma. *New England Journal of Medicine.* Vol.279, No.1, (January 1968), pp. 171-175, ISSN 1759-4790

Zimmermann, C.; Avery, W., Finelli, A., Farwell, M., Fraser, C. & Borisy, A. (2009). Selective Amplification of Glucocorticoid Anti-inflammatory Activity through Synergistic Multi-target Action of a Combination Drug. *Arthritis Research and Therapy*. Vol.11, No.1, (January 2009), pp. 12-26, ISSN 1759-4790

8

A Rabbit Model of Systemic Lupus Erythematosus, Useful for Studies of Neuropsychiatric SLE

Rose G. Mage[1] and Geeta Rai[2]
[1]Laboratory of Immunology, NIAID, National Institutes of Health
[2]Department of Molecular and Human Genetics, Faculty of Science
Banaras Hindu University, Varanasi
[1]US
[2]India

1. Introduction

The aim of this review is to present in one place a summary of the development of a rabbit model of SLE conducted using pedigreed rabbits bred and selected at the National Institute of Allergy and Infectious Diseases (NIAID), NIH. We provide an overview of the knowledge gained by using rabbits *(Oryctolagus cuniculus)* as models for SLE, and eliciting autoantibodies typical of those produced by patients with SLE. We present here summaries of work by ourselves and coauthors that can contribute to improved understanding of neuropsychiatric SLE (NPSLE) (Sanches-Guerro et al., 2008). Our gene expression studies (Rai, et al., 2010) and extensive evaluations of autoantibody responses coupled with observed clinical symptoms of animals immunized against peptides from the Smith antigen (Sm) or the NMDA glutamate receptor have shown promise to improve understanding NPSLE.

An overview of immune system development, genetic diversity of immunoglobulin genes and somatic diversification during B-cell development in rabbits can be found in a review by Mage et al., (2006) and reference therein. Investigations of autoantibodies found in patients with NPSLE and the problems of diagnosis and specific treatments are addressed in other chapters in this volume.

2. Our model

2.1 Earlier studies of SLE models by other laboratories using rabbit

We set out to develop a model of SLE in pedigreed rabbits because an earlier report showed that immunization of non-pedigreed rabbits with peptides such as PPPGMRPP, derived from the Sm B/B′ subunit of the spliceosomal Smith autoantigen led to epitope spreading, SLE-like autoantibody production and clinically observed seizures. This peptide sequence is one of the major regions of reactivity in SLE patients and may mimic the peptide PPPGRRP from the EBNA-1 component of Epstein-Barr virus (EBV) (James et al., 1995). Another study attempted to reproduce this report but only found some evidence for epitope spreading with no suggestion of induced autoimmunity (Mason et al., 1999). We hypothesized that the different results may have been obtained because small numbers of rabbits were studied, and there may have been different genetic susceptibilities among outbred rabbits studied by the two groups. Since our work already depended on breeding and maintenance of immunoglobulin allotype-defined pedigreed rabbits, we were in a position to pursue this idea further. In addition to using the MAP-8-PPPGMRPP immunogen used in these previous studies (termed SM-MAP-8 in the following sections), we chose a new immunogen termed GR-MAP-8 based on a report by DeGiorgio et al (2001) that some anti-DNA antibodies cross-react with the NMDA glutamate receptor.

2.2 The model in pedigreed rabbits

We established a rabbit model of Systemic Lupus Erythematosus (SLE) in which peptide immunization led to lupus-like autoantibody production including anti-Sm, -RNP, -SS-A, -SS-B and -dsDNA. Some neurological symptoms in form of seizures and nystagmus were observed (Rai et al., 2006). The animals were selectively bred within the colony of pedigreed, immunoglobulin allotype-defined but non-inbred rabbits at the NIAID. We continued breeding responders from the first three groups studied (Rai et al., 2006, 2010, Puliyath et al., 2008, Yang et al., 2009a,b). Details about genetics, gene expression and cellular studies are in the sections below. The genetic heterogeneity of the pedigreed animals studied may correspond to that found among patients of a given ethnicity.

2.2.1 Methods

Rabbits: All rabbit experimentation and immunization protocols were reviewed and approved by the Animal Care and Use committees of the NIAID, NIH and of Spring Valley Laboratories where the animals were bred, housed and monitored. The animals' designations, sexes, and allotypes at the V_H a immunoglobulin heavy chain and Cκ b light chain loci are summarized in Tables 1A and B. Rabbits of groups 1, 3, 4, 5 and 6 received peptides (SM or GR) synthesized on MAP-8 branched lysine backbones and rabbits of group 2 received the peptides on MAP-4. BB indicates control rabbits that received backbone alone. SM animals received MAP-peptide derived from the sequence of the Smith antigen spliceosomal B/B' complex. GR animals received MAP-peptide derived from the NMDA glutamate receptor sequence.

Antigens: The peptide immunogens "GR" and "SM" used for the initial rabbit immunizations (Rai et al., 2006), were synthesized on branched lysine MAP-8 and MAP-4 backbones (BB) (AnaSpec) The SM peptide sequence PPPGMRPP corresponds to major antigenic regions at 191-198, 216-223 and 231-238 of the nuclear protein Sm B/B' (James et al, 1995). The GR peptide sequence DEWDYGLP corresponds to a known rabbit sequence of an extracellular epitope of the NR2b subunit of neuronal postsynaptic NMDA receptor. The MAP-BB without peptide was used as a control antigen. For subsequent studies, (Puliyath et al., 2008, Yang et al., 2009b, Rai et al. 2010), MAP-8 was the BB of choice because it appeared to elicit more diverse autoantibody responses.

Immunization: Rabbits each received subcutaneous (s.c.) injections of one of the MAP-peptides or control BB (0.5 mg/0.5 ml, in borate buffered saline, pH 8.0) emulsified with 0.5 ml of complete Freund's adjuvant (CFA). Boosts were given s.c. at 3-week intervals with the same antigen concentration emulsified with incomplete Freund's adjuvant (IFA). Controls that received only CFA followed by IFA were included in one study (Yang et al., 2009b). Sera collected immediately before immunization (pre-immune) and 1 week after each boost (post-boost) were stored at -20°C in multiple aliquots for assays.

Rabbit ID	Rabbit no.	Allotype	Sex
Group 1			
SM1	XX129-3	a1/1, b4/5	M
SM2	2XX127-4	a1/1, b5/5	F
SM3	2XX288-2	a1/1, b9/9	M
SM4	1XX288-4	a1/1, b5/9	F
SM5	2XX127-2	a1/1, b9/9	M
SM6	2XX92-06	a1/1, b9/9	F
GR7	XX129-5	a1/1, b4/5	M
GR8	2XX127-5	a1/1, b9/9	F
GR9	1XX288-3	a1/1, b5/5	M
GR10	2XX288-6	a1/1, b5/9	F
BB11	2XX127-1	a1/1, b5/5	M
BB12	1XX78-8	a1/1, b9/9	F
Group 2			
SM13	LL191-1	a1/1, b4/5	M
SM14	LL191-2	a1/1, b5/5	F
SM15	2LL179-1	a1/1, b9/9	M
SM16	1LL163-3	a1/1, b9/9	F
SM17	LL164-4	a1/1, b9/9	F
GR18	1LL178-2	a1/1, b9/9	M
GR19	1LL178-3	a1/1, b4/4	F
GR20	1LL178-4	a1/1, b9/9	F
GR21	1LL178-5	a1/1, b4/9	M
GR22	1LL178-6	a1/1, b4/9	F
GR23	1LL178-8	a1/1, b4/4	F
BB24	LL164-1	a1/1, b9/9	M
BB25	LL164-3	a1/1, b9/9	F
BB26	2LL179-3	a1/1, b5/9	M
BB27	1LL163-4	a1/1, b5/9	F
Group 3			
GR28	LL108-1	a1/1, b5/9	M
GR29	LL108-3	a1/1, b5/5	F
GR30	LL108-4	a1/1, b9/9	F
BB31	2LL179-2	a1/1, b9/9	M
Group 4			
SM32	1QQ299-2	a1/1, b5/5	M
SM33	1QQ299-3	a1/1, b4/5	F
SM34	6QQ299-1	a1/1, b4/9	M
SM35	6QQ299-2	a1/1, b4/5	F
GR36	3QQ299-1	a1/1, b4/5	M
GR37	3QQ299-2	a1/1, b5/9	M
GR38	3QQ299-4	a1/1, b5/9	M
GR39	4QQ299-1	a1/1, b5/9	M
GR40	5QQ299-2	a1/1, b5/9	F
GR41	5QQ299-3	a1/1, b5/5	F
BB42	1QQ299-1	a1/1, b5/5	M
BB43	5QQ299-4	a1/1, b5/5	F
BB44	6QQ299-3	a1/1, b4/9	F
PB45	1QQ173-1	a1/1, b5/9	M
PB46	1QQ173-2	a1/1, b5/5	M
PB47	1QQ173-3	a1/1, b5/5	M

Table 1. A. Designations of sexes and allotypes of Groups 1-4.
PB45, 46, and 47 received injections with phosphate buffered saline only.

Group 5			
GR 48	UA345-1	a2/2, b9k/9k	M
GR49	1UA344-1	a1/2, b9k/9k	M
GR50	1UA344-5	a1/2, b9k/9k	F
GR51	1YY119-6	a1/1, b9/9	F
GR52	1YY119-8	a1/1, b9/9	F
GR53	2YY119-6	a1/1, b9/9	M
GR54	2YY299-5	a1/1, b4/9	F
GR55	2YY299-3	a1/1, b4/9	F
GR56	UA345-2	a1/2, b4/9k	M
GR57	1UA344-2	a1/2, b5/9k	M
GR58	1UA344-6	a2/2, b5/9k	F
GR59	1YY119-7	a1/1, b9/9	F
GR60	1YY327-2	a1/1, b5/9	M
GR61	2YY327-9	a1/1, b4/5	F
GR62	2YY299-4	a1/1, b4/9	F
GR63	2YY119-8	a1/1, b9/9	F
BB64	UA345-4	a2/2, b9k/9k	F
BB65	2UA344-1	a1/2, b9k/9k	F
BB66	1UA344-3	a2/2, b5/9k	M
BB67	2YY327-8	a1/1, b4/5	M
BB68	UA345-6	a1/2, b4/9k	F
BB69	1YY327-4	a1/1, b5/9	F
BB70	1YY119-5	a1/1, b9/9	M
BB71	2YY119-7	a1/1, b9/9	M
Group 6			
GR72	UA345-5	a2R3/2R3, 4/9k	F
GR73	UA269-3	a1/1, b4/9k	F
BB74	6YY328-4	a1/1, b5/9	M
BB75	2YY125-6	a1/2, b9k/9k	M
CF1	6YY328-3	a1/1, b5/9	M
CF2	1UA161-1	a1/1, b9/9	M
GR76	2YY119-9	a1/1, b9/9	F
GR77	UA269-1	a1/1, b4/5	M
BB78	YY118-6	a1/1, b9/9	M
BB79	1UA161-2	a1/1, b9/9	M
CF3	1YY125-4	a2/2, b4/9k	M
CF4	2YY125-4	a2/2, b5/9k	M
GR80	XA345-1	a1/2, b9/9k	F
GR81	2UA14-2	a1/1, b5/9	F
BB82	XA346-2	a1/1, b9/9	M
BB83	2UA14-3	a1/1, b5/9k	F
CF5	XA345-2	a1/2, b9/9k	F
GR84	XA234-2	a1/2, b5/9	F
GR85	XA346=1	a1/1, b9/9	M
BB86	XA234-2	a1/2, b5/9	M
B87	3XA203-2	a1/ali	M
CF6	2XA344-2	a1/1, b9/9	F
CF7	1XA344-1	a1/1, b9/9	M

Table 1. B. Designations of sexes and allotypes of Groups 5 and 6.

Clinical Assessments: Rabbits were housed in a separate room equipped with video surveillance so that abnormal behavior such as seizure activity and other neurological dysfunctions could be detected. They were observed daily and also received periodic complete health evaluations. Hematology using a Bayer Advida, model 120 hematology analyzer and blood chemistry assessments of each rabbit were carried out in a Veterinary diagnostic laboratory (Antech Diagnostics, Lake Success NY).

ELISA for anti-peptide antibodies, anti-dsDNA and autoantibodies to nuclear antigens: Serum antibody responses to the MAP-peptides and control immunogens were measured by solid phase ELISA as previously described (Rai et al 2006). "Polystyrene 96-well plates (Corning Inc, Corning, NY, Cat # 3590) were coated with 50 μl/well of either SM-, GR- or BB- (MAP-8 or MAP-4) at 10 μg/ml in bicarbonate buffer, (pH 9.6) and incubated overnight at 4ºC. Plates were washed three times with PBS (pH 7.2) containing 0.1% Tween 20 and blocked with 100 μl blocking solution for 1 hr at 37ºC (Quality Biological Inc, Gaithersburg, MD). Wells were then incubated 1 hr, at 37ºC with 50 μl/well of sera titrated by four-fold dilutions in blocking solution, washed 5 times, incubated for 1 hr at 37ºC with 50 μl of a 1:2000 dilution (0.4 ng/μl) of affinity-purified horseradish peroxidase conjugated (HRP) goat anti-rabbit IgG (H+L) secondary antibody (Jackson Immunoresearch Laboratories Inc., West Grove, PA), developed with 3, 3', 5, 5'- tetramethylbenzidine (TMB) (Inova Diagnostics, Inc., San Diego, CA) and the resulting OD read at 450 nm."

Commercially available human diagnostic kits (INOVA Diagnostics) were adapted and used to assay serum autoantibodies to total extractable nuclear Ags (ENA) and to component Ags Sm, Rnp, SS-A, SS-B. Assays for autoantibodies to calf thymus dsDNA were adapted similarly using two different commercially available kits (Vidia, Vestec (Kit A); Zeus scientific, NJ (Kit B). Briefly, 100 μl rabbit sera diluted 1:100 in the proprietary sample diluents were added to antigen-coated wells and incubated for 60 min. at 37°C (Kit A) or 30 min. at RT (Kit B). Wells were then washed, incubated for 60 min. at 37°C (Kit A) or 30 min at RT (Kit B) with secondary antibody HRP-goat anti-rabbit IgG Fc (Jackson Immunoresearch Laboratories, Inc.) and developed with TMB for reading OD at 450 nm. For groups 5 and 6, anti-dsDNA, -ANA, -RNP and -Sm were assayed with the Quantalite kits (Inova Diagnostics) substituting affinity purified HRP-goat anti-rabbit IgG Fc for the anti-human secondary reagent (Puliyath et al., 2008, Yang et al., 2009b).

Detection of anti-nuclear antibodies (ANA) by indirect immunofluorescence: Commercially available slides coated with fixed Hep-2 cells (Antibodies Inc., Davis, CA) were incubated with rabbit antisera diluted 1:20 in 5% goat serum (Jackson Immunoresearch Laboratories Inc.) for 30 min. at RT. ANA binding was detected by fluorescence microscopy following 30 min incubation at RT with 12.5 ng/μl of FITC-goat anti-rabbit IgG Fc (Southern Biotech Inc., Birmingham, AL). Fluorescent binding patterns were compared with reference pictures provided by Antibodies, Inc.

Flow cytometry: Anti-human antibodies that cross reacted with rabbit B-cell activation factor (BAFF) (biotin conjugated goat anti-human BAFF polyclonal antibody), transmembrane activator and CAML interactor (TACI) (biotin conjugated goat anti-human TACI polyclonal antibody)(Antigenix, America, Inc.), BAFF receptor (BR3) (purified goat anti-human BR3 antibody) (R&D systems) were used for staining. Briefly, purified PBMCs were incubated on ice for 40 min with primary antibody before washing twice with cold PBS containing 1% FCS, then subsequent incubation with various secondary reagents or secondary antibodies. For BR3 detection, a biotinylated donkey anti-goat IgG was used as secondary antibody. Biotinylated antibodies were visualized by PE-conjugated streptavidin (Jackson ImmunoResearch laboratories, Inc.). After washing, cells were analyzed using a FACS-Calibur flow cytometer (BD Pharmingen) and FlowJo analytical software (Tree Star). Cells were gated on the side scatter x forward scatter (SSCxFSC) profiles to include both small and large lymphocytes, as well as monocytes but exclude red blood cells and granulocytes; dead cells were excluded by propidium iodide staining. Rabbit IgM+ B cells were detected by FITC-conjugated goat anti-rabbit IgM (Southern Biotechnology Associates).

Gene Expression studies: *RNA extraction and synthesis of cDNA and cRNA*
Peripheral white blood cells (PWBCs) were lysed with TRIzol (Invitrogen, CA) and total RNA was extracted using RNAeasy Mini columns following the manufacturer's instructions (Qiagen, CA). The cRNA probes were prepared from mRNA using the Affymetrix gene chip eukaryotic small sample target labeling protocol assay version II (Affymetrix, Santa Clara, CA) using 2 cycles of cDNA synthesis and *in vitro* transcription (IVT) reactions. The cRNA thus obtained was used in the final IVT cycle for obtaining biotinylated cRNA using CTP and UTP (EnzoBioarray, Enzo Life Sciences, Farmingdale, NY) (Rai et al 2010).
Microarray analysis Affymetrix U95A human microarray chips were used and hybridization of the labeled cRNA was carried out according to the manufacturer's recommended protocol. Non-normalized MAS5 signals were used to compare raw probeset intensity values between human and rabbit samples. Final rabbit study analyses were conducted with expression values summarized using dChip, log2 transformed and Loess normalized using an R package (http://www.elwood9.net/spike). Analyses of the gene sets were done using Database for Annotation, Visualization and Integrated Discovery (DAVID) (http://david.abcc.ncifcrf.gov/knowledgebase/) and Ingenuity Pathways Analysis (IPA) (Ingenuity Systems, Mountain View, CA; www.ingenuity.com).

Quantitative real time PCR: Quantitative real time PCR analysis of mRNAs was performed on a 7900HT Sequence Detection System (Applied Biosystems). The cDNA synthesized from isolated PWBCs was directly used as template for real-time PCR by using TaqMan 2x PCR Master Mix Reagents Kit (Applied Biosystems). Each sample from three independent experiments was run in duplicate. The unit number showing relative mRNA levels in each sample was determined as a value of mRNA normalized against Peptidylprolyl isomerase A (PPIA). RT-PCR data were analyzed by using the $2^{-\Delta\Delta C_T}$ method. Based on its uniform expression among rabbit groups in the microarray analysis, rabbit peptidylprolyl isomerase A (*PPIA*; cyclophilin A) was selected as the housekeeping gene control and used for the calculation of ΔC_T. Where rabbit sequences were unavailable, primers were designed after searching for rabbit sequences with corresponding human gene sequences in the database containing the trace archives of the whole genome shotgun sequence of the rabbit (*Oryctolagus cuniculus*) generated by the Broad Institute of MIT and Harvard University (NCBI trace archive: cross- species Megablast at http://www.ncbi.nlm.nih.gov/blast/tracemb.shtml) and in assemblies of rabbit scaffolds at Ensembl and UCSC (see NCBI Rabbit Genome Resources site) at: http://www.ncbi.nlm.nih.gov/projects/genome/guide/rabbit/

2.2.2 Genetics and autoantibody responses
Figure 1 shows the pedigree and an overview of antibody responses of the rabbits immunized and selectively bred during the project to develop a rabbit model of SLE. There were 31 1- to 2-year-old rabbits in the initial studies (Rai et al., 2006). Rabbits of groups 2 or

3 were descendants of rabbits of groups 1 or 2 and/or their siblings. Rabbits that did not respond with autoantibody production after immunization during this initial study by Rai et al., (2006) are not shown. The fourth group was described in Rai et al., (2010) and their mRNA included along with mRNA from the first three groups for gene expression profiling of a total of 46 pedigreed control- or immunized-rabbits as detailed below (section 2.2.3). Controls that received only phosphate buffered saline are designated PB. Because the GR peptide generally elicited better autoantibody responses than the SM peptide, the two subsequent groups [5 (Puliyath et al., 2008) and 6 (Yang et al., 2009b)] were immunized with GR-MAP-8 or control BB-MAP-8. The final 6th group also included controls that received complete followed by incomplete Freund's adjuvant but no MAP-BB or MAP-peptide, to investigate whether adjuvants alone led to any autoantibody production (designated CF).

An overview of autoantibody responses, and the relationships of males (squares) and females (circles) in six immunization groups is shown in Figure 1. The four quadrants indicate post-immunization elevations of levels of anti-dsDNA (upper left), anti-Sm and/or anti-RNP (lower left), ANA by IFA (upper right) and ANA by ELISA (lower right). For the 5th (Puliyath et al. 2008) and 6th groups (Yang et al., 2009b), darker shades indicate high autoantibody responses. The large circles and squares represent the 6th group developed from selective breeding using responders from earlier groups. Figure originally published by Yang et al., (2009b) Investigations of a rabbit (*Oryctolagus cuniculus*) model of systemic lupus erythematosus (SLE), BAFF and its receptors. *PLoS ONE* Vol. 4, 2009.

The selective breeding led to subsequent progeny (groups 5 and 6) exhibiting more consistent autoantibody production. In the pedigree, we can trace the ancestry of some responder rabbits back to the first high responders (SM1 and GR9) that also exhibited seizures. For example, GR54 and GR55 from litter 2YY299 had high-responder grandsires SM1 and SM15 (Puliyath et al. 2008). The model developed using selectively bred pedigreed rabbits remains a promising one for further genetic investigations.

As is found in human sera (Li et al., 2011), some rabbits had detectable pre-immune anti-nuclear antibodies (ANA) by ELISA. ANA of sixteen of twenty-four rabbits in group 5, including four immunized with only MAP-8 backbone had an increased ELISA value (delta OD) above pre-immune of 1.0 or more optical density units after the third boost. Anti-dsDNA increased in 12/24 rabbits after the fifth or seventh boost (Puliyath et al., 2008). Figure 2 shows examples of indirect immunofluorescence (ANA-IFA) studies of some sera from group 6 (Yang et al. 2009b). As in human SLE sera, the ANA-IFA patterns reflect responses to one or more autoantigens in different individuals. Littermates that received GR peptide such as UA269-3 and -1 (GR73 and GR77) developed similar patterns after the 3rd boost. ANA staining with sera of littermates XA346-1 and -2 (GR85 and BB82) resulted in different patterns. GR85 serum exhibited some cytoplasmic and peripheral nuclear staining not seen with the serum of BB82. Puliyath et al., (2008) also noticed that GR-immunized littermates had similar ANA-IFA staining patterns but that BB immunized animals' patterns generally differed.

2.2.3 Gene expression studies

We extended the information about the rabbit model of SLE by microarray-based expression profiling of mRNA from peripheral blood leukocytes following peptide immunization (Rai et al., 2010). Data obtained in studies of gene expression in the first four groups of immunized rabbits were deposited in the Gene Expression Omnibus and became

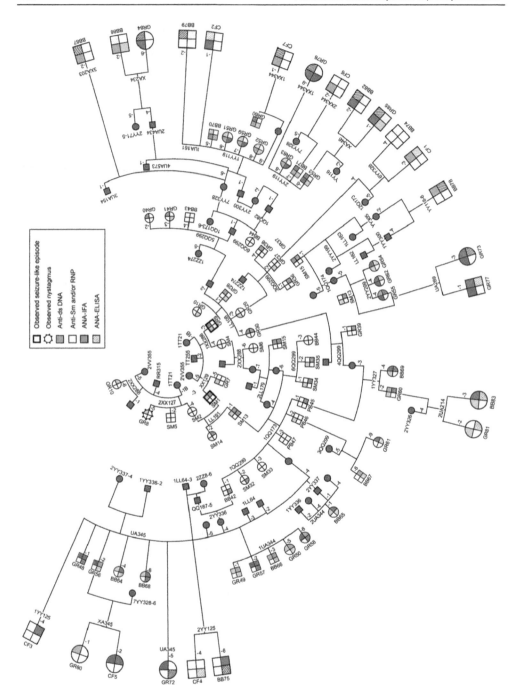

Fig. 1. Pedigree and summary of autoantibody responses.

public on Jul 23, 2010 at the NCBI website: http://www.ncbi.nlm.nih.gov/geo/query/acc.cgi?acc=GSE23076
Experiment type: Expression profiling by array. GEO accession: Series GSE23076 Query DataSets for GSE23076

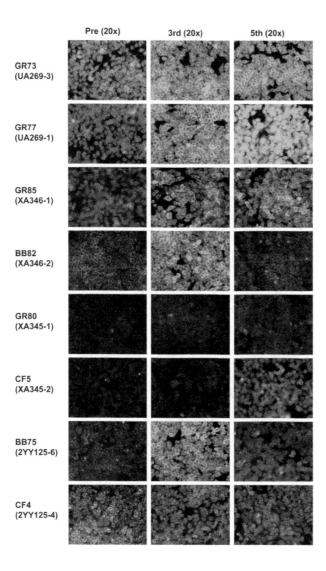

Fig. 2. Examples of indirect ANA-IFA assays of pre- and post-immune sera. Figure originally published by Yang et al., (2009b) Investigations of a rabbit (*Oryctolagus cuniculus*) model of systemic lupus erythematosus (SLE), BAFF and its receptors. *PLoS ONE* Vol.4, 2009.

At the time of the gene expression studies, microarrays specific for study of gene expression profiles were not available for rabbits. We therefore first conducted comparisons of identically prepared rabbit and human cRNA binding to the Affymetrix U95 microarray available for human gene expression analyses. We showed that the human microarray could be used with rabbit cRNA to yield information on genetic pathways activated and/or suppressed in autoantibody-producing immunized rabbits. After demonstrating that human expression arrays could be used with rabbit RNA to yield information on molecular pathways, we designed a study evaluating gene expression profiles in a total of 46 rabbits from 4 groups of the pedigreed control and immunized rabbits. We discovered unique gene expression changes associated with lupus-like serological patterns in immunized rabbits. Our results also demonstrated that caution must be applied when choosing the structure of the carrier Multiple Antigen Peptide (MAP-peptide) for immunization. We discovered that using MAP-4 rather than MAP-8 significantly altered patterns of immune response and gene expression.

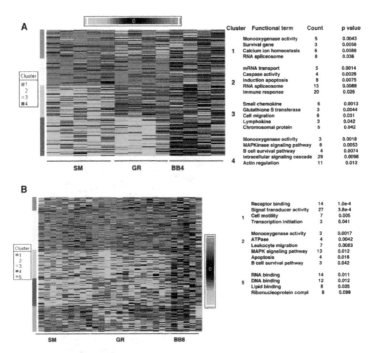

Fig. 3. Gene expression patterns differ when the backbone of immunogen is MAP-4 (A) or MAP-8 (B). In panel A, Cluster 1 genes were overrepresented in the SM group, Cluster 2 were common to both, Cluster 3 genes were overexpressed in the GR group and Cluster 4 genes were decreased in expression in both groups. Count indicates the number of different genes associated with each functional term. Figure modified from one originally published in The Journal of Immunology. Rai, G., Ray S., Milton, J., Yang, J., Ren, P., Lempicki, R., and Mage, R.G. 2010. Gene expression profiles in a rabbit model of systemic lupus erythematosus autoantibody production. J. Immunol. 185:4446-4456. Copyright © [2010] The American Association of Immunologists, Inc.

Figure 3 shows that distinct patterns and clusters of functionally related genes were found to be upregulated when peptides SM or GR on MAP-4 backbone (A) were used as immunogens compared to when MAP-8 backbone was used (B) (Rai et al., 2010). Validation of gene expression data by quantitative real-time PCR was conducted for two genes for which primer sequences were available beta2-microglobulin (B2M) and p-21-protein (Cdc42/Rac)-activated kinase 1 (PAK1) (Figure 6 in Rai et al., 2010). These genes appear in the interactive pathway shown in Figure 4 below. Among the genes significantly upregulated in SLE rabbits were those associated with NK cytotoxicity, antigen presentation, leukocyte migration, cytokine activity, protein kinases, RNA spliceosomal ribonucleoproteins, intracellular signaling cascades, and glutamate receptor activity (Rai et al., 2010).

Functional Annotation	p-Value	Number of molecules
Inflammatory Disorder	1.6E-11	25
Immunological Disorder	3.1E-11	23
Rheumatic Disease	5.4E-11	19
Autoimmune Disease	2.7 E-08	18
Rheumatoid Arthritis	1.7E-06	13
Glomerulonephritis	2.6E-06	5
Inflammation	2.5E-05	7
Lupus Nephritis of Mice	3.2E-04	3

Table 2. The top functional annotations found using Ingenuity Pathways Analysis (IPA) in comparisons of upregulated genes of rabbits making anti-dsDNA to those only making other anti-nuclear antibodies.

Figure 4 and Table 2 summarize the patterns of upregulated gene expression found in the rabbits from the three groups immunized with MAP-8-peptides that made anti-dsDNA compared to those that only made other anti-nuclear antibodies. Twenty-five genes associated with inflammatory disorders were significantly upregulated in expression. Subsets of these were associated with various immunological disorders in the IPA databases including Autoimmune, Rheumatic, and inflammatory diseases. The results linked increased immune activation with up-regulation of components associated with neurological and anti-RNP responses, demonstrating the utility of the rabbit SLE model to uncover biological pathways related to SLE-induced clinical symptoms, including NPSLE. We suggested that our finding of distinct gene expression patterns in rabbits that made anti-dsDNA should be further investigated in subsets of SLE patients with different autoantibody profiles (Rai et al., 2010). In Figure 4, the connecting lines indicate direct interactions among the products of these genes. The shapes classify the proteins found as transmembrane receptors e.g. CD 40, cytokines/growth factors, e.g. CCL2, kinases, e.g. TYK2, peptidases, e.g. MMP9, other enzymes, e.g. ARF1 and transcriptional regulators, e.g. STAT5B. Genes shown were common to the pathways listed in Table 2 that were upregulated in the anti-dsDNA positive rabbits. Figure 4 was modified from one originally published in the Journal of Immunology. Rai, G., Ray S., Milton, J., Yang, J., Ren, P., Lempicki, R., and Mage, R.G. 2010. Gene expression profiles in a rabbit model of systemic lupus erythematosus autoantibody production. J. Immunol. 185:4446-4456. Copyright © [2010] The American Association of Immunologists, Inc.

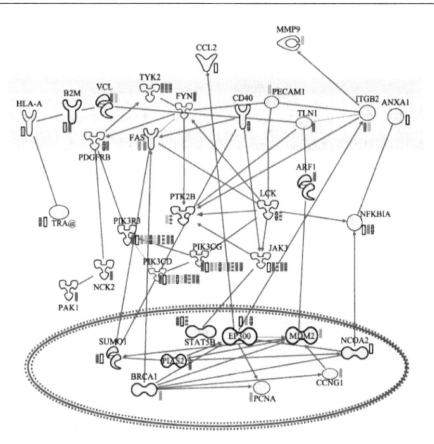

Fig. 4. Interactive pathway network of upregulated genes in anti-dsDNA positive rabbits.

2.2.4 Rabbit BAFF

Our laboratory described the expression and localization of rabbit B-cell activating factor (BAFF also termed BLys, TNFSF13b TALL1, zTNF4) and its receptor BR3 in cells and tissues of the rabbit (Yang et al., 2009a). In addition to its important role in B-cell development and survival, disease activity in human lupus patients has been reported to correlate with serum BAFF levels (reviewed in Groom et al., 2007) and with elevated expression of mRNA for BAFF and two BAFF receptors, BR3 and transmembrane activator and CAML interactor (TACI) in PBMC of lupus patients (Petri et al, 2008). We therefore also investigated BAFF and its receptors in our rabbit model of SLE (Yang et al., 2009b). We previously concluded that BAFF detected on B cells by flow cytometry represented BAFF bound to its receptors on the cells (Yang et al, 2009a). An independent study (Yeramilli, & Knight, 2010) also reported that BAFF-binding receptors on rabbit B-cells are occupied by endogenous soluble BAFF. These authors' studies also suggested that B cells in rabbit could produce BAFF. With the small number of total animals available in group 6 (Table 1B), and no reagents available to detect levels of serum BAFF, we could only measure BAFF on cell surfaces by flow cytometry. These studies found decreased surface expression of BAFF, BR3 and TACI after immunization and boosting in most animals. However, two rabbits that produced high anti-dsDNA responses (GR76 and GR77) developed higher percentages of BAFF/CD14 and BR3/CD14 positive cells. We did observe consistently lower mean fluorescence intensities of staining of TACI on PBMC and lower percentages of TACI positive cells. We suggested that since TACI is a negative regulator of B cells in mouse and man, perhaps the decrease in TACI in the rabbits producing autoantibodies had allowed autoreactive B cells to escape regulation.

At the time these studies were conducted, clinical trials targeting BAFF/BLys and its receptors were in progress. With the FDA approval of Benlysta® (belimumab) in March, 2011, this monoclonal antibody, that inhibits binding of BLys/BAFF to receptors on B cells, became the first United States FDA approved treatment for SLE in over fifty years. Unfortunately, the clinical trials did not include SLE patients with severe active central nervous system lupus or nephritis. Post-approval trials will be required before this treatment can be recommended for these cohorts of patients.

2.3 Future prospects

2.3.1 Detection of autoantibodies to other antigens including neuroantigens in the rabbit model

In our rabbits, the development of severe symptoms may not yet have occurred because many were euthanized to make room for immunization and testing of their progeny and for tissue collection. For example, although nephritis was not observed, our gene expression studies identified upregulation of genes associated with Glomerulonephritis and also found in mice with Lupus Nephritis (Table 2 and Figure 4). Protein arrays containing microbial and autoantigens have been used to extend information on patients' serum profiles beyond the standard tests used in diagnosis (see for example, Robinson et al., 2002; Quintana et al., 2004; Li et al., 2005; Fattal et al. 2010). Recently, Li et al, (2011) used protein microarrays to determine risk factors for ANA positivity in healthy persons and concluded that serum profiles of autoantibodies can potentially identify healthy individuals with potential to develop lupus and other autoimmune diseases. Their observations extended the widely quoted earlier observations by Arbuckle et al, (2003) that autoantibodies develop as much as ten years before the clinical onset of SLE. In a NOD mouse model of cyclophosphamide-accelerated diabetes, Quintana et al (2004) used a protein microarray to predict from autoantibody repertoires, resistance or susceptibility to the development of diabetes before the induction with cyclophosphamide. Recently Fattal et al, (2010) applied the same technology to studies of SLE patients and controls. They reported highly specific SLE profiles that typically show increases in IgG binding to dsDNA, single-stranded DNA, Epstein–Barr virus, and hyaluronic acid. Interestingly, a healthy control subject who had the SLE antibody profile was later found to develop clinical SLE. Decreases in some specific IgM reactivities to autoantigens observed in this and earlier studies (Li et al., 2005) suggest that some natural IgM autoantibodies may play a protective role. A project to determine the antibody profiles of the rabbits' serum IgG and IgM, purified anti-dsDNA, and anti-peptide on protein microarrays carrying microbial and self antigens including those from the central and peripheral nervous system is in progress.

2.3.2 NPSLE and anti-NMDA glutamate receptors

The suggestion from extensive studies in the laboratory of Betty Diamond that some anti-dsDNA antibodies may react with the NMDA receptor and contribute to neurological manifestations in some lupus patients (DeGiorgio et al. 2001; Kowal et al, 2004), has led to numerous follow-up studies by the Diamond group, (Diamond & Volpe, 2004) and others. A recent editorial (Appenzeller, 2011) provides an updated overview of controversies in the field and discusses the accompanying paper by Gono et al., (2011) who report new analyses of 107 patients' sera for cross-reactivities of anti-dsDNA with a peptide derived from the sequence of the human NMDA receptor 2A (NR2A) compared with the similar peptide from human NR2B. They suggest that the sensitivity for detection of autoantibodies is greater with the NR2A peptide although their ELISA results directly comparing serum reactivities with each peptide were correlated with high significance (r = 0.94; P<0.0001). They conclude that assays of sera for anti-NR2A antibodies may be a better predictor of NPSLE than assays for NR2B and suggest that mixed results from other similar studies may be explained by small numbers of patients (Husebye et al., 2005) or less sensitive assays. We chose the GR peptide used in our immunization protocol based on the human sequence of NR2B because the rabbit sequence was not yet known. However, we knew that this sequence was highly conserved in several species including mouse, rat, dog, cow and chicken.

2.3.3 Rabbit genomics

Future studies of rabbit autoimmune and infectious diseases will benefit from the availability of a high quality draft rabbit genome sequence and assembly at ~7 x coverage recently completed at the Broad Institute, Boston (OryCun2.0). The donor was from a partially inbred strain. NCBI maintains a Rabbit Genome Resources website: http://www.ncbi.nlm.nih.gov/projects/genome/guide/rabbit/

Rabbit genomic sequences and assemblies from the ENCODE Project, with ~ 1% of rabbit genomic sequence from a different, outbred NZW animal are also available in GenBank. The selection of peptides for future immunization studies in rabbits can benefit from searching these resources.

3. Conclusion

The work described in this review documents that rabbits have a strong genetic component that leads to predisposition to production of autoantibodies similar to those found in SLE patients including those with NPSLE. Breeding and selection for consistent autoantibody production in the rabbit model can be accomplished over a few generations. When one of us (RGM) retired to Emeritus status at NIAID, the pedigreed colony was no longer maintained. Some animals related to those studied were distributed to others. In addition, although the pedigreed colony was dispersed, there is sperm available from two male breeders rabbits LL191-1 (SM13) and 1UA344-1 (GR49). In particular male SM13 and his progeny in the breeding scheme shown in Figure 2 generated numerous responders that made autoantibodies similar to those found in human Lupus patients. Cryovials of sperm from these animals are currently stored at the Twinbrook 3 facility of the Comparative Medicine Branch (CMB) of NIAID in liquid nitrogen storage tanks, and monitored weekly by their personnel. Further contact information can be obtained at the website of the CMB, of the NIAID, NIH at: http://www.niaid.nih.gov/LabsAndResources/labs/aboutlabs/cmb/Pages/default.aspx.

4. Acknowledgment

This research was supported by the Intramural Research Program of the NIH, NIAID. All coauthors of the papers from the laboratory made valuable contributions to the current understanding of the rabbit model of SLE. We appreciate the major contributions of Cornelius Alexander, Laboratory of Immunology, NIAID as well as the veterinary staff at Spring Valley Laboratories who provided invaluable technical assistance. We thank Jeff Skinner for statistical analyses, Mariam Quiñones for help with IPA analyses and figures, and Folake Soetan and Rami Zahr for assistance with preparation of some figures. We dedicate this chapter to the memory of Dr. Barbara A. Newman who was a major contributor to this research.

5. References

Appenzeller, S.; (2011) NR2 antibodies in neuropsychiatric systemic lupus erythematosus. *Rheumatology (Oxford).* Vol. 50 (February 2011) Epub ahead of print doi:10.1093/rheumatology/ker015

Arbuckle, M.R.; McClain. M.T., Rubertone, M. V., Scofield, R. H., Dennis, M.D., James, J.A., & Harley, J.B. (2003) Development of autoantibodies before the clinical onset of systemic lupus erythematosus. *N. Engl. J. Med.*, Vol. 349, No. 16 pp. 1526-1533.

DeGiorgio, L. A.; Konstantinov, K. N, Lee, S. C., Hardin, J. A., Volpe, B. T. & Diamond, B. (2001) A subset of lupus anti-DNA antibodies cross-reacts with the NR2 glutamate receptor in systemic lupus erythematosus. *Nat. Med.* Vol.7, No.11 (November 2001), pp. 1189–1193.

Diamond, B.; & Volpe, B. T. (2004). Cognition and immunity: antibody impairs memory. *Immunity* Vol.21 No.2, (August 2004). pp. 179–188.

Fattal, I.; Shental, N,, Mevorach, D., Anaya, J.M., Livneh, A., Langevitz, P., Zandman-Goddard, G., Pauzner, R., Lerner, M., Blank, M., Hincapie, M.E., Gafter, U., Naparstek, Y., Shoenfeld, Y., Domany, E., & Cohen IR. (2010) An antibody profile of systemic lupus erythematosus detected by antigen microarray. Immunology. 2010 Vol.130, No.3, (July 2010) pp. 337-343.

Groom, J.R.; Fletcher, C.A., Walters, S.N., Grey, S.T., Watt, S.V., Sweet, M.J., Smyth, M.J., Mackay, C.R., & Mackay, F. (2007) BAFF and MyD88 signals promote a lupuslike disease independent of T cells. *J. Exp. Med.* Vol. 204, No. 8, (August 2007) pp.1959-1971.

Gono, T.; Kawaguchi, Y., Kaneko, H., Nishimura, K., Hanaoka, M., Kataoka, S., Okamoto, Y., Katsumata, Y., & Yamanaka, H. (2011) Anti-NR2A antibody as a predictor for neuropsychiatric systemic lupus Erythematosus. *Rheumatology* Vol.50 (January 2011) Epub ahead of print. doi:10.1093/rheumatology/keq408 ISSN 1462-0332.

Husebye, E. S.; Z. M. Sthoeger, M. Dayan, H. Zinger, D. Elbirt, M. Levite, & E. Mozes. (2005). Autoantibodies to a NR2A peptide of the glutamate/NMDAreceptor in sera of patients with systemic lupus erythematosus. *Ann. Rheum. Dis.* 64, No.8 (August 2005) pp. 1210–1213.

James, J. A.; Gross, T., Scofield, R. H. & Harley, J. B. (1995). Immunoglobulin epitope spreading and autoimmune disease after peptide immunization: Sm B/B -derived PPPGMRPP and PPPGIRGP induce spliceosome autoimmunity. *J. Exp .Med.* Vol.181, No.2 (February 2005), pp. 453–461.

Kowal, C.; DeGiorgio, L. A., Nakaoka, T., Hetherington, H., Huerta, P. T., Diamond, B. & Volpe, B. T. (2004). Cognition and immunity: antibody impairs memory. *Immunity* Vol.21 No.2, (August 2004). pp. 179–188.

Li Q.Z.; Xie C., Wu, T., Mackay, M., Aranow, C., Putterman, C., & Mohan, C. (2005) Identification of autoantibody clusters that best predict lupus disease activity using glomerular proteome arrays. *J Clin Invest.* Vol.115, No. 12, (December 2005) pp.3428–3439.

Li, Q.Z.; Karp, D.R., Quan, J., Branch, V.K., Zhou. J., Lian, Y., Chong, B.F., Wakeland, E.K., & Olsen, N.J. (2011). Risk factors for ANA positivity in healthy persons. *Arthritis Research & Therapy* 2011 13 No.2 (March 2011):R38.

Mage, R.G.; Lanning,D., & Knight, K.L. (2006). B cell and antibody repertoire development in rabbits: the requirement of gut-associated lymphoid tissues. *Develop. Comp. Immunol.* Vol.30, No.1-2, (January February 2006) pp.137-153.

Mason, L.J.; Timothy, L.M., Isenberg, D.A., & Kalsi, J.K. (1999) Immunization with a peptide of Sm B/B' results in limited epitope spreading but not autoimmune disease. *J. Immunol.* Vol.162, No.9, (May, 1999) pp. 5099-5105.

Petri, M.; Stohl, W., Chatham, W., McCune, W.J., Chevrier, M., Ryel, J., Recta, V., Zhong, J., & Freimuth, W. (2008) Association of plasma B lymphocyte stimulator levels and disease activity in systemic lupus erythematosus. *Arthritis Rheum.* Vol.58, No. 8 (August, 2008) pp.2453-2459.

Puliyath, N.; Ray, S., Milton, J., & Mage R. G. (2008) Genetic contributions to the autoantibody profile in a rabbit model of systemic lupus erythematosus (SLE). *Vet. Immunol. Immunopathol.* Vol.125, No.3-4, (October 2008), pp. 251-267.

Quintana, F.J.; Hagedorn, P.H., Elizur. G., Merbl. Y., Domany, E., & , Cohen I.R. (2004) Functional immunomics: microarray analysis of IgG autoantibody repertoires predicts the future response of mice to induced diabetes. *Proc Natl Acad Sci USA* Vol.101, Suppl 2 (October 2004) pp. 14615-14621.

Rai, G.; Ray, S., Shaw, R. E., DeGrange, P. F., Mage, R. G., & Newman, B. A. (2006). Models of systemic lupus erythematosus: Development of autoimmunity following peptide immunizations of noninbred pedigreed rabbits. *J. Immunol.* Vol.176, No.1 (January 2006), pp. 660-667.

Rai, G.; Ray S., Milton, J., Yang, J., Ren, P., Lempicki, R., & Mage, R.G. (2010). Gene expression profiles in a rabbit model of systemic lupus erythematosus autoantibody production. *J. Immunol.* Vol.185, No.7 (October 2010), pp. 4446-4456.

Robinson, W.H.; DiGennaro, C., Hueber, W., Haab, B.B., Kamachi, M., Dean, E.J., Fournel, S., Fong, D., Genovese, M.C., de Vegvar, H.E., Skriner, K., Hirschberg, D.L., Morris, R.I., Muller, S., Pruijn, G.J., van Venrooij, W.J., Smolen, J.S., Brown, P.O., Steinman, L., & Utz, P.J. (2002) Autoantigen microarrays for multiplex characterization of autoantibody responses. Nature Medicine Vol. 8, No. (March 2002), pp. 295-301.

Sanchez-Guerrero, J.; Aranow, C., Mackay, M., Volpe, B. & Diamond, B.(2008) Neuropsychiatric systemic lupus erythematosus reconsidered. *Nature Clinical Practice Rheumatology* Vol 4. No. 3 (March 2008) pp. 112-113.

Yang, J.; Pospisil, R. & Mage, R.G. (2009a). Expression and localization of rabbit B-cell activating factor (BAFF) and its specific receptor BR3 in cells and tissues of the rabbit immune system. *Develop. Comp. Immunol.* Vol.33, No.5 (May 2009), pp. 697-708.

Yang, J.; Pospisil, R., Ray, S., Milton, J., & Mage, R. G. (2009b) Investigations of a rabbit (*Oryctolagus cuniculus*) model of systemic lupus erythematosus (SLE), BAFF and its receptors. *PLoS ONE* Vol.4, No.12, (December 2009) e8494, Open Access online.

Yeramilli, V.A. & Knight, K.L (2010) Requirement for BAFF and APRIL during B Cell Development in GALT. *J. Immunol.* Vol. 184, No. 10 (May 2010) pp. 5527-5536.

9

Embryonic and Placental Damage Induced by Maternal Autoimmune Diseases - What Can We Learn from Experimental Models

Zivanit Ergaz[1] and Asher Ornoy[2]
[1]Laboratory of Teratology, Israel Canada Institute of Medical Research
Hebrew University Hadassah Medical School, Jerusalem
Department of Neonatology, Hadassah-Hebrew University Hospital
Mount Scopus, Jerusalem
[2]Laboratory of Teratology, Israel Canada Institute of Medical Research, Hebrew University
Hadassah Medical School, Jerusalem, Israel and Israeli Ministry of Health
Israel

1. Introduction

Autoimmune diseases may have an adverse effect on reproduction and pregnancy outcome. Systemic Lupus Erythematosus (SLE) is associated with a wide variety of antibodies to different cell body components, mostly antiphospholipid antibodies. These are a heterogeneous group of antibodies that bind to negatively charged phospholipids and/or serum phospholipid binding proteins. Antiphospholipid syndrome (APLs) may occur as primary APLs or in association with autoimmune diseases. During normal pregnancy maternal immunity and hormones allow fetal survival, but when these mechanisms are impaired it may have a detrimental effect on the fetus. Pregnancies in women with APLs can be complicated by a high rate of pregnancy loss, pre-eclampsia, fetal growth restriction, prematurity and fetal distress. Disease flare during pregnancy predicts adverse fetal outcome (Kwok et al., 2011). The mechanisms underlying the recurrent abortions and fetal loss among women suffering from SLE are not completely elucidated. Thrombotic placental events may explain only some of the miscarriages. In vitro cell culture of placental trophoblast cell lines with IgG from patients suffering from APLs showed that APLs/ anti-β2-glycoprotein I antibodies / anti-β 2 globulin antibodies might disrupt the annexin coverage of thrombogenic anionic surfaces on the trophoblast and endothelial cell monolayers and lead to Factor X and prothrombin activation (Rand et al., 1997). However histopathological findings suggestive of thrombosis cannot be detected in the majority of the placentas from women suffering from APLs (Levy et al., 1998, Meroni et al., 2008). It has been suggested that antiphosholipids may be responsible for a local acute inflammatory response mediated by complement activation and neutrophil infiltration that eventually leads to fetal loss. Circulating antiphospholipid antibodies occurring at about 40% of SLE patients are associated with fetal loss. Some investigators regard APLs as a marker for recurrent abortions and not necessarily as their primary cause. Lupus anticoagulants, anticardiolipin and anti-β2-glycoprotein I antibodies are typically found among the patients. Complement activation was shown to play a role in antiphospholipid antibody - mediated fetal loss associated with inflammatory process, when C4d, a degradation product of C4 was demonstrated in human placenta of SLE patients (Cohen et al., 2011), as well as diminished number of T regulatory cells, associated with pregnancy loss and pre-eclampsia (Tower et al., 2011). Circulating microparticles that expose phospholipids in the outer membrane and induce coagulation via tissue factor have been associated with lupus anticoagulants and poor obstetric outcome (Alijotas-Reig et al., 2009). Other reports indicate that enhanced oxidative stress could be linked to autoimmune diseases; however, there is lack of data about anti oxidant status of the placenta and embryos during pregnancy in women suffering from autoimmune diseases.

2. The role of experimental animal studies in evaluation of pregnancy complications among women suffering from autoimmune diseases

As more than one mechanism of pathogenesis exists for fetal damage in autoimmune diseases, experimental animal models can be used to isolate the different causative effects. Evaluation of the role of different antibodies and molecules can be obtained by direct injection or induction of antibodies production in the pregnant animals and evaluation of the resultant effect on the embryos and fetuses. In such case the effect is evaluated in normal animals rather than being secondary to an autoimmune disease.

Previous published studies revealed fetal damage induced by various antibodies. A smaller litter size was demonstrated after the injection to pregnant BALB/C mice with a human cytomegalovirus -peptide-induced monoclonal antiphospholipid (Gharavi et al., 2004). Fetal heart block and bradycardia were evidenced in a murine model as a result of maternal autoantibodies to Ro and La antigen induced by maternal immunization (Suzuki et al., 2005). In addition maternal immunization with DNA memitope in mice led to the induction of autoantibodies that bind DNA and the N-methyl-D-aspartate receptor in the maternal circulation leading to increased neocortical cell death in the fetal brain and subsequent delayed acquisition of neonatal reflexes and cognitive impairments in the adult offspring. In this model the antibodies that were detected in the fetal neocortex outside of blood vessels evidenced their transport through fetal circulation until binding to the fetal brain (Lee et al., 2009). We previously found that the immunization of BALB /C mice with mouse laminin-1 was followed by the development of anti-laminin-1 antibodies. A double fetal resorption rate and lower fetal and placental weight was found in the laminin-1 immunized group compared with controls. Resorption rate was highest in the subgroup of animals with very high levels of anti-laminin-1 (Matalon et al., 2003). Other molecules were also found to have direct embryotoxic effects. The injection of a low-molecular weight fraction of boiled human serum containing antiphospholipid antibodies that had been obtained from women with antiphospholipid syndrome to pregnant rats at day 5 - 6 of pregnancy resulted in increased embryonic apoptosis 2 to 4 hours after the injection (Halperin et al., 2008).

3. In vitro systems to evaluate sera toxicity in autoimmune diseases

To try to evaluate the different mechanisms that lead to poor obstetric outcome we practiced three in vitro systems that use sera obtained from patients suffering from autoimmune diseases and recurrent abortions as culture media.

3.1 In vitro development of pre-implantation mice embryos in culture

Mouse blastocysts obtained from the uterine horns before implantation at 3.5 days of gestation can be cultured for up to 10 days and reach the developmental stage equivalent of 9.5 to 10 days of gestation in utero, or one-half of the total gestational period. At that early somite stage, the blood circulation in the yolk sac is not yet established and the anterior neuropore is open. The limb buds and the primordia of the lung, liver, and pancreas are not yet present (Chen & Hsu, 1982).

The technology in brief: Female mice are treated with gonadotropins followed 48 h later by Human Chorionic Gonadotropin in order to cause super-ovulation. The mice are mated with males and insemination is verified the following morning by the finding of a copulation plug in the vagina (day 0). Late morula-early blastocyst stages are obtained by flushing the uterine horns with culture medium 3 days after mating. Embryos are removed from several mice, pooled in an embryological watchglass, washed and transferred to fresh medium. A group of 8-10 embryos are placed in drops with Eagle's medium supplemented with 50% or 80% human serum. L Glutamine is added to the medium in a concentration of 2 mM/cc. Embryos are cultured in a humidified atmosphere in unaerobic conditions under paraffin drops. They are checked before incubation, after 24 and 72 hours or other incubation times under an inverted microscope to determine the developmental stage. The parameters used as criteria for assessing the rate of development and differentiation of embryos are namely, hatching of blastocysts from the zona pellucida, their adhesion to the substratum, and outgrowth and spreading on the surface (Abir et al., 1990).

Using this method, one can examine direct effects of the sera from women with recurrent abortions on early pre-implantation embryos.

3.2 In vitro development of early somite stage rat embryos in culture

The early somite rat embryo culture allows the investigation of the embryotoxicity of various teratogens in face of the difficulty to perform studies on mammalian embryos while in utero (New et al., 1976). It is an in vitro method to evaluate teratogenicity of various chemicals (i.e. different drugs and chemicals) as the tested compounds are added to the culture medium and the embryos cultured during organogenesis (New et al., 1976). The various agents can be evaluated either individually or in combination. Adverse embryonic outcomes (malformations or embryolethality) were shown to be directly related to the serum concentration of the compound being tested and can be compared to the serum concentration in the human. Moreover, as embryos can also be cultured directly on human serum, it may serve as a tool to investigate the direct effects of sera from women with different diseases on embryonic development. Additionally, the early somite rat embryo culture model can allow the evaluation of success of various treatment modalities and thus may be an important tool to predict the outcome of the pregnancy. This can be achieved due to the yolk sac (the chorioallantoic placental equivalent at this stage in rat pregnancy) which provides a large surface area for nutritional and respiratory exchange between the embryo and the culture medium. Previous studies proved that rat conceptuses explanted at 9.5-12.5 days, when the embryo develops from the early neurula to the late tail bud stage, can be maintained in vitro for 48 hours with almost 100% survival and growth that is indistinguishable from that occurring in vivo.

The technology in brief: Pregnant female rats are euthanized on day 9.5 to 12.5 of pregnancy when sperm finding is considered to be day 0. The embryos are cultured for 28-48 hours at

37°C in rotating bottles, and supplemented with gas mixtures: day-1: 20% Oxygen, 75% N2, 5% CO2, and day-2: 40% oxygen, 55% N2, and 5% CO2. After 28-48 hours of culture the embryos are examined under a dissecting microscope and scored according to the method described by Brown et al (Brown & Fabro, 1981) and us (Abir & Ornoy, 1996, Abir et al., 1994). Only embryos with a beating heart are examined for yolk sac size and circulation, axial rotation, neural tube closure, presence of telencephalic vesicles, optic and otic vesicles, number of somites, body size, and presence of gross anomalies. The use of morphological scoring system provides an index for embryonic development proportional to the embryonic age and aids in the detection of anomalies induced by the different teratogens. The embryos and yolk sacs are kept for different morphological, biochemical and molecular studies.

The possible direct effects of the sera from women with autoimmune diseases can be examined on cultured rat embryos using sera or IgG obtained from women with SLE/APLs as the culture medium, and analyzing the effects these sera has on embryonic growth, rate of anomalies, and ultrastructural yolk sac damage compared to sera from control healthy women and control rats.

3.3 Human placental explants in culture

The use of first trimester chorionic villi explants cultures has the advantage over cell culture of being the in vivo source of extravillous trophoblast and the preservation of topological and functional villous-extravillous trophoblast inter-relationships. It was demonstrated that first trimester villous explants maintained on Matrigel or rat tail collagen support the villous explants differentiation, migration and hormone production in 98 per cent of cultures (Genbacev et al., 1992). The study of placental explants in culture, where no blood circulation exists, enabled the evaluation of the direct effects of different sera on the placenta, thus exposing the mechanisms of placental damage other than placental infarcts, thrombosis and vasculopathy.

The technique in brief: Placental tissue of 5.5–7.5 weeks of gestation are transferred on sterile gauze in an ice-cold phosphate-buffered saline and then removed to a Petri dish and rinsed in phosphate buffered saline. Placental tissue is dissected from deciduas and fetal membranes for inspection under a dissecting microscope. Explants of approximately 10 mg wet weight are transferred into Millicell-CM culture dish insert (Millipore, Bedford, MA), which has been previously layered with polymerized Matrigel® (Collaborative Research, Bedford, MA). The inserts are then placed in 24-well culture dishes. Explants are placed in incubator (5% CO2) for 60 min at 39°C to evaporate phosphate buffered saline droplets to assist in villi adherence to the thin layer of Matrigel®. Cultures are incubated overnight in an incubator with 5% CO2. Twelve hours from the initiation of culture 400 μl of different types of different sera enriched with 1 mg glucose/ml are added directly to the inserts. Both the media from the insert (top) and the well (bottom) are changed every 48 hr, collected, and stored at -20°C until assayed. Villous explants are inspected daily using an inverted phase-contrast microscope for general cellular integrity, cellular proliferation, and outgrowth. The explants remain in culture for 4 days. At the end of the experiment, villi with supporting Matrigel® are dissected out using surgical blades and kept for morphological, immunohistochemical biochemical and molecular studies, and the media is removed for the analysis of major hormones secreted by the placental tissue.

To evaluate the possibility that in SLE/APLs at least some of the antibodies may directly damage placental trophoblastic cells, consequently causing fetal damage that may lead to intrauterine growth restriction or fetal death and to evaluate therapeutic interventions we used human placental explants in culture.

4. In vitro studies of embryotoxicity of sera from women with recurrent abortions on pre-implantation mice in culture

4.1 The embryotoxicity of sera from women with recurrent abortions on pre-implantation mice in culture

Mouse blastocysts 3.5-day-old at late morula stage and inside the zona pellucida, were cultured for 72 h in 50% or 80% sera from women with recurrent abortions. In embryos cultured in sera from women with recurrent abortions, 53.2% did not reach blastocystic development, compared to 33.6% of the embryos grown on sera from women after only one miscarriage and 8.2% and 12% on control sera from women following delivery of a normal infant or on sera obtained from women in the second trimester of a normal pregnancy respectively. When sera from women with miscarriages were divided into "high risk'"(50% or more embryotoxicity) and "low risk"(less than 50% embryotoxicity) sera, the "high risk" sera from two or more miscarriages caused an average of 72.1% undevelopment (i.e. not reaching the blastocystic stage), while the "low risk" sera from the same group caused 33.6% undevelopment. The "high risk" sera from one miscarriage were embryotoxic to 55.8% of the blastocysts and the "low risk" sera from the same group caused only 8.7% undevelopment similar to the controls (Abir et al., 1990).

4.2 The limitations of the pre-implantation rat culture

The limitations of this method is that it is impossible to evaluate even early post-implantation periods that equivalents early organogenesis. It cannot be used for the study of growth restriction and for the effects of teratogens which affect the embryo in later stage. In addition, the small embryonic size limits the possibility to perform various biochemical and genetic studies and does not allow the investigation of the effect of the different chemicals on isolated organs.

In conclusion: More pre-implantation mouse blastocytes failed to reach blastocystic development when cultured in sera obtained from women with recurrent abortions compared to those cultured in control sera.

5. In vitro studies of the embryotoxicity of sera from patients suffering from systemic lupus erythematosus/antiphospholipid syndrome on early somite rat embryos in culture

5.1 The role of IgG antibodies in recurrent abortions

To test the hypothesis that IgG antibodies from women with recurrent abortions may be responsible for the miscarriage, sera from women one day after an abortion were used as culture media for 10.5 days old embryos and compared to human control sera obtained from women either during a second trimester of a normal pregnancy or a day after normal delivery. Anomalies rate increased from 22% among controls to 47% among embryos cultured in sera from women who had a history of one abortion and to 54% among embryos cultured in sera from women who had a history of two abortions or more. Anomalies included mainly microcephaly, open neural tube, lack of eyes and cardiac anomalies. The difference between the sera was more prominent when the sera were classified as low- less than 50% anomalies compared to high-more than 50%. The high rate of anomalies was particularly characteristic to the highly teratogenic sera while in the other sera anomalies rate was similar to controls. This difference may indicate a basic difference between the two sera groups: one that has a factor(s) that is teratogenic in this model and the other that induces abortions in a different mechanism that is not relevant to this model.

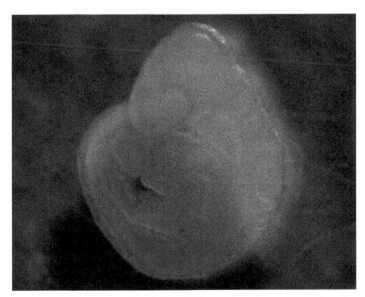

Fig. 1. Early somite 10.5 days rat embryo after 28 hours in culture: normal embryo

To further evaluate whether the embryotoxic factor in this model is IgG, we used high risk sera and control sera, separated the IgG fraction and exchanged it between the sera. We defined three groups: one in which IgG from controls corrected the anomalies induced by the toxic sera, and the IgG from toxic sera induced anomalies in the embryos cultured in the control sera, the second in which control sera did not reduce the rate of anomalies but the IgG induced anomalies in the controls, and the third in which no effect was demonstrated after IgG exchange. We assumed that in these embryos a different factor was responsible for the teratogenicity. When the yolk sacs were evaluated by transmission electron microscopy we found a morphological damage represented by fewer microvilli and more inclusions in the entodermal epithelial cell in the sacs from embryos cultured in high risk sera (Abir et al., 1993).

5.2 The role of IgG antibodies in intra-uterine growth restriction
Besides recurrent abortions and fetal death, a main morbidity among infants of mothers suffering from autoimmune diseases is intra-uterine growth restriction. To investigate the role of the IgG antibodies on embryonic and fetal growth we evaluated the effect of high levels of antiphospholipid and anti DNA antibodies on 11.5 days rat embryos in culture, a stage when most of the organs have already been formed. Reduced fetal growth and yolk

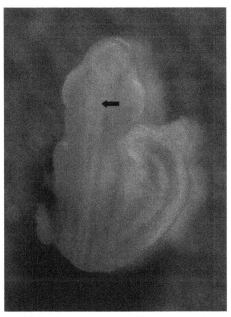

Fig. 2. Early somite 10.5 days rat embryo after 28 hours in culture: arrow-open neural tube

sac diameter were found in embryos cultured in media containing IgG from women suffering from SLE / recurrent abortions, compared to IgG from controls or medium without IgG. When we evaluated the role of the different IgG fractions (anticardiolipin-β2 glycoprotein, antiphosphatidylserine, anti-double stranded DNA, anti-laminin, anti-thyroglobulin and anti-pyruvate dehydrogenase) compared to controls, only embryos that were cultured in sera positive for anti-cardiolipin were significantly smaller than the embryos cultured in sera containing normal IgG fractions. The embryos cultured in medium containing anticardiolipin/ anti DNA/ antiphosphatidylserine had a smaller yolk sac. However, embryos cultured in sera from SLE patients with a history of recurrent abortions were also smaller even when they were negative for antiphosphatydilserine. In spite of the fact that in these experiments the embryos were cultured towards the end of organogenesis when many of the organs have already been formed, 15.6% of the embryos exposed to IgG purified from women suffering from SLE / recurrent abortions had anomalies, while only 8.7% of the embryos exposed to IgG purified from sera of healthy women were malformed. There was a significant difference in the development of the brain and branchial bars between embryos that were exposed to patients' IgG and those exposed to IgG that was purified from healthy women. There was also a significant reduced somite number among the experimental group embryos (Matalon et al., 2002).

5.3 The effect of IgG antibodies on the yolk sac

The embryos at the early somite stage are surrounded by their yolk sac and by their ectoplacental cone which is the trophoblastic part of the cellular complex at the embryonic pole of the blastocyst. The ectoplacental cone is responsible for the invasion into the decidua. To evaluate the mechanism by which IgG affects the yolk sac, 11.5 days old embryos were cultured in two human IgG2 monoclonal antiphosphatidylserine antibodies

(HL5B, RR7F). The antiphosphatidylserine antibodies were associated with implantation failure in previous studies with mainly trophoblastic injury by inhibition of syncytium formation, decreased human chorionic gonadatropin (hCG) production, and disturbed trophoblast invasion (McIntyre, 2003). The HL5B monoclonal antibody was generated from a primary antiphospholipid syndrome patient with multiple central ischemic events and the RR7F monoclonal antibody was generated from SLE patient with high titers of circulating antiphosphatidylserine and anticardiolipin antibodies, with no history of thrombosis or fetal loss. Both antibodies showed reactivity against phosphatidylserine and cross-reactivity with cardiolipin but lacked reactivity against β2-glycoprotein and did not have a lupus anticoagulant activity. Embryos cultured in both sera had reduced yolk sac diameter without significant difference in the rate of anomalies. Apoptotic processes were found in some of the giant cells and in most of the cells located in the area between the mature giant cells to the small cytotrophoblastic mononuclear cells. More apoptotic cells were counted within the ectoplacental giant cells exposed to anti phosphatidylserine in comparison with cells that were exposed to the control human IgG. More than 19% of the giant cells that were exposed to HL5B (from the patient with multiple ischemic events) underwent apoptosis, while only 12.7%of the cells exposed to RR7F (from the patient with high titers of circulating antiphosphatidylserine and anticardiolipin, with no thrombosis neither fetal loss) and 7.3 and 9.6% of the cells exposed to the control IgG or the experimental medium alone underwent apoptosis. Both antibodies stained the ectoplacental cone in the rat embryos most strongly with the moderately larger cell layer. Cytotrophoblastic mononuclear cells, which are located in the center of the ectoplacental cone, were not stained. The control antibodies did not stain the ectoplacental cone at all. Immunofluorescence staining proved that the anti phosphatidylserine monoclonal antibodies, reacted with 11.5-day ectoplacental cone cells (Matalon et al., 2004).

5.4 The embryotoxicity of oxidative stress

The role of oxidative damage in disease activity among patients suffering from autoimmune diseases has become more evident in the last decade (Wang et al., 2010). Reactive Oxygen Species (ROS) have been implicated in causing immunogenic modifications in the DNA and causing oxidative damage that may lead to various autoimmune and degenerative diseases. Excessive ROS production which disturbs redox status, may damage macromolecules and modulate the expression of a variety of immune and inflammatory molecules leading to inflammatory processes and affecting tissue damage (Nathan, 2002).

The role of oxidative stress in SLE was demonstrated in various studies including: an association of the oxidative stress parameters with the pro-inflammatory cytokines (Shah et al., 2011b); exposure of purified human dsDNA resulting in ROS production that led to changes in the primary structure of the dsDNA that rendered it highly immunogenic when injected into rabbits (Al Arfaj et al., 2007); a positive correlation between apoptotic cell numbers and ROS production and increased numbers of apoptotic cells positively correlating with lipid peroxidation in SLE patients (Shah et al., 2011a). The Conflicting results on antioxidant enzyme activities may be due to continued oxidative stress and measurement of different components of the antioxidant system at different disease stages (Ames et al., 1999, Whitaker & Knight, 2008, Zaken et al., 2000). However the role of oxidative stress in recurrent fetal death and growth restriction is unclear.

Despite medical treatment, women with autoimmune diseases suffer from increased rate of pregnancy complication. We tried to determine if during remission there is a relation between

the clinical history of the SLE patients (i.e. recurrent abortions and/or thromboembolic event)
and the morphologic and functional damage which their sera induce on the 10.5 days rat
embryos and yolk sac in culture. We used as culture media sera from SLE /APLs patients
during remission (The APLs patients were at least one year free of clotting events and the SLE
patients had SLEDAI (Systemic lupus erythematosus disease activity index-a commulative
clinical and laboratory index with higher scores representing increased disease activity) 2000
less than 4 and compared it to control human sera. The survival of the embryos cultured in
sera of SLE /APLs women decreased significantly from 87.5% to 70.9% in comparison to
embryos cultured in control sera. There was a positive correlation between survival rate, the
neurological developmental stage (calculated by summing the score given for the caudal
neural tube, hind, mid and forebrain) and number of somites. Additionally a significant
positive correlation between the growth parameters was demonstrated among the embryos
cultured in sera from patients and controls: the larger embryos had larger yolk sacs; had
higher general and neurologic developmental score and more somites, implying more mature
embryos. (Ergaz et al., 2010). A high rate of anomalies in embryos cultured in sera from
women with recurrent spontaneous abortions (Abir et al., 1994) or following the addition to
the culture medium of purified IgG from SLE and APLs patients (Abir & Ornoy, 1996),
differed from the study using sera obtained from non-pregnant patients in remission, where
there was no increase in the rate of anomalies compared to controls. It can be speculated
therefore, that the teratogenicity of the sera reflected the patient's high-activity disease state
(Clowse et al., 2005). Delayed neurological system development when the brain structures
development were behind the other embryonic systems was the predominant finding in
correlation with clinical studies published in the medical literature that reported learning and
memory impairment among offspring of mothers with SLE (Urowitz et al., 2008, Ross et al.,
2003) and the finding that the main anomalies in our previous studies were neural tube defects
(Abir et al., 1994). We speculate that the low activity of the disease allowed high survival and
low anomalies rate in most of the sera but some sera remained teratogenic due to factors that
were still active despite remission. We defined two sera groups: "toxic" sera with over-all
survival rate under ⅔ and those cultured in "non-toxic" sera with over-all survival above ⅔. In
order to define the characteristics of the "toxic" sera we analyzed the correlations between the
survival rate, the growth parameters, maternal laboratory findings regarding APLs and the
clinical history of the patients. We did not find a correlation between sera toxicity and: the
diagnosis of APLs; The levels of the specific antibodies (anti-double stranded DNA, anti-single
stranded DNA and the antiphospholipid antibodies: anti cardiolipin, anti-$\beta2$ glycoprotein,
antiphosphatidylserine, antiphosphatidylcholine and antiphosphatidylethanolamine) which
were high compared to human controls. There was no significant correlation between the
survival rate and any specific antibody measured in those sera, the history of recurrent
abortions and toxemia and the history of thrombo-embolic attacks. The yolk sac function was
evaluated by measuring the 14C sucrose endocytic index which did not differ between the
controls and SLE/APLs non toxic sera, this is explained by the fact that we studied the index
only in "non toxic" sera.

To evaluate the antioxidant defense mechanisms which include a variety of intracellular
enzymes we evaluated superoxide dismutase, catalase like activity, and low molecular
weight antioxidants. The low molecular weight antioxidants includes lypophilic and
hydrophilic molecules like glutathione, carnosine, ascorbate (vitamin C), tocopherol
(vitamin E), carotenoids (vitamin A), bilirubin, uric acid and flavonoids, which act directly
with various reactive oxygen species, DNA repair enzymes and methionine sulphoxide

reductase that repair or remove reactive oxygen species-damaged biomolecules (Ornoy et al., 1999). Our previous studies on the reducing power of the low molecular weight antioxidants in control rat embryos and yolk sacs revealed only one peak 1 at 560-620 mvolts on 9.5-11.5 days of gestation and an additional peak (peak 2) at 950-970 mvolts first appearing on day 11.5 of gestation (Zaken et al., 2000), which is the day we ended our culture. The major components of peak 1 as measured by HPLC are ascorbic and uric acids, Tryptophan, carnosine, melatonine (Beit-Yannai et al., 1997) and thioacetic acid (Chevion et al., 2000) were found to be the major components of peak 2 in the rat brain . The low molecular weight antioxidants were evaluated by cyclic voltametry (Zaken et al., 2000). Most of the embryos cultured in the "toxic" SLE /APLs sera did not have the peak 2 of the low molecular weight antioxidants. The lack of the peak 2 in the present study may be the reflection of the delayed embryonic maturation as the embryos were smaller and less developed. This is similar to our finding of decreased low molecular weight antioxidants demonstrated by the absence of peak 2, in 10.5 days embryos cultured for 28 hours under diabetic conditions (Zaken et al., 2000). There was also a positive correlation between a lower peak 1 of low molecular weight antioxidants and recurrent abortions in the embryos cultured in the SLE / APLs sera that was not related to sera toxicity. Catalase and superoxide dismutase activity did not vary between the groups. It is unknown whether the oxidative insult has a similar effect on the different developing organs. We evaluated the oxidative stress in the total embryo, while the different organs and systems in the rat embryo may have different expressions under similar circumstances (Dubnov et al., 2000). The normal levels of the anti oxidant enzymes evaluated may indicate that sera toxicity is not related to oxidative stress. We did not find any past clinical history or laboratory finding that was in correlation with the sera embryotoxicity. The possible causes for the high embryotoxicity of about half of the sera in remission are currently unknown.

5.5 The effect of maternal medical treatment on sera teratogenicity
The role of some treatment modalities was evaluated by rat embryo cultures in sera from women with and without medications. We examined 10.5 days old embryos cultured in sera from women suffering from SLE complicated by recurrent abortions, either untreated women, or treated with steroids and aspirin and compared the results to embryos cultured in sera from control women and to a pool of control rat sera. Untreated sera resulted in 45.1% death rate compared to 29.8% in treated sera, 3.9% in control human and 5.1% in control rat serum. Malformation rate decreased from 73.3% in untreated sera to 37.5% in treated sera, 10.2% in human controls and 5.4% in rat controls. Malformations were mostly in the heart, brain, limbs and tail (Ornoy et al., 1998). Thus, treatment that improves pregnancy outcome also reduces the embryotoxic effects of the sera.

5.6 The effect of maternal medical treatment on the extent of yolk sac damage
Transmission electron microscopy of the yolk sacs revealed an increase in intracellular inclusions and decrease in microvilli number in both experimental groups, embryos cultured in sera from treated or untreated patients compared to controls. Scanning electron microscope revealed abnormally large entodermal cells, a decreased number of microvilli with sometimes crater formation (Ornoy et al., 1998). The anticoagulant treatment reduced fetal anomalies rate but did not improve yolk sac damage implying that yolk sac damage is only a component in the different factors leading to fetal damage.

5.7 The limitations of the early somite rat embryo culture system

By using the early somite rat embryo culture system we evaluated the direct effect of sera
from patients suffering from autoimmune diseases and analyzed the levels of the different
sera variables during flare and remission. The impact of the different sera was not universal,
and only some of the sera caused embryonic damage. Since the antiphospholipid antibodies
were proven as the cause of embryotoxic effect only in some of the sera, we believe that
other mechanisms are involved in the teratogenic effect and growth restriction as well. A
disadvantage of this in vitro testing are also the limited culture time and limited period of
embryogenesis that is undertaken in the commonly used culture system which restricts the
range of embryotoxicity that can be induced. It may, therefore, render the testing system
unsuitable for teratogens that are likely to exert their major toxicological effect very early or
late in gestation (Webster et al., 1997). Additionally we evaluated embryonic growth,
structural anomalies and yolk sac function. Infants of mothers who suffer from SLE
experience mainly intra-uterine growth retardation, which may be more prominent at the
final pregnancy stages not in correlation with the pregnancy stage of early somite rat
embryos. The lack of change in oxidative stress parameters may reflect the evaluation of the
embryo as a whole. It is unknown whether the oxidative insult has a similar effect on the
different developing organs. The different organs and systems in the rat embryo may have
different expressions under similar circumstances as shown in another murine model
(Dubnov et al., 2000).

In conclusion: Early somite rat embryos cultured in sera from women who suffered from
autoimmune diseases had lower survival rate, increase anomalies rate and delayed
maturation as reflected by their lower morphological score and less developed anti-oxidant
system. The damage was related to IgG antibodies only in some of the embryos.
Morphologic yolk sac damage was constant and did not improve with maternal medical
treatment.

6. Placental explants studies

6.1 The effect of SLE/APLs sera on placental explants

At the early somite stage the yolk sac is the equivalent of the human chorioallantoic
placenta. The inhibition of yolk sac growth even without inhibition of embryonic growth, as
well as ultrastructural damage to the yolk sac endothelial cells may indicate that the
primary insult or at least a major insult in SLE /APLs and recurrent abortions may be
damage to the placenta.

We therefore examined the effects of sera from the patients on early human placental explants
obtained from interruptions of normal 5.5 to 7.5 week-old pregnancies (because of
psychosocial reasons), and compared to the effects of sera from healthy women and of a
chemically defined medium. Placental explants cultured on sera from untreated non-pregnant
women with SLE/APLs demonstrated a significant decrease in the trophoblastic cell
proliferation rate compared with non-pregnant control women (Ornoy et al., 2003). Placental
extracts cultured in SLE/APLs had a higher rate of apoptosis, and reduced βhCG secretion in
correlation with antiphospholipid antibodies levels. The sera were analyzed for the presence
and quantification of anti-double stranded DNA, anti-single stranded DNA and
antiphospholipid antibodies (anti cardiolipin, anti-β2glycoprotein, antiphosphatidylserine,
antiphosphatidylcholine and antiphosphatidylethanolamine) and Anti-Ro and anti-La. High
levels of all the different antiphospholipid atibodies and both anti-dsDNA and anti-ssDNA

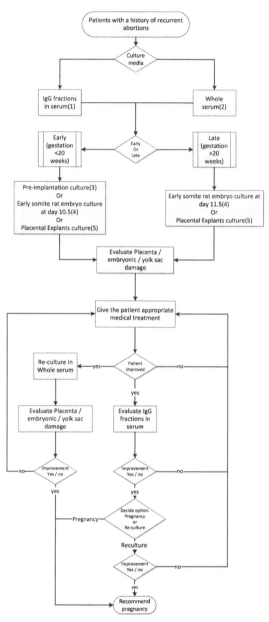

(1) More specific, embryotoxic in 2/3 of the sera.
(2) Less specific but allows to investigate the multi factorial mechanisms of embryotoxicity.
(3) Evaluate blastocystic development.
(4) Evaluate: Embryonic survival, score, anomalies rate and yolk sac apoptosis.
(5) Evaluate trophoblastic cell proliferation, apoptosis and βhCG secretion.

Fig. 3. In vitro cultures as an aid in clinical decisions making for recurrent abortions

showed a trend towards reduction in βhCG secretion by the placental extracts in culture. Titers of anti-Ro and anti-La did not correlate with a reduction in the βhCG levels, probably because anti-Ro and anti-La antibodies exert their effect on pregnancy by a passively transferred autoimmune disease in fetuses or newborns, causing neonatal lupus and not through placental damage. There was no specific single antibody that could be identified to cause the placental damage, but rather a combination of different antibodies was responsible for the cumulative damage, in accordance with the inconsistent findings of the effects of the different antiphospholipid antibodies (Schwartz et al., 2007).

6.2 The effect of maternal medical treatment on the degree of damage induced in placental explants

When we evaluated the impact of maternal treatment with steroids and/or aspirin on placental explants, treatment significantly increased proliferation rate compared with the untreated group but remained significantly lower than that found in the control non-pregnant women. Additionally, a significant increase in the rate of the trophoblastic cell apoptosis was demonstrated compared to explants cultured in sera from treated or control women. The apoptotic rate, however, was still significantly higher in the treated group than that found in the control human group (Yacobi et al., 2002).

6.3 The limitations of the placental explants culture system

The placental explants system allows the investigation of the direct effect of sera on trophoblastic proliferation. This system where only young human placental explants are cultured does not seem to enable the investigation of late pregnancy damage induced by the various mechanisms. Additionally it does not allow the investigation of growth parameters which tend to impact the fetus at later pregnancy stages.

In conclusion: Placental explants culture in SLE/APLs sera had decreased trophoblastic cells proliferation, a higher rate of apoptosis, and reduced βhCG secretion in correlation with antiphospholipid antibodies levels, and increased yolk sac trophoblastic cell apoptosis.

7. Conclusions

The pathophysiology of fetal loss and growth restriction among patients suffering from SLE/APLs is still an open question that needs to be studied. The pre-implantation murine and early somite rat embryo culture offers a model for evaluation of the direct effect of the different antibodies and molecules on survival and growth at different time points during pregnancy. The concomitant evaluation of the yolk sac function allows the investigation of those molecules on the rodent's placental equivalent. The addition of the human early placental extracts culture improves the understanding of the disturbance to early placental differentiation, migration and hormone production induced by similar teratogens.

8. Future research possibilities

New molecules associated with fetal death, embryotoxicity and growth failure were discovered in the last years. The direct effect of those molecules can be evaluated in vitro on placental explants, murine pre-implantation embryos and on early somite rat embryos in culture in order to isolate the impact that each molecule has, solely or in combination with other molecules on pregnancy outcome. The evaluation of the pathological, immunological and biochemical parameters of the cultured embryos may add more clues to the multi-factorial mechanism of fetal damage among women suffering from autoimmune diseases. The understanding of those mechanisms may help to develop new treatment modalities which can also be evaluated in this model.

9. References

Abir R, Zusman I, Ben Hur H, Yaffe P, & Ornoy A. The effects of serum from women with miscarriages on the in vitro development of mouse preimplantation embryos. Acta Obstet Gynecol Scand. 1990;69(1):27-33.

Abir R, Ornoy A, Ben Hur H, Jaffe P, & Pinus H. IgG exchange as a means of partial correction of anomalies in rat embryos in vitro, induced by sera from women with recurrent abortion. Toxicol In Vitro. 1993 Nov;7(6):817-26.

Abir R, Ornoy A, Ben Hur H, Jaffe P, & Pinus H. The effects of sera from women with spontaneous abortions on the in vitro development of early somite stage rat embryos. Am J Reprod Immunol. 1994 Sep;32(2):73-81.

Abir R, & Ornoy A. Teratogenic IgG from sera of women with spontaneous abortions seem to induce anomalies and yolk sac damage in rat embryos. A possible method to detect abortions of immunologic origin. Am J Reprod Immunol. 1996 Feb;35(2):93-101.

Al Arfaj AS, Chowdhary AR, Khalil N, & Ali R. Immunogenicity of singlet oxygen modified human DNA: implications for anti-DNA antibodies in systemic lupus erythematosus. Clin Immunol. 2007 Jul;124(1):83-9.

Alijotas-Reig J, Palacio-Garcia C, & Vilardell-Tarres M. Circulating microparticles, lupus anticoagulant and recurrent miscarriages. Eur J Obstet Gynecol Reprod Biol. 2009 Jul;145(1):22-6.

Ames PR, Alves J, Murat I, Isenberg DA, & Nourooz-Zadeh J. Oxidative stress in systemic lupus erythematosus and allied conditions with vascular involvement. Rheumatology (Oxford). 1999 Jun;38(6):529-34.

Beit-Yannai E, Kohen R, Horowitz M, Trembovler V, & Shohami E. Changes of biological reducing activity in rat brain following closed head injury: a cyclic voltammetry study in normal and heat-acclimated rats. J Cereb Blood Flow Metab. 1997 Mar;17(3):273-9.

Brown NA, & Fabro S. Quantitation of rat embryonic development in vitro: a morphological scoring system. Teratology. 1981 Aug;24(1):65-78.

Chen LT, & Hsu YC. Development of mouse embryos in vitro: preimplantation to the limb bud stage. Science. 1982 Oct 1;218(4567):66-8.

Chevion S, Roberts MA, & Chevion M. The use of cyclic voltammetry for the evaluation of antioxidant capacity. Free Radic Biol Med. 2000 Mar 15;28(6):860-70.

Clowse ME, Magder LS, Witter F, & Petri M. The impact of increased lupus activity on obstetric outcomes. Arthritis Rheum. 2005 Feb;52(2):514-21.

Cohen D, Buurma A, Goemaere NN, Girardi G, le Cessie S, Scherjon S, et al. Classical complement activation as a footprint for murine and human antiphospholipid antibody-induced fetal loss. J Pathol. 2011 Mar 10.

Dubnov G, Kohen R, & Berry EM. Diet restriction in mice causes differential tissue responses in total reducing power and antioxidant compounds. Eur J Nutr. 2000 Feb;39(1):18-30.

Ergaz Z, Mevorach D, Goldzweig G, Cohen A, Patlas N, Yaffe P, et al. The embryotoxicity of sera from patients with autoimmune diseases on post-implantation rat embryos in culture persists during remission and is not related to oxidative stress. Lupus. 2010 Dec;19(14):1623-31.

Genbacev O, Schubach SA, & Miller RK. Villous culture of first trimester human placenta-- model to study extravillous trophoblast (EVT) differentiation. Placenta. 1992 Sep-Oct;13(5):439-61.

Gharavi AE, Vega-Ostertag M, Espinola RG, Liu X, Cole L, Cox NT, et al. Intrauterine fetal death in mice caused by cytomegalovirus-derived peptide induced aPL antibodies. Lupus. 2004;13(1):17-23.

Halperin R, Elhayany A, Ben-Hur H, Gurevich P, Kaganovsky E, Zusman I, et al. Pathomorphologic and immunohistochemical study on the devastation of rat embryos by antiphospholipid antibody positive serum. Am J Reprod Immunol. 2008 Dec;60(6):523-8.

Kwok LW, Tam LS, Zhu T, Leung YY, & Li E. Predictors of maternal and fetal outcomes in pregnancies of patients with systemic lupus erythematosus. Lupus. 2011 May 4.

Lee JY, Huerta PT, Zhang J, Kowal C, Bertini E, Volpe BT, et al. Neurotoxic autoantibodies mediate congenital cortical impairment of offspring in maternal lupus. Nat Med. 2009 Jan;15(1):91-6.

Levy RA, Avvad E, Oliveira J, & Porto LC. Placental pathology in antiphospholipid syndrome. Lupus. 1998;7 Suppl 2:S81-5.

Matalon ST, Shoenfeld Y, Blank M, Yacobi S, Blumenfeld Z, & Ornoy A. The effects of IgG purified from women with SLE and associated pregnancy loss on rat embryos in culture. Am J Reprod Immunol. 2002 Nov;48(5):296-304.

Matalon ST, Blank M, Matsuura E, Inagaki J, Nomizu M, Levi Y, et al. Immunization of naive mice with mouse laminin-1 affected pregnancy outcome in a mouse model. Am J Reprod Immunol. 2003 Aug;50(2):159-65.

Matalon ST, Shoenfeld Y, Blank M, Yacobi S, von Landenberg P, & Ornoy A. Antiphosphatidylserine antibodies affect rat yolk sacs in culture: a mechanism for fetal loss in antiphospholipid syndrome. Am J Reprod Immunol. 2004 Feb;51(2):144-51.

McIntyre JA. Antiphospholipid antibodies in implantation failures. Am J Reprod Immunol. 2003 Apr;49(4):221-9.

Meroni PL, Gerosa M, Raschi E, Scurati S, Grossi C, & Borghi MO. Updating on the pathogenic mechanisms 5 of the antiphospholipid antibodies-associated pregnancy loss. Clin Rev Allergy Immunol. 2008 Jun;34(3):332-7.

Nathan C. Points of control in inflammation. Nature. 2002 Dec 19-26;420(6917):846-52.

New DA, Coppola PT, & Cockroft DL. Comparison of growth in vitro and in vivo of post-implantation rat embryos. J Embryol Exp Morphol. 1976 Aug;36(1):133-44.

Ornoy A, Yacobi S, Avraham S, & Blumenfeld Z. The effect of sera from women with systemic lupus erythematosus and/or antiphospholipid syndrome on rat embryos in culture. Reprod Toxicol. 1998 Mar-Apr;12(2):185-91.

Ornoy A, Zaken V, & Kohen R. Role of reactive oxygen species (ROS) in the diabetes-induced anomalies in rat embryos in vitro: reduction in antioxidant enzymes and low-molecular-weight antioxidants (LMWA) may be the causative factor for increased anomalies. Teratology. 1999 Dec;60(6):376-86.

Ornoy A, Yacobi S, Matalon ST, Blank M, Blumenfeld Z, Miller RK, et al. The effects of antiphospholipid antibodies obtained from women with SLE/APS and associated pregnancy loss on rat embryos and placental explants in culture. Lupus. 2003;12(7):573-8.

Rand JH, Wu XX, Andree HA, Lockwood CJ, Guller S, Scher J, et al. Pregnancy loss in the antiphospholipid-antibody syndrome--a possible thrombogenic mechanism. N Engl J Med. 1997 Jul 17;337(3):154-60.

Ross G, Sammaritano L, Nass R, & Lockshin M. Effects of mothers' autoimmune disease during pregnancy on learning disabilities and hand preference in their children. Arch Pediatr Adolesc Med. 2003 Apr;157(4):397-402.

Schwartz N, Shoenfeld Y, Barzilai O, Cervera R, Font J, Blank M, et al. Reduced placental growth and hCG secretion in vitro induced by antiphospholipid antibodies but not by anti-Ro or anti-La: studies on sera from women with SLE/PAPS. Lupus. 2007;16(2):110-20.

Shah D, Aggarwal A, Bhatnagar A, Kiran R, & Wanchu A. Association between T lymphocyte sub-sets apoptosis and peripheral blood mononuclear cells oxidative stress in systemic lupus erythematosus. Free Radic Res. 2011a May;45(5):559-67.

Shah D, Wanchu A, & Bhatnagar A. Interaction between oxidative stress and chemokines: Possible pathogenic role in systemic lupus erythematosus and rheumatoid arthritis. Immunobiology. 2011b Apr 13.

Suzuki H, Silverman ED, Wu X, Borges C, Zhao S, Isacovics B, et al. Effect of maternal autoantibodies on fetal cardiac conduction: an experimental murine model. Pediatr Res. 2005 Apr;57(4):557-62.

Tower C, Crocker I, Chirico D, Baker P, & Bruce I. SLE and pregnancy: the potential role for regulatory T cells. Nat Rev Rheumatol. 2011 Feb;7(2):124-8.

Urowitz MB, Gladman DD, MacKinnon A, Ibanez D, Bruto V, Rovet J, et al. Neurocognitive abnormalities in offspring of mothers with systemic lupus erythematosus. Lupus. 2008;17(6):555-60.

Wang G, Pierangeli SS, Papalardo E, Ansari GA, & Khan MF. Markers of oxidative and nitrosative stress in systemic lupus erythematosus: correlation with disease activity. Arthritis Rheum. 2010 Jul;62(7):2064-72.

Webster WS, Brown-Woodman PD, & Ritchie HE. A review of the contribution of whole embryo culture to the determination of hazard and risk in teratogenicity testing. Int J Dev Biol. 1997 Apr;41(2):329-35.

Whitaker BD, & Knight JW. Mechanisms of oxidative stress in porcine oocytes and the role of anti-oxidants. Reprod Fertil Dev. 2008;20(6):694-702.

Yacobi S, Ornoy A, Blumenfeld Z, & Miller RK. Effect of sera from women with systemic lupus erythematosus or antiphospholipid syndrome and recurrent abortions on human placental explants in culture. Teratology. 2002 Dec;66(6):300-8.

Zaken V, Kohen R, & Ornoy A. The development of antioxidant defense mechanism in young rat embryos in vivo and in vitro. Early Pregnancy. 2000 Apr;4(2):110-23.

Permissions

The contributors of this book come from diverse backgrounds, making this book a truly international effort. This book will bring forth new frontiers with its revolutionizing research information and detailed analysis of the nascent developments around the world.

We would like to thank Dr. Hani Almoallim, for lending his expertise to make the book truly unique. He has played a crucial role in the development of this book. Without his invaluable contribution this book wouldn't have been possible. He has made vital efforts to compile up to date information on the varied aspects of this subject to make this book a valuable addition to the collection of many professionals and students.

This book was conceptualized with the vision of imparting up-to-date information and advanced data in this field. To ensure the same, a matchless editorial board was set up. Every individual on the board went through rigorous rounds of assessment to prove their worth. After which they invested a large part of their time researching and compiling the most relevant data for our readers. Conferences and sessions were held from time to time between the editorial board and the contributing authors to present the data in the most comprehensible form. The editorial team has worked tirelessly to provide valuable and valid information to help people across the globe.

Every chapter published in this book has been scrutinized by our experts. Their significance has been extensively debated. The topics covered herein carry significant findings which will fuel the growth of the discipline. They may even be implemented as practical applications or may be referred to as a beginning point for another development. Chapters in this book were first published by InTech; hereby published with permission under the Creative Commons Attribution License or equivalent.

The editorial board has been involved in producing this book since its inception. They have spent rigorous hours researching and exploring the diverse topics which have resulted in the successful publishing of this book. They have passed on their knowledge of decades through this book. To expedite this challenging task, the publisher supported the team at every step. A small team of assistant editors was also appointed to further simplify the editing procedure and attain best results for the readers.

Our editorial team has been hand-picked from every corner of the world. Their multi-ethnicity adds dynamic inputs to the discussions which result in innovative outcomes. These outcomes are then further discussed with the researchers and contributors who give their valuable feedback and opinion regarding the same. The feedback is then collaborated with the researches and they are edited in a comprehensive manner to aid the understanding of the subject.

Apart from the editorial board, the designing team has also invested a significant amount of their time in understanding the subject and creating the most relevant covers. They scrutinized every image to scout for the most suitable representation of the subject and create an appropriate cover for the book.

The publishing team has been involved in this book since its early stages. They were actively engaged in every process, be it collecting the data, connecting with the contributors or procuring relevant information. The team has been an ardent support to the editorial, designing and production team. Their endless efforts to recruit the best for this project, has resulted in the accomplishment of this book. They are a veteran in the field of academics and their pool of knowledge is as vast as their experience in printing. Their expertise and guidance has proved useful at every step. Their uncompromising quality standards have made this book an exceptional effort. Their encouragement from time to time has been an inspiration for everyone.

The publisher and the editorial board hope that this book will prove to be a valuable piece of knowledge for researchers, students, practitioners and scholars across the globe.

List of Contributors

Jose Miguel Urra
Immunology Service, General Hospital Ciudad Real, Ciudad Real, Spain

Miguel De La Torre
Nephrology Service, Cabueñes Hospital, Asturias, Spain

Suad M. AlFadhli
Kuwait University, Kuwait

Daniel N. Clark and Brian D. Poole
Brigham Young University, USA

Cynthia A. Leifer and James C. Brooks
College of Veterinary Medicine, Cornell University, USA

Roberto Paganelli, Alessia Paganelli and Maria C. Turi
Department of Medicine and Sciences of Aging, University "G. d'Annunzio" of Chieti-Pescara and Ce.S.I.- U.d'A. Foundation, Chieti scalo (CH), Italy

José Delgado Alves
Systemic Immunomediated Diseases Unit, Department of Medicine IV, Hospital Prof. Doutor Fernando Fonseca, Amadora, Italy
CEDOC-Centro de Estudos de Doenças Crónicas Faculdade de Ciências Médicas, Universidade Nova de Lisboa, Portugal

Isabel Ferreira
Systemic Immunomediated Diseases Unit, Department of Medicine IV, Hospital Prof. Doutor Fernando Fonseca, Amadora, Italy

I. T. Rass
Center of Theoretical Pharmacology, Russian Academy of Sciences, Moscow, Russia

Rose G. Mage
Laboratory of Immunology, NIAID, National Institutes of Health, US

Geeta Rai
Department of Molecular and Human Genetics, Faculty of Science, Banaras Hindu University, Varanasi, India

Zivanit Ergaz
Laboratory of Teratology, Israel Canada Institute of Medical Research, Hebrew University Hadassah Medical School, Jerusalem, Israel
Department of Neonatology, Hadassah-Hebrew University Hospital Mount Scopus, Jerusalem, Israel

Asher Ornoy
Laboratory of Teratology, Israel Canada Institute of Medical Research, Hebrew University, Hadassah Medical School, Jerusalem, Israel and Israeli Ministry of Health, Israel

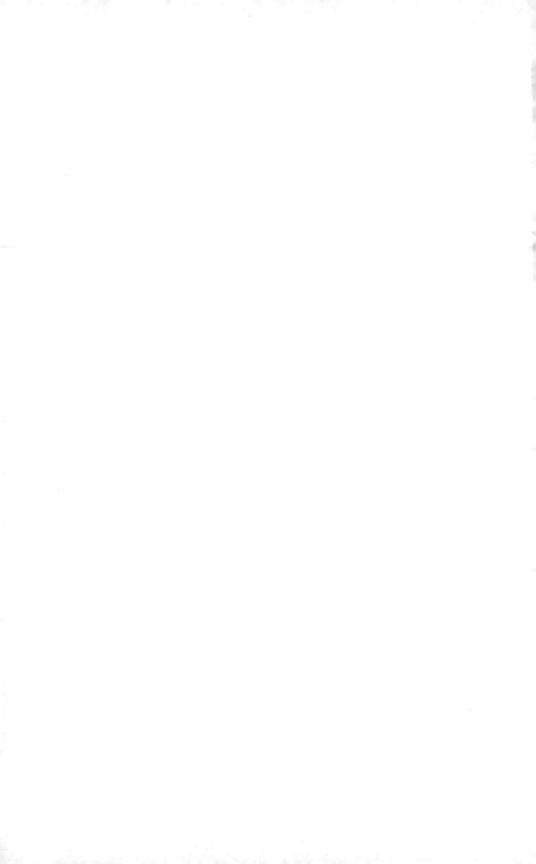